ANTHONY F. DePALMA, M.D.

PROFESSOR OF ORTHOPEDIC SURGERY,
JEFFERSON MEDICAL COLLEGE,
THOMAS JEFFERSON UNIVERSITY

WITH 2850 ILLUSTRATIONS BY
BARBARA B. FINNESON and WILLIAM A. OSBURN

VOLUME TWO

SECOND EDITION

The management of FRACTURES and DISLOCATIONS

an atlas

W. B. SAUNDERS COMPANY

PHILADELPHIA • LONDON • TORONTO • 1970

W. B. Saunders Company: West Washington Square
Philadelphia, Pa.

12 Dyott Street
London W.C.1

1835 Yonge Street
Toronto 7, Ontario

The Management of Fractures and Dislocations

Print No.:   1   2   3   4   5   6   7   8   9

CONTENTS

CONTENTS

Dislocations of the Hip and Fractures of the Acetabulum

Fractures of the Femur

Injuries of the Soft Tissues and Bony Elements of the Knee Joint

CONTENTS

Fractures of the Tibia and Fibula

Injuries of the Ankle: Sprains, Dislocations and Fractures

Fractures and Fracture-Dislocations of the Bones of the Foot

CONTENTS

FRACTURES AND DISLOCATIONS IN THE REGION OF THE WRIST

EXTENSION FRACTURES OF THE LOWER END OF THE RADIUS

These lesions result from a fall on the dorsiflexed and pronated hand. On striking the ground the hand becomes fixed but the momentum of the body produces two forces, a twisting force that causes excessive supination of the forearm and a compression force that acts vertically through the carpus to the radius.

The lunate in the proximal carpal row acts as the apex of a wedge against the articular surface of the radius. Depending upon the age of the patient the following lesions may occur:

a. In very young children, the mechanism usually results in a greenstick fracture of the distal end of the radius with or without a fracture of the distal end of the shaft of the ulna.

b. In older children and adolescents, separation of the lower epiphysis with dorsal displacement or crushing of the radial epiphysis may occur.

c. In adults, a fracture usually occurs within 1 inch of the wrist joint. The distal fragment may or may not be displaced upward and backward. It may or may not be comminuted. In young adults the distal fragment generally is not comminuted; in older individuals, especially the elderly, the distal fragment usually shows varying degrees of comminution.

d. In displaced fractures, the styloid process may be avulsed or there may be a fracture through the lower end of the ulna.

e. The lesion may be complicated by injury to the median or sensory branch of the radial nerve.

f. It also may be complicated by a fracture of the scaphoid bone or a dislocation of the lunate bone.

EPIDEMIOLOGY OF EXTENSION FRACTURES OF THE LOWER END OF THE RADIUS

REMARKS

This lesion occurs in all age groups — in my series the age ranged from 15 to 86 years.

Sixty to 65 per cent of all fractures of the radius involve the distal end and are of the extension type.

This fracture occurs more frequently in women (76 per cent) than in men (24 per cent).

The left forearm is involved more frequently (55 per cent) than the right arm (45 per cent).

Open fracture is rare; it occurs in approximately 1 per cent of the cases. Some of the late complications are:

1. Malunion—this is a rather common complication and it definitely relates to the functional results: the greater the deformity, the greater the impairment of function.

2. Nonunion—this is indeed a rare complication but it may occur. I have seen three instances of nonunion.

3. Pain over the region of the ulnar styloid due to nonunion or malunion. Fracture of the styloid process of the ulna occurs in approximately 50 to 55 per cent of the cases and of these approximately 25 per cent develop nonunion.

4. Traumatic arthritis or subluxation of the distal radio-ulnar joint. Although this may occur, in general, the disability secondary to osteoarthritis or subluxation is insignificant.

5. Rupture of the tendon of the extensor pollicis longus—this is not a common complication. It may occur while the patient is still in plaster (within three or four weeks after injury) or it may occur late (four to 12 months after injury).

Although even rarer than rupture of the extensor tendons of the thumb, rupture of the flexor tendons may occur many months after an extension fracture of the distal end of the radius.

6. Growth deformities resulting from injuries to the lower radial epiphysis may occur; always warn the parents of such a possibility.

7. Carpal tunnel syndrome—this is not a frequent complication; it is a late complication.

Accurate reduction is essential in order to obtain a good functional result. It is true that many patients with marked deformity have very few complaints and the result, subjectively, is good. However, these are usually elderly people who are more willing to adjust themselves to the residual impairment. This is not true of the young adults who make strenuous demands on the wrist and who are not willing to accept a malformation of the wrist.

Anatomic reduction is readily achieved by manipulation and in the noncomminuted types it is maintained by plaster fixation. This is not true in the comminuted type in which displacement of the fragments frequently occurs during the healing period.

A true Colles fracture comprises a transverse fracture of the radius 4 cm. proximal to the wrist joint with upward, backward and outward displacement of the distal fragment; this lesion is rare. Today the designation "Colles fracture" is loosely applied to most of the complete fractures of the distal end of the radius.

Extension Fracture of the Lower End of the Radius without Comminution

Typical Deformity (Dinner-Fork Deformity)

1. Abrupt dorsal prominence.
2. Gently rounded volar prominence.
3. The wrist is broadened.
4. The hand is deviated outward.

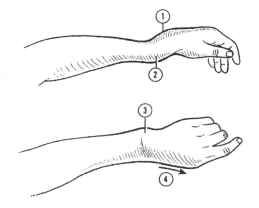

X-Ray Appearance of Normal Wrist

1. Styloid process of the radius extends 1 cm. beyond that of the ulna.

2. The articular surface of the radius projects proximally and toward the ulna 15 to 30 degrees (average 23 degrees).

3. The plane of the radial articular surface slopes downward and forward 1 to 23 degrees (average 11 degrees).

Note: Compare these anatomic features with those noted in a Colles fracture.

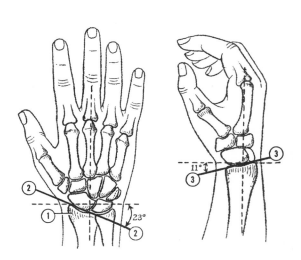

Prereduction X-Ray

1. The distal radial fragment is displaced proximally. (The radial styloid may be on the same plane as the ulnar styloid or proximal to it.)

2. The distal radial fragment is displaced upward and backward.

3. The plane of the articular surface of the radial fragment projects backward. (This angle varies greatly with each case.)

4. The carpus and the hand deviate toward the radius.

5. The ulnar styloid may or may not be fractured.

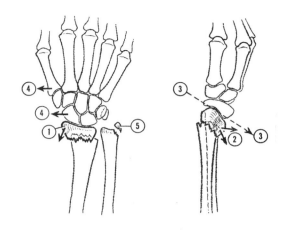

Reduction by Traction and Manipulation

PREFERRED METHOD (GENERAL ANESTHESIA)

The patient assumes the supine position on a fracture table.

1. Apply finger traction, using the Weinberg finger traction apparatus.

2. The elbow is flexed to a right angle.

3. The forearm is fully supinated.

4. Counter traction is made by muslin bandage secured to the bottom of the table.

5. Apply finger traction until the radial styloid is distal to the ulnar styloid.

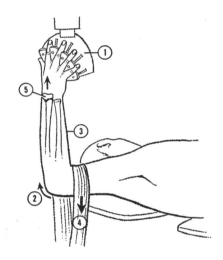

1. Now turn the forearm into a position of pronation. (This corrects the supination twist of the distal fragment.)

2. With the fingers of both hands on the volar side of the forearm and both thumbs just behind the proximal fragment on the dorsum of the wrist, flex the wrist strongly and at the same time with both thumbs push the distal fragment forward and toward the ulna.

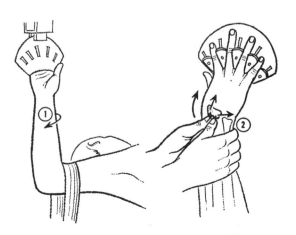

Reduction by Traction and Manipulation (Continued)

While the position of flexion and ulnar deviation is maintained by an assistant, apply a circular cast over very little padding.

1. The cast extends from just below the elbow to proximal to the metacarpal heads on the dorsal side and to the middle palmar crease on the volar side.

Just before the plaster sets, remove the traction apparatus.

2. Hold the wrist in a position of flexion and ulnar deviation with one hand.

3. Mold the plaster well along the radial concavity with the other hand.

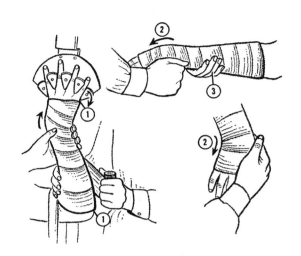

ALTERNATE METHOD

(Local anesthesia may be used.)

To reduce a fracture of the right radius:

1. Grasp the distal fragment with the right hand.

2. Grasp the wrist above the level of the fracture with the left hand.

3. Make steady traction in the angle of displacement of the distal fragment.

While traction is maintained,

4. Flex and pronate the distal fragment with the right hand, using

5. The index finger of the left hand on the volar surface which acts as the fulcrum; at the same time,

6. Push the distal fragment forward and downward with the thumb of the left hand.

7. Take a new grip on the wrist with the right hand. The thenar eminence is placed against the radial styloid.

8. Grasp the forearm with the left hand.

9. With the right hand, push the distal fragment toward the ulna.

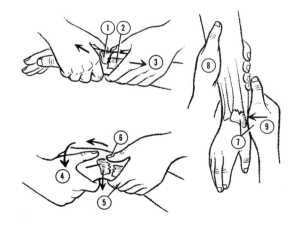

Reduction by Traction and Manipulation *(Continued)*

While an assistant maintains traction on the thumb and fingers, apply a plaster cast over very little padding from just below the elbow to proximal to the metacarpal heads. While the plaster is setting, hold the position of

1. Flexion;
2. Ulnar deviation;
3. Pronation; and
4. Mold the plaster along the radial concavity.

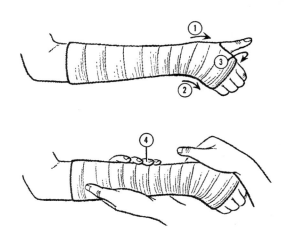

Postreduction X-Ray

1. The normal length of the radius has been restored. The radial styloid is distal to the ulnar styloid.
2. The articular plane of the radius now is directed toward the ulna.
3. The articular surface of the radius is directed downward, forward and inward.

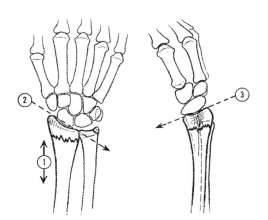

Postreduction Management

Take x-rays immediately after the application of the cast; if reduction is not satisfactory, another attempt to achieve accurate reduction should be made.

The cast should be applied tightly enough to prevent loss of position of the fragments but not so tightly as to cause circulatory embarrassment. If there is any evidence of circulatory embarrassment, split the cast along the dorsum for its entire length. (Be sure to cut any constricting padding beneath the cast.)

Elevate the arm with the fingers pointing toward the ceiling for the first 24 hours and apply ice bags.

After the first 24 to 48 hours, allow free use of the arm, elbow and fingers.

Page 909

Take x-rays again on the fifth and tenth days. Check for maintenance of position.

If the cast becomes loose after about ten days, apply a new cast to prevent redisplacement of the fragments.

If moderate flexion was necessary to maintain reduction, remove the cast after two weeks, bring the wrist to a neutral position, and apply another cast.

During the healing period, insist on a regulated regimen of shoulder, elbow and finger exercises. The sling should be discarded after the first 24 to 48 hours.

Remove the plaster cast after six weeks. (In older persons it may be necessary to maintain plaster immobilization longer.)

Institute physical therapy, heat, gentle massage, underwater massage and active exercises for the fingers, wrist, elbow and shoulder.

Extension Fractures of the Lower End of the Radius with Comminution

REMARKS

These are common lesions in the elderly.

If the comminuted distal fragment is displaced backward and upward, the typical "dinner-fork" deformity is present.

In many instances there is no backward displacement; the comminuted fragment is driven directly upward or outward.

The ulnar styloid is frequently pulled off or the distal end of the ulna fractured and displaced.

The inferior radio-ulnar joint may be disrupted or the triangular fibro-cartilage of this joint displaced.

Traction and manipulative maneuvers readily achieve a satisfactory reduction but redisplacement is the rule while in a plaster cast.

Redisplacement is prevented by transfixion of the fragments as depicted below.

Check for deficit of the median nerve or the sensory branch of the radial nerve.

The ligamentous apparatus and capsule remain intact permitting the reduction demonstrated below.

Prereduction X-Rays of Some of the Types of Fractures Encountered

X-RAY

1. The distal radial fragments are severely comminuted.

2. The radial fragments are displaced upward and backward.

3. The length of the radius is decreased; the tip of the ulnar styloid is almost on the same plane as the radial styloid.

4. The plane of the articular surface of the radial fragments projects upward and backward.

5. The tip of the ulnar styloid is pulled off.

X-RAY

1. There is severe comminution of the distal radial fragment with impaction.

2. The distal radial fragments are displaced directly upward (and not backward).

3. The length of the radius is shortened.

X-RAY

1. There is comminution of the distal radial fragment.

2. Moderate backward and upward displacement of the radial fragments is present.

3. The radial and ulnar styloid are almost on the same plane.

4. There is fracture with comminution of the distal end of the ulna.

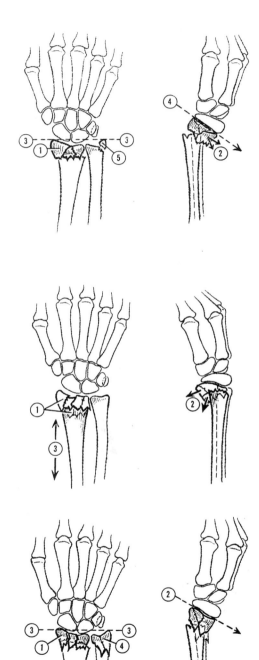

Preferred Method of Management

(Reduction by traction, manipulation and transfixion pin, with general anesthesia.)

The patient assumes the supine position on a fracture table.

1. Apply Weinberg finger traction apparatus.

2. The elbow is flexed 90 degrees.

3. The forearm is fully supinated.

4. Make counter traction by muslin bandage secured to the bottom of the table.

5. Now apply finger traction until the radial styloid is distal to the ulnar styloid process.

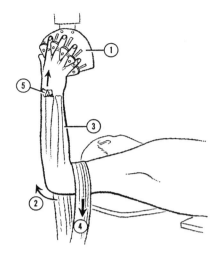

1. Now turn the forearm into a position of pronation.

2. Place the fingers of both hands on the volar side of the forearm and

3. Both thumbs on the dorsal aspect of the wrist just behind the proximal fragments; flex the wrist and at the same time with the thumbs push the distal fragments forward and toward the ulna.

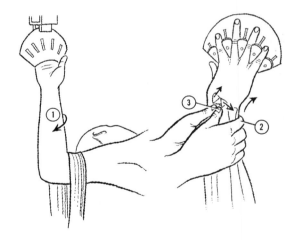

Preferred Method of Management
(Continued)

1. While an assistant holds this position of flexion and ulnar deviation, the operator compresses the wrist between the heels of his hands. This molds the radial fragments into place.

2. While traction and the position of flexion and ulnar deviation are maintained by an assistant,

3. Pass a threaded wire (7/64 inch) through the ulna into the radial styloid. The wire enters the ulna 4 to 5 cm. proximal to the tip of its styloid and is directed slightly forward toward the radial styloid making an angle of approximately 45 degrees with the ulna.

Note: If the distal end of the ulna is fractured, the wire enters the proximal fragment of the ulna about 2 cm. proximal to the fracture line.

4. Cut the wire below the level of the skin.

Note: The wire acts like a tent-pole — suspending the fragments on the radial styloid process.

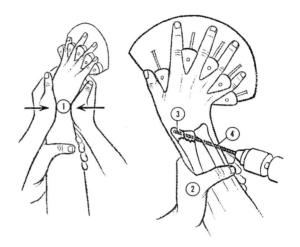

While traction is still maintained, apply a circular cast over very little padding.

1. The cast extends from the middle of the arm to the metacarpal heads.

Just before the plaster sets, remove the traction apparatus and

2. Hold the wrist in a position of slight flexion, pronation and ulnar deviation with one hand and

3. Mold the plaster well along the radial concavity with the other hand.

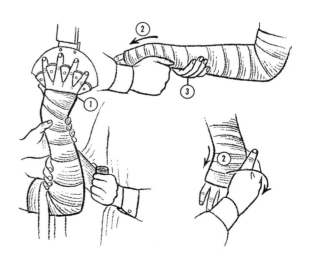

Postreduction X-Ray

In all three instances:

1. Radial length is restored. The radial styloid is more distal than the ulnar styloid.

2. The plane of the articular surface of the radius is now directed inward, forward and downward.

3. The fragments of the distal radial segment are accurately approximated.

4. A transfixion wire maintains the length of the radius and prevents redisplacement of the distal radial fragments.

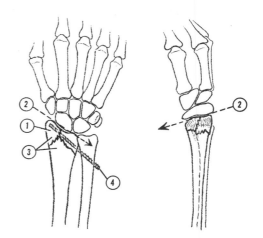

Postreduction Management

Take an x-ray immediately after insertion of the wire. If reduction is not satisfactory, the entire procedure should be repeated. (This is rarely necessary.)

The cast should be applied over very little padding but not so tightly as to cause circulatory embarrassment. If at any time signs (pallor, cyanosis, swelling) and symptoms (pain, paralysis) manifest themselves, split the cast along the dorsum for its entire length and cut any constricting padding beneath the cast.

Elevate the arm with the fingers pointing toward the ceiling for the first 24 hours and apply ice bags.

Support the arm in a triangular sling.

Take x-rays again on the fifth and tenth days and then at the end of the fourth and sixth weeks. Check for maintenance of position.

If the cast becomes loose, apply a new cast.

Encourage the patient to use the fingers and thumb freely and to exercise the fingers and shoulder on a regulated program.

Under local anesthesia, remove the cast and wire at the end of six to eight weeks depending on the state of healing. (Older people heal more slowly and may require eight to ten weeks of internal fixation.)

Institute physical therapy: heat, gentle massage, underwater massage and active exercises for the fingers, wrist, elbow and shoulder.

Note: Occasionally the patient may develop a shoulder-arm-hand syndrome at any time during the healing period. This can often be avoided by active use of the shoulder and fingers. When the syndrome is present, blocking of the cervical sympathetic ganglion by procaine (1 per cent) every four or five days gives relief of pain and may terminate the syndrome.

The goal of this method of treatment is to correct the components of this type of fracture, namely (1) the supination twist of the distal fragment, (2) radial deviation of the distal fragments, (3) alterations in the angle of inclination of the articular surface of the radius and (4) shortening of the radius. If these components are restored to normalcy an excellent result can be anticipated. If not, impairment of function is in proportion to the severity of the residual deformity. Also disability is greater with increasing age. The most frequent defect in motion is palmar flexion; next is dorsiflexion. About one-third of the patients will have some impairment of rotation and one-half some impairment of lateral motion. Approximately 30 to 35 per cent complain of some weakness in the grip.

FLEXION FRACTURES OF THE LOWER END OF THE RADIUS

Without Comminution (Reversed Colles Fracture; Smith's Fracture)

REMARKS

A true Smith's fracture is very rare; it comprises a fracture of the entire thickness of the distal end of the radius one-half to one inch above the wrist; the lower end of the radius is displaced forward and upward.

This lesion may be sustained by direct trauma, as a fall on the back of the hand as described by Smith. This mechanism is rare. More frequently it is caused by an indirect mechanism, as when the patient falls backward on the outstretched hand in supination. On striking the ground the hand locks in supination but the body momentum and its direction force the arm into hyperpronation thus producing a typical pronation injury.

In reduction of these fractures, the hand must be markedly supinated—maintenance of the position can be achieved only by holding the position of supination in plaster. Failure to do this will invariably result in redisplacement of the fragments and impairment of function. Maintenance of the supinated position for six weeks will not be followed by permanent restriction of pronation except in the unusual case.

The deformity (garden-spade deformity) is the reverse of the dinner-fork deformity of a Colles fracture.

The lower fragment may be comminuted—this type is most frequently encountered in the elderly, mostly women—and the ulnar styloid process is usually avulsed.

Typical Deformity (Garden-Spade Deformity)

1. Dorsal prominence of the distal end of the proximal fragment.
2. Fullness of the wrist on the volar side due to the displaced distal fragment.
3. Deviation of the hand toward the radial side.

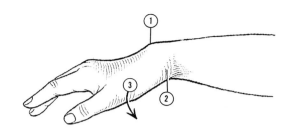

Prereduction X-Ray

1. The distal fragment is displaced forward and upward.
2. The fracture line runs obliquely from below upward and forward.
3. The distal fragment comprises the entire thickness of the shaft of the radius.
4. The distal fragment and the hand are deviated toward the radial side.

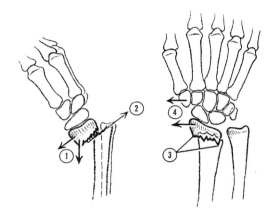

Reduction by Traction and Manipulation (General Anesthesia)

1. Apply Weinberg finger traction apparatus.
2. The elbow is flexed at a right angle.
3. The forearm is supinated fully.
4. Counter traction is made by muslin bandage secured to the bottom of the table.
5. Apply finger traction until the radial styloid is distal to the ulnar styloid.

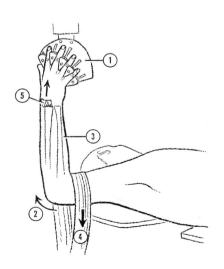

Page 917

Reduction by Traction and Manipulation (General Anesthesia) (Continued)

While traction is maintained:

1. The fingers of both hands steady the lower end of the proximal fragment while

2. Both thumbs on the volar aspect of the wrist push the distal fragment upward and backward.

3. The wrist is forced into dorsiflexion and ulnar deviation.

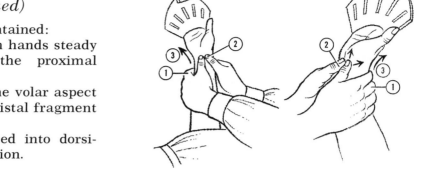

1. While the position of slight dorsiflexion and ulnar deviation is maintained by an assistant, apply a circular cast from the middle of the arm to just proximal to the metacarpal heads; the elbow is flexed 90 degrees and the arm is fully supinated.

While the plaster is setting, remove the traction apparatus.

2. Hold the wrist in slight dorsiflexion and in ulnar deviation and supination.

3. Apply even pressure over the front of the lower end of the radius and carpus.

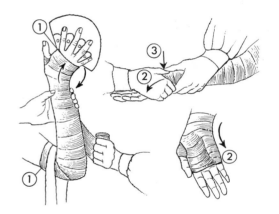

Postreduction X-Ray

1. The radial styloid is distal to the ulnar styloid.

2. The distal fragment is restored to its normal relation to the proximal fragment.

3. Radial deviation of the lower fragment and hand has been corrected.

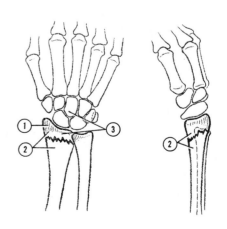

Postreduction Management

Take x-rays immediately after application of the cast; if reduction is not satisfactory, another attempt to achieve accurate reduction of the fracture should be made.

The cast should be applied tightly enough to prevent loss of position of the fragments but not so tightly as to cause circulatory embarrassment. If there is any evidence of circulatory embarrassment, split the cast along the dorsum for its entire length. (Be sure to cut any constricting padding beneath the cast.)

Elevate the arm with the fingers pointing toward the ceiling for the first 24 hours and apply ice bags.

After the first 24 or 48 hours, allow free use of the arm, elbow and fingers.

Take x-rays again on the fifth and tenth days. Check maintenance of position.

If the cast becomes loose after about ten days, apply a new cast to prevent redisplacement of the fragments.

During the healing period, insist on a regulated regimen of shoulder and finger exercises. The sling should be discarded after the first 24 to 48 hours.

Remove the plaster cast after six weeks. (In older individuals it may be necessary to maintain plaster immobilization longer.)

Institute physical therapy: heat, gentle massage, underwater massage and active exercises for the fingers, wrist, elbow and shoulder.

Flexion Fractures of the Lower End of the Radius with Comminution

REMARKS

These lesions are more likely to be encountered in the elderly.

Redisplacement of the fragments is the rule unless some continuous traction is maintained during the healing period.

As in the extension type of fracture, the ulnar styloid may be avulsed or the distal radio-ulnar joint may be disrupted.

Prereduction X-Ray

1. The distal radial fragment is comminuted.
2. Displacement is upward and forward.
3. The distal fragments are deviated radially.
4. The styloid process of the ulna is avulsed and is more distal than the radial styloid.

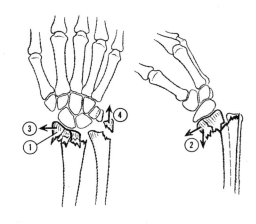

Reduction by Traction, Manipulation and Transfixion Pin (General Anesthesia)

1. Apply Weinberg finger traction apparatus.
2. The elbow is flexed 90 degrees.
3. The forearm is supinated fully.
4. Make counter traction by muslin bandage secured to the bottom of the table.
5. Now apply traction until the radial styloid is distal to the ulnar styloid.

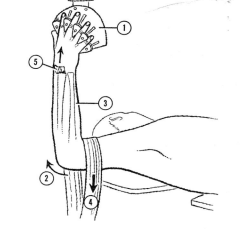

1. Place the fingers of both hands on the dorsum of the wrist.
2. Place the thumbs just proximal to the distal fragments on the volar aspect of the wrist.
3. Dorsiflex the wrist and at the same time push the distal fragment upward, backward and ulnarward with both thumbs.
4. While an assistant holds the position of slight dorsiflexion and ulnar deviation, the operator compresses the wrist between the heels of his hands.

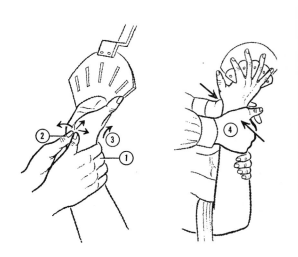

Reduction by Traction, Manipulation and Transfixion Pin (General Anesthesia) (Continued)

1. While an assistant holds the position of dorsiflexion and ulnar deviation,

2. Pass a threaded wire (7/64 inch) through the ulna into the styloid process of the radius.

The wire enters the ulna 4 to 5 cm. proximal to the tip of its styloid process and is directed slightly forward and upward making an angle of 45 degrees with the shaft of the ulna.

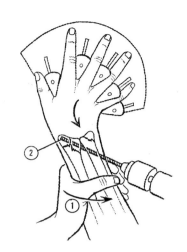

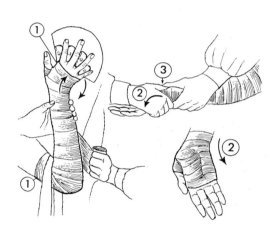

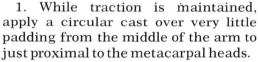

1. While traction is maintained, apply a circular cast over very little padding from the middle of the arm to just proximal to the metacarpal heads.

Just before the plaster sets, remove the traction apparatus.

2. Hold the wrist in slight dorsiflexion, supination and ulnar deviation.

3. Press firmly against the volar aspect of the distal fragments and carpus.

Postreduction X-Ray

1. The radial styloid is distal to the ulnar styloid.

2. The articular surface of the radius is now restored to its normal plane of inclination.

3. The fragments of the distal segment are accurately approximated.

4. A transfixion wire maintains the length of the radius and prevents redisplacement of the radial fragments.

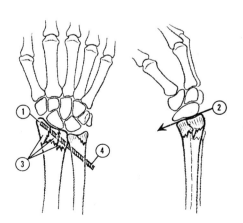

Page 921

Postreduction Management

Take x-rays immediately after insertion of the wire. If the reduction is not satisfactory, the entire procedure should be repeated. (This is rarely necessary.)

The cast should be applied over very little padding but not so tightly as to cause circulatory embarrassment. If at any time signs (pallor, cyanosis, swelling) and symptoms (pain, paralysis) manifest themselves, split the cast along the dorsum for its entire length and cut any constricting padding beneath the cast.

Elevate the arm with the fingers pointing toward the ceiling for the first 24 hours and apply ice bags.

Support the arm in a triangular sling.

Take x-rays again on the fifth and tenth days and then at the end of the fourth and sixth weeks. Check for maintenance of position.

If the cast becomes loose, apply a new cast.

Encourage the patient to use the fingers and the thumb freely and to exercise the fingers and the shoulder on a regulated program.

Under local anesthesia remove the cast and the wire at the end of six to eight weeks depending on the state of healing. (Older people heal more slowly and may require eight to ten weeks of internal fixation.)

Institute physical therapy: heat, gentle massage, underwater massage and active exercises for the fingers, wrist, elbow and shoulder.

Note: Occasionally the patient may develop a shoulder-arm-hand syndrome at any time during the healing period. This can often be avoided by active use of the shoulder and fingers. When the syndrome is present, blocking of the cervical sympathetic ganglion by procaine (1 per cent) every four to five days gives relief of pain and may terminate the syndrome.

POSTERIOR AND ANTERIOR MARGINAL FRACTURES OF THE LOWER END OF THE RADIUS

REMARKS

Both types include a portion of the articular surface of the radius.

In most instances of the anterior type, the hand and carpus is displaced forward with a large anterior marginal fragment of the articular surface.

In both instances varying degrees of comminution of the radial fragment may exist.

Posterior marginal fractures are frequently overlooked and are responsible for late rupture of the extensor pollicis longus; the fracture line involves the groove of this tendon; subsequent incongruity of this groove may cause fraying of the tendon.

The anterior type is produced by a pronation mechanism; therefore the fracture should be held in supination. Also, this fracture will slip if placed in dorsiflexion—it should be put in a position of slight flexion.

The posterior type is produced by a supination mechanism.

A. Prereduction X-Ray of Anterior Marginal Fracture

1. A large fragment of the anterior articular surface of the radius is displaced forward and upward.

2. The carpus follows the radial fragment.

3. Some comminution of the radial fragment exists.

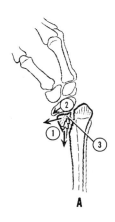

A

Page 923

B. Prereduction X-Ray of Posterior Marginal Fracture (Barton's Fracture)

1. Oblique fracture of the posterior lip of the distal end of the radius directed upward and backward.

Note: There is considerable confusion in the designation of the anterior marginal fracture. It is often referred to as Barton's fracture and also as a type of Smith's fracture. Remember that both names refer to the same fracture – an anterior marginal fracture.

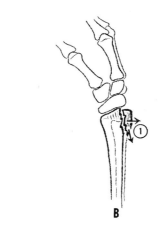

Reduction by Traction and Manipulation (For Both Types) (Under General Anesthesia)

1. Apply Weinberg finger traction apparatus.
2. The elbow is flexed 90 degrees.
3. The forearm is placed in supination for anterior marginal fractures, and in pronation for posterior marginal fractures.
4. Make counter traction by muslin bandage secured to the bottom of the table.
5. Now apply strong upward traction.

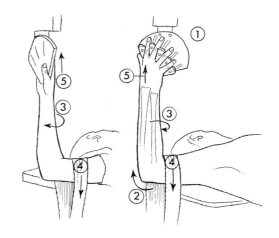

1. While traction is maintained, compress the wrist firmly with the heels of both hands.

Apply a circular cast from the middle of the arm to just proximal to the metacarpal heads.

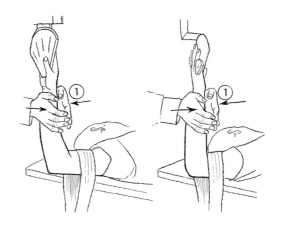

Reduction by Traction and Manipulation (For Both Types) (Under General Anesthesia) (Continued)

For anterior marginal fractures:
1. The hand is in supination.
2. The wrist is slightly flexed.

Note: Dorsiflexion will displace the carpus and radial fragment volarly.

For posterior marginal fractures:
3. The hand is in midposition.
4. The wrist is in the neutral position.

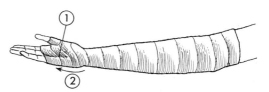

For anterior marginal fractures

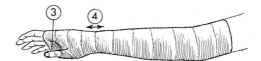

For posterior marginal fractures

A. Postreduction X-ray of Anterior Marginal Fracture

1. The anterior lip is restored to its anatomic position.
2. Displacement of the carpus is corrected.
3. The length of the radius is restored.

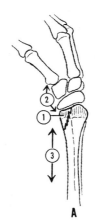

A

B. Postreduction X-Ray of Posterior Margin Fracture

1. The posterior lip is restored to its normal position.
2. The articular surface of the radius shows no incongruity.

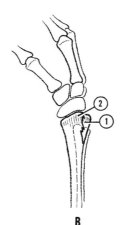

B

Postreduction Management

Take x-rays immediately after the application of the cast. If the reduction is not satisfactory, another attempt to achieve accurate reduction of the fracture should be made.

The cast should be applied tightly enough to prevent loss of position of the fragments but not so tightly as to cause circulatory embarrassment. If there is any evidence of circulatory embarrassment, split the cast along the dorsum for its entire length. (Be sure to cut any constricting padding beneath the cast.)

Elevate the arm with the fingers pointing toward the ceiling for the first 24 hours and apply ice bags.

After the first 24 or 48 hours, allow free use of the arm and fingers.

Take x-rays again on the fifth and tenth days. Check for maintenance of position.

If the cast becomes loose after ten days, apply a new cast to prevent redisplacement of the fragments.

During the healing period, insist on a regulated regimen of shoulder and finger exercises. The sling should be discarded after the first 24 to 48 hours.

Remove the plaster cast after six weeks. (In older individuals it may be necessary to maintain plaster immobilization longer.)

Institute physical therapy: heat, gentle massage, underwater massage and active exercises for the fingers, wrist, elbow and shoulder.

FRACTURE OF THE RADIAL STYLOID PROCESS (CHAUFFEUR'S FRACTURE)

REMARKS

This lesion is important because it implicates the articular surface of the radius.

In most instances there is no displacement of the radial fragment; hence simple immobilization in a plaster cast for four to six weeks is all that is required.

If there is displacement and reduction fails to restore perfect anatomic congruity of the articular surface, open reduction and fixation with a screw is indicated.

Prereduction X-Ray

1. The fracture line is directed upward and outward.
2. The articular surface of the radius is involved.
3. The carpus is shifted slightly to the radial side with the radial fragment.

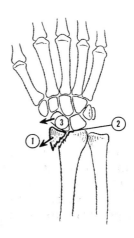

Reduction by Traction and Manipulation (Under General Anesthesia)

1. Apply Weinberg finger traction apparatus.
2. The elbow is flexed 90 degrees.
3. The forearm is in midposition as regards rotation.
4. Make counter traction by muslin bandage secured to the bottom of the table.
5. Now apply strong upward traction.

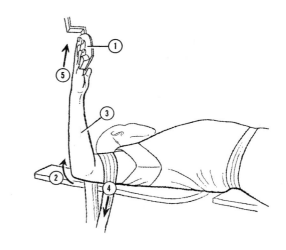

While traction is maintained:
1. Compress the fragment firmly with the heels of both hands; first compress the fragment laterally, then
2. Compress the volar and dorsal surfaces.

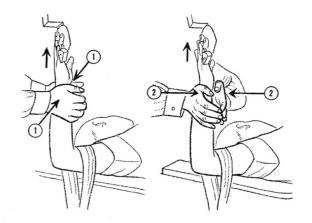

While an assistant holds the forearm in midposition and the wrist in ulnar deviation, apply a plaster cast.
1. The cast extends from below the elbow to just proximal to the metacarpal heads.
2. The forearm is in midposition.
3. The hand is deviated toward the ulna.

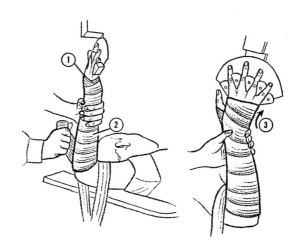

Postreduction X-Ray

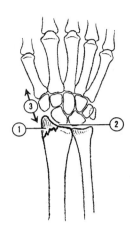

1. The radial fragment is restored to its anatomic position.
2. The articular surface of the radius is congruous.
3. The radial shift of the carpus is corrected.

Postreduction Management

Take x-rays immediately after application of the cast. If the reduction is not satisfactory, another attempt to achieve accurate reduction of the fracture should be made.

The cast should be applied tightly enough to prevent loss of position of the fragments but not so tightly as to cause circulatory embarrassment. If there is any evidence of circulatory embarrassment, split the cast along the dorsum for its entire length. (Be sure to cut any constricting padding beneath the cast.)

Elevate the arm with the fingers pointing toward the ceiling for the first 24 hours and apply ice bags.

After the first 24 to 48 hours, allow free use of the arm, elbow and fingers.

Take x-rays again on the fifth and tenth days. Check for maintenance of position.

If the cast becomes loose after about ten days, apply a new cast to prevent redisplacement of fragments.

During the healing period, insist on a regulated regimen of shoulder, elbow and finger exercises. The sling should be discarded after the first 24 to 48 hours.

Remove the plaster cast after six weeks. (In older individuals it may be necessary to maintain plaster immobilization longer.)

Institute physical therapy; heat, gentle massage, underwater massage and active exercises for the fingers, wrist, elbow and shoulder.

Page 929

Alternate Method

(To be employed if reduction fails to approximate the fragments to their anatomic position.)

1. The articular surfaces are congruous.
2. Fixation is maintained with a screw.

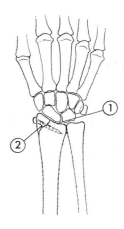

ISOLATED INJURIES OF THE ARTICULAR DISC OF THE WRIST WITHOUT SUBLUXATION OR DISLOCATION OF THE INFERIOR RADIO-ULNAR JOINT

REMARKS

Injury to the articular disc of the wrist is known to occur with subluxation, dislocation of the inferior radio-ulnar joint or with fractures in this region.

It is not generally recognized that severe injury to the disc may occur without associated lesions of the joint.

The most common pathologic condition found is tearing of the disc from its attachment to the margin of the ulnar notch of the radius — rarely the disc may be torn from its attachment to the base of the ulnar styloid process. Occasionally the disc may be just scored and fragmented.

MECHANISM OF INJURY

The primary function of the triangular disc is to prevent lateral displacement of the ulna. During all phases of rotation the disc is taut so that forceful movements in excess of the normal range of rotation in either direction (pronation or supination) are capable of traumatizing the disc.

The most common mechanism is one of extreme dorsiflexion and pronation of the hand; less frequently the mechanism is extreme hyperextension and supination. The mechanisms are also capable of producing a dorsal or volar dislocation of the head of the ulna.

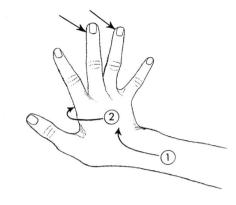

1. The wrist is dorsiflexed (extended).
2. The wrist is forced in extreme pronation.

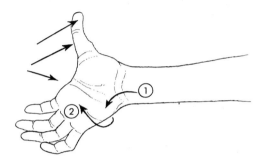

1. The wrist is hyperextended.
2. The hand is forced in extreme supination.

Pain is localized to the dorsum of the wrist over the radio-ulnar joint. Pronation or supination against resistance causes pain; occasionally a click occurs on rotation of the wrist. X-ray examination is negative.

Management

For lesions caused by a pronation mechanism:

Apply a plaster cast from the middle of the arm to just proximal to the metacarpal heads.

1. The elbow is flexed 90 degrees.
2. The hand is supinated.

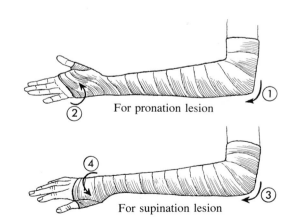

For pronation lesion

For supination lesion

For lesions caused by a supination mechanism:

3. The elbow is flexed 90 degrees.
4. The hand is pronated.

The cast is maintained for three weeks. After removal of the cast permit free use of the limb but avoid forceful rotatory movements, especially against resistance, such as the use of a screwdriver.

OPERATIVE MANAGEMENT (EXCISION OF THE ARTICULAR DISC)

REMARKS

This procedure is employed in cases that fail to respond to conservative management.

Excision of the disc relieves symptoms in cases not associated with fracture or dislocation of the inferior radio-ulnar joint. Simple excision of the disc in cases associated with dislocation or fracture may prove very disappointing.

The diagnosis is readily established by a previous history of injury and localized pain and tenderness over the radio-ulnar joint associated with a click on rotation. No abnormal configuration of the joint is present.

Operative Procedure

1. Make a transverse incision on the ulnar side of the dorsum of the wrist, at the level of the distal end of the radius.

2. Expose the common extensor tendons and the tendon of the extensor digiti minimi.

3. Make a vertical incision on the outer side of the common extensor tendons—through the sheath of the extensor digiti minimi.

4. Expose the capsule of the joint.

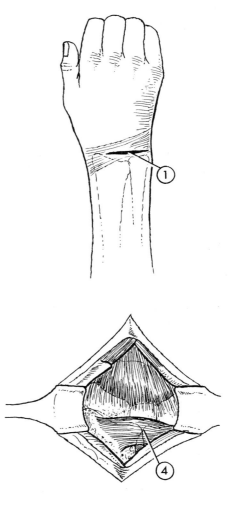

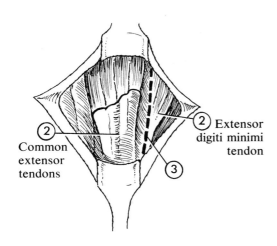

Common extensor tendons

② Extensor digiti minimi tendon

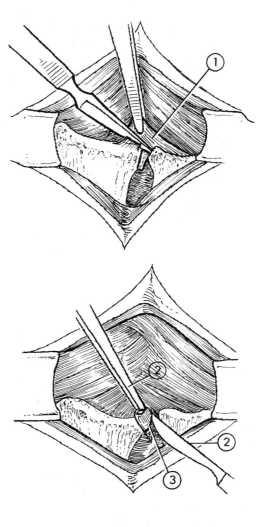

Operative Procedure (Continued)

1. By sharp dissection separate the capsule from the articular disc.

2. Grasp the disc with a Kocher clamp and, with a thin bladed scalpel,

3. Dissect the disc free from the surrounding soft tissue. (Close the capsule and the sheath of the extensor digiti minimi.)

Immobilization

Apply a plaster splint on the volar aspect of the arm.

The hand and forearm are in neutral position.

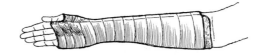

Postoperative Management

Remove the cast after two weeks.
Allow free use of the limb within the patient's tolerance.
Avoid forceful movements of rotation, especially against resistance.

TRAUMATIC DISLOCATION OF THE DISTAL END OF THE ULNA (WITHOUT AN ASSOCIATED FRACTURE)

Dislocation or subluxation of the distal end of the ulna associated with fractures of the radius either at its distal or proximal end are well known. However, acute traumatic dislocation or subluxation of the head of the ulna without an associated fracture is not well known and such disorders are frequently not recognized either clinically or by x-ray.

The head of the ulna may be displaced anteriorly or posteriorly depending on the responsible mechanism.

Occasionally the lesions are the result of a direct blow on the ulnar border of the forearm; more often indirect mechanisms are responsible.

Extreme extension and extreme pronation of the hand and wrist produce a dorsal dislocation of the head of the ulna.

1. The wrist and hand are forcefully extended and
2. Pronated.
3. Dorsal dislocation results.

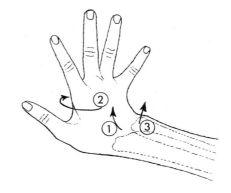

Extreme extension and extreme supination of the hand and wrist produce a volar dislocation of the head of the ulna.

Page 935

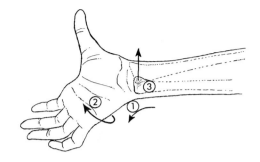

1. The wrist and hand are forcefully extended and
2. Supinated.
3. Volar dislocation results.

Clinical Features of Dorsal Dislocation

Marked prominence of the head of the ulna on the dorsum of the wrist.
Hand is locked in pronation.
Transverse diameter of wrist appears narrower than normal.
Any attempt to supinate the hand elicits severe pain.

Note: There is always a history of recent acute injury.

Clinical Features of Volar Dislocation

Normal prominence of head of ulna on dorsum of the wrist is absent.
Hand is locked in supination.
Prominence of head of ulna on volar aspect of the wrist.
Transverse diameter of the wrist is narrower than normal.
Any attempt to pronate the hand is painful.

Essential Pathologic Conditions

Rupture of the volar and dorsal ligaments of the inferior radio-ulnar joint and rupture or detachment of the triangular articular disc.

These three structures are responsible for the stability of the wrist. If the attachments of the disc hold, avulsion of the styloid process of the ulna results. This is a relatively common occurrence.

In extreme pronation the dorsal ligament becomes taut and then ruptures; in extreme supination the anterior volar ligament becomes taut and then ruptures.

X-Ray Appearance

The interpretation is often erroneous. Always take x-rays of the opposite wrist for comparison. Oblique views may be necessary to demonstrate the lesion.

Volar Dislocation

ANTEROPOSTERIOR VIEW

1. The head of the ulna has shifted radially.

LATERAL VIEW

2. The head of the ulna is displaced anteriorly.

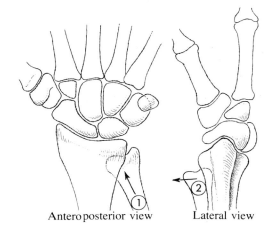

Anteroposterior view   Lateral view

Posterior Dislocation

ANTEROPOSTERIOR VIEW

1. Some lateral shift of the ulna.

LATERAL VIEW

2. The head of the ulna is displaced dorsally.

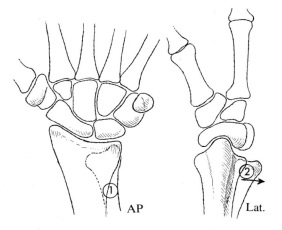

AP   Lat.

Manipulative Reduction (General Anesthesia)

To reduce a volar dislocation of the right wrist:

1. Grasp and steady the patient's supinated forearm with your left hand.

2. With your right hand grasp the patient's hand and place your thumb over the prominence of the head of the ulna.

3. While making firm backward pressure on the head of the ulna,

4. Forcefully pronate the hand and wrist.

Note: Reduction is usually accompanied by a loud click.

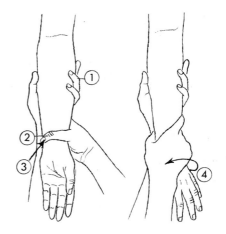

To reduce a dorsal dislocation of the right wrist:

1. Grasp and steady the patient's pronated forearm with your left hand.

2. With your right hand grasp the patient's hand and place your thumb over the prominence of the head of the ulna.

3. While making steady firm forward pressure on the head of the ulna,

4. Forcefully supinate the hand and wrist.

Note: A click usually accompanies the reduction.

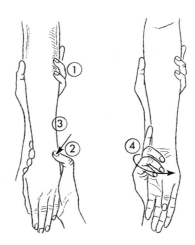

Immobilization

For volar dislocation:
Apply a plaster cast from the middle of the arm to just proximal to the metacarpal joints.
  1. The elbow is flexed 90 degrees.
  2. The forearm is fully pronated.

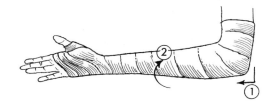

For dorsal dislocation:
  1. The elbow is flexed 90 degrees.
  2. The forearm is fully supinated.

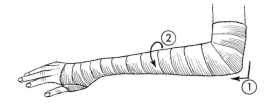

The cast is maintained for three to four weeks.

After removal of the cast allow free use of the limb within the patient's tolerance.

Avoid any forceful rotation of the hand and wrist, especially against resistance.

Habitual or Recurrent Subluxation of the Inferior Radio-Ulnar Joint

REMARKS

This disorder follows inadequately treated acute traumatic dislocations of the head of the ulna.

There is always a history of an acute traumatic injury.

In the reduced state the joint exhibits pronounced anteroposterior laxity.

A click accompanies the subluxation.

The disorder may be very disabling because of the associated pain and weakness of the wrist. In anterior habitual dislocations supination is weakened whereas in posterior dislocations pronation is weakened.

Occasionally the disorders produce no significant impairment of function; these cases should not be treated.

Excision of the head of the ulna is the procedure of choice for painful and disabling lesions.

Reconstruction procedures designed to repair the ligaments of the joint generally fail.

For excision of the head of the ulna, see page 837 for technique and postoperative management.

GROWTH DISTURBANCES FOLLOWING INJURIES TO THE DISTAL RADIAL EPIPHYSIS

REMARKS

Crushing injuries of the epiphyseal plate cause premature closure of the disc and arrest of growth of the radius.

The amount of arrest of growth and the variety and degree of the angular deformity that may develop are unpredictable.

Fractures of the radial epiphysis should be checked by x-ray every six months to determine the fate of the cartilaginous disc.

In young children, growth inequality may be minimized by resection of the distal ulnar epiphyseal disc. This should not be done in children approaching skeletal maturity.

When growth inequality is present, the deformity is corrected by resection of 1 inch of the distal end of the ulna. This procedure should not be performed in children.

In children, if growth inequality cannot be prevented, wait until skeletal maturity is achieved (18 to 19 years of age); then resect the distal end of the ulna.

Preoperative X-Ray

1. Premature closure of the distal radial epiphyseal disc.

2. The radius is shortened.

3. The ulna extends distal to the radius.

4. The distal radio-ulnar joint is dislocated.

5. The hand deviates to the radial side.

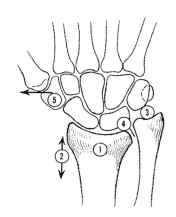

Operative Correction

1. Make a 2 inch incision along the medial aspect of the ulna, beginning at the tip of the styloid and extending upward.

2. Expose the distal end of the ulna by subperiosteal dissection.

3. One inch above the tip of the styloid, make several drill holes in the ulna and divide the bone obliquely at this level.

4. Preserve the ulnar collateral ligament.

5. Reef the periosteal sleeve and ligament to make a continuous structure.

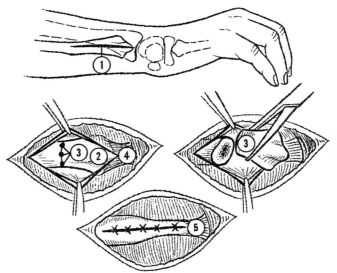

Postoperative X-Ray

1. The distal end of the ulna has been resected.

2. The hand is now in the neutral position.

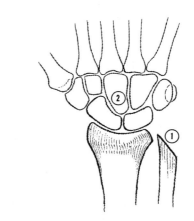

Immobilization

Apply an anterior plaster slab to the forearm and wrist extending distally as far as the proximal palmar crease.

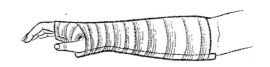

Postoperative Management

Remove the plaster slab after seven days and institute exercises to restore normal function in the wrist and fingers.

MALUNITED FRACTURE OF THE DISTAL END OF THE RADIUS

REMARKS

Many gradations of malunited fractures are encountered.

Many cases with only minor deformity give rise to no dysfunction; these should be accepted and require no surgical intervention.

In cases with marked deformity and dysfunction, incongruity of the distal radio-ulnar joint is always present in varying degrees, and is the prime source of pain.

Simple osteotomy of the radius without excision of the distal 1 inch of the ulna is justified only in those cases with a residual dorsal tilt of the radius, with little or no loss of length of the radius and with minimal or no implication of the distal radio-ulnar joint.

Malunion with gross deformity and marked implications of the radio-ulnar joint are best treated by osteotomy of the distal end of the radius and excision of the distal 1 inch of the ulna.

Occasionally, in the elderly, malunion is complicated by a reflex dystrophy of the hand and at times the entire arm (Sudeck's bone atrophy). In these cases no surgical intervention is justifiable until the symptoms and other clinical features are static and definite evidence of improvement is manifested.

Manipulative maneuvers with forceful traction as previously described may be attempted in cases of malposition up to two or three weeks following the fresh fracture. After this period of time, these conservative measures invariably fail and operative intervention is indicated.

The indications for osteotomy of the radius and for osteotomy of the radius plus excision of the distal 1 inch of the ulna are applicable to malunions of both extension and flexion types of fractures.

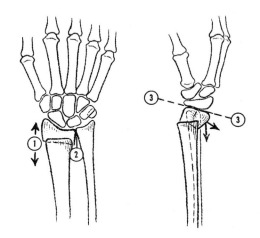

Preoperative X-Ray (Extension Fracture)

1. The radius is shortened.
2. Relations of the radio-ulnar joint are disturbed.
3. The articular surface of the radius is directed upward and backward.

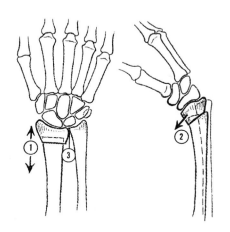

Preoperative X-Ray (Flexion Fracture)

1. The radius is shortened.
2. The distal fragment is displaced anteriorly.
3. The normal relations of the radio-ulnar joint are altered.

Operative Correction

1. Make a 3 inch incision extending upward in the midline of the dorsal aspect of the radius beginning at the level of the wrist joint.

2. Divide the deep fascia and expose the tendons of the extensor carpi radialis longus and the extensor carpi radialis brevis as they emerge from under the extensor pollicis brevis on the lateral side of the wound and the extensor pollicis longus on the medial side.

3. Make a longitudinal incision in the periosteum of the radius in the interval between the extensor carpi radialis brevis and the extensor pollicis longus.

4. By subperiosteal dissection, expose the distal 2½ inches of the radius as far as its articular surface.

5. With a thin sharp osteotome, sever transversely the radius approximately ¾ to 1 inch distal to its articular surface.

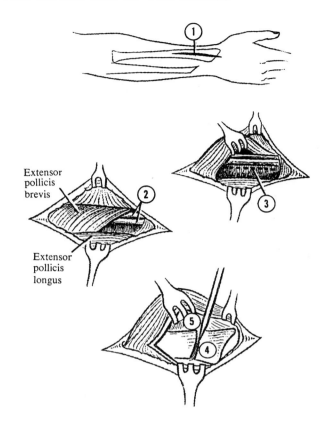

1. Next make a 2 inch incision along the medial aspect of the ulna beginning at the tip of its styloid process and extending upward.

2. Expose the distal end of the ulna by subperiosteal dissection.

3. Divide the ulna 1 inch above the tip of the styloid process and remove it by sharp dissection, leaving the ulnar collateral ligament intact.

4. On closure, the periosteal tube of the ulna should be continuous with the collateral ligament.

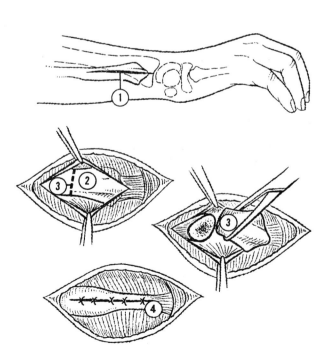

Operative Correction
(Continued)

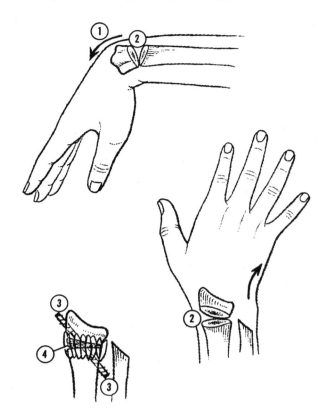

FOR EXTENSION FRACTURES

1. Flex the wrist acutely and bring the hand into ulnar deviation.

2. Open the defect on the dorsal and lateral aspect of the radius sufficiently to restore the articular plane of the radius to its normal plane of inclination.

3. While the corrected position is maintained and the hand is deviated toward the ulna, pass a ³/₁₆ inch threaded wire through both fragments. The wire enters the distal fragment just proximal to its styloid process and is directed obliquely toward the ulna and engages the ulnar side of the proximal radial fragment. The wire is cut below the level of the skin.

4. Pack the defect in the radius with cancellous bone chips previously obtained from the crest of the ilium.

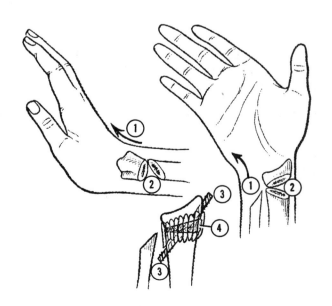

FOR FLEXION FRACTURES

1. Extend the wrist acutely and bring the hand into ulnar deviation.

2. Open the defect on the lateral and volar aspect of the radius sufficiently to restore the articular plane of the radius to its normal plane of inclination.

3. Transfix the fragments with ³/₁₆ inch threaded wire. The wire is cut below the level of the skin.

4. Pack the defect in the radius with cancellous bone chips.

Postoperative X-Ray: Extension and Flexion Fractures

1. The distal end of the ulna is resected.
2. The articular surface of the radius is restored to its normal plane of inclination.
3. The length of the radius is increased.

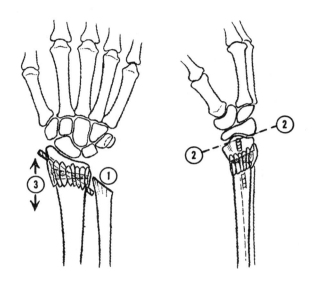

Immobilization

EXTENSION FRACTURES

Apply a circular cast from the metacarpophalangeal joints to below the axilla.

1. The forearm is in midposition.
2. The wrist is slightly flexed.
3. The hand is deviated toward the ulna.

FLEXION FRACTURES

1. The forearm is in midposition.
2. The wrist is slightly dorsiflexed.
3. The hand is deviated slightly toward the ulna.

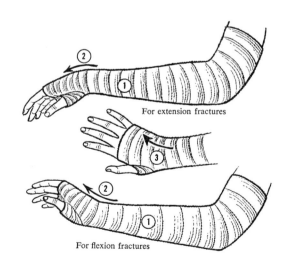

For extension fractures

For flexion fractures

Postoperative Management

Take check x-rays after the first and second weeks. Check for maintenance of position of the fragments.

If after ten to 14 days the plaster cast becomes loose, reapply the cast.

Usually at the end of six to eight weeks healing is advanced enough to permit removal of the threaded wire.

Immobilize for two more weeks after the removal of the wire. Immobilization should be continued until there is x-ray and clinical evidence of bony union. This may mean ten to 16 weeks.

After removal of the cast, institute physical therapy and exercises to restore motion in all joints.

During the period of immobilization, the fingers and shoulder should be exercised continuously.

NONUNION OF THE DISTAL END OF THE RADIUS

REMARKS

This is a rare complication following Colles fractures.

There is always shortening of the radius and disalignment at the distal radio-ulnar joint.

The treatment of choice is resection of the distal 1 inch of the ulna, realignment of the radial fragment, internal fixation by a transfixion wire, and bone grafting.

Preoperative X-Ray

1. Radial deviation of the wrist and hand.

2. The radius is shortened.

3. The distal end of the ulna extends distal to the styloid of the radius.

Operative Management

1. Make a 2 inch incision along the medial aspect of the ulna beginning at the tip of the styloid and extending upward.

2. Expose the distal end of the ulna by subperiosteal dissection.

3. Divide the ulna obliquely 1 inch above the tip of the styloid process and remove the distal segment by sharp dissection, preserving the ulnar collateral ligament.

4. On closure of the wound, the periosteal tube of the ulna should be continuous with the ulnar collateral ligament.

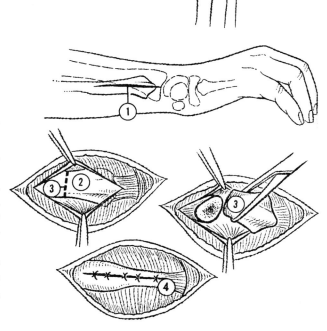

Operative Management
(Continued)

1. Make a 3 inch incision extending upward in the midline of the dorsal aspect of the radius, beginning at the level of the wrist joint.

2. Divide the deep fascia and expose the tendons of the extensor carpi radialis longus and the extensor carpi radialis brevis as they emerge from under the extensor pollicis brevis on the lateral side of the wound and the extensor pollicis longus on the medial side.

3. Make a longitudinal incision in the periosteum of the radius in the interval between the extensor carpi radialis brevis and the extensor pollicis longus.

4. Cut out the fibrous tissue between the fragments, freshen the ends of the fragments and realign the distal to the proximal fragment.

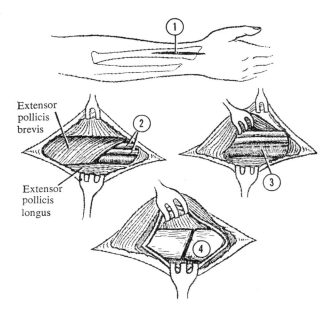

Extensor pollicis brevis

Extensor pollicis longus

1. With the hand in ulnar deviation and the fragments in the corrected position, transfix the fragments with a $\frac{3}{16}$ inch threaded wire. It enters the distal fragment in the region of the radial styloid and is directed obliquely upward and toward the ulna.

2. Cut the wire below the level of the skin.

3. Surround the fracture site with slabs of cancellous bone.

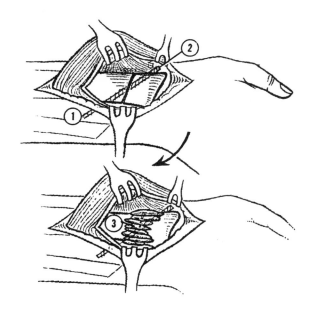

Immobilization

EXTENSION FRACTURES

Apply a circular cast from the meta-carpophalangeal joints to below the axilla.

1. The forearm is in midposition.
2. The wrist is slightly flexed.
3. The hand is deviated toward the ulna.

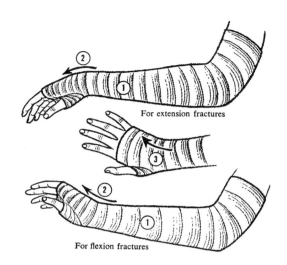

For extension fractures

For flexion fractures

FLEXION FRACTURES

1. The forearm is in midposition.
2. The wrist is slightly dorsiflexed.
3. The hand is deviated slightly toward the ulna.

Postoperative Management

Take check x-rays after the first and second week. Check for maintenance of the position of the fragments.

If after ten to 14 days the plaster cast becomes loose, reapply the cast.

Usually at the end of six to eight weeks healing is advanced enough to permit removal of the threaded wire.

Immobilize for two more weeks after the removal of the wire. Immobilization should be continued until there is x-ray and clinical evidence of bony union. This may mean ten to 16 weeks.

After removal of the cast, institute physical therapy and exercises to restore motion in all joints.

During the period of immobilization the fingers and shoulder should be exercised continuously.

FRACTURES AND DISLOCATIONS OF THE CARPAL BONES

REMARKS

Injuries to the wrist implicating the carpal bones are common lesions in all age groups, particularly in young adults.

Comprehension of the factors involved in the production of many of these lesions and of the rationale of the treatment instituted requires knowledge of some of the pertinent anatomic features of the wrist.

ANATOMIC CONSIDERATIONS

The wrist comprises the interval between the distal end of the radius and ulna and the proximal end of the metacarpal bones. Within this area is a very complex system of articulations which work in unison to provide almost a global range of motion at the wrist joint.

There are eight carpal bones of different size and shape; they are all fitted to one another to form a compact powerful unit. They are arranged in two rows: the distal row articulates with the proximal surface of the metacarpal bones and the proximal row with the distal end of the radius and the triangular fibrocartilage at the distal end of the ulna; the ulna does not articulate with the carpus.

The bones in the proximal row are arranged in a smooth arc which articulates on its convex side with the articular surface of the radius and the fibrocartilage covering the distal end of the ulna.

There are five large joint cavities in addition to the intercarpal joint spaces. These are:

The radiocarpal joint.

The distal radio-ulnar joint.

The midcarpal joint.

The large carpometacarpal joint (between the carpus and the second, third, fourth and fifth metacarpals).

The small carpometacarpal joint (between the first metacarpal and the trapezium).

As depicted in the accompanying figure, some of these joint cavities are continuous with one another while others are separated from one another. Note that the radiocarpal joint is not continuous with the inferior radio-ulnar joint and that the large carpometacarpal joint is separate and distinct from the small carpometacarpal joint. On the other hand, the midcarpal joint is continuous with the intercarpal joints between the proximal and distal rows of carpal bones and the carpometacarpal joints are continuous with the distal intercarpal joints and the intermetacarpal joints.

Volar and Dorsal Aspects of the Wrist

1. Scaphoid.
2. Lunate.
3. Triquetrum.
4. Pisiform.
5. Trapezium.
6. Trapezoid.
7. Capitate.
8. Hamate.
9. Intra-articular disc.

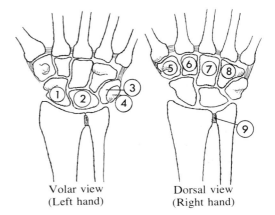

Volar view
(Left hand)

Dorsal view
(Right hand)

The proximal row forms a smooth arc; its convex side articulates with the radius and the fibrocartilage of the ulna while the capitate and hamate fit snugly into the concave side of the arc. Although the carpal bones are of different size and shape they fit together into a strong compact unit.

Joint Cavities of the Wrist

1. Radiocarpal joint.
2. Distal radio-ulnar.
3. Midcarpal joint.
4. Intercarpal joints.
5. Large carpometacarpal joint.
6. Small carpometacarpal joint.

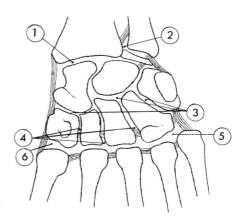

Most of the motion at the wrist joint occurs between the radius and the carpal bones, which function as a single unit. However, there is independent motion between the proximal and distal row of carpal bones and in the intercarpal joints.

The proximal row moves as a single unit and separately from the distal row. The greater part of the total motion is between the radius and the proximal row; considerably less motion occurs between the proximal and distal row. The amount of motion between the distal row and the metacarpal bones is insignificant.

When the wrist is extended the proximal row glides forward and lies against the anterior lip of the distal articular surface of the radius while the distal row rotates dorsally.

When the wrist is flexed the proximal row of the carpal bones glides backward, abutting against the dorsal lip of the distal articular surface of the radius; the distal row shifts forward.

When the hand is deviated toward the radius, the scaphoid, the lunate and the triquetrum glide as a unit toward the ulna while the distal row, together with the metacarpal bones, moves toward the radius. When the hand is deviated toward the ulna, the proximal row moves toward the radius while the distal row and the metacarpals move toward the ulna. The scaphoid, which lies in both rows, is related in function to both the radial and ulnar side of the midcarpal joint.

The radial portion of the midcarpal joint comprises the distal half of the scaphoid, the trapezium and trapezoid rotating around the radial side of the capitate.

The ulnar portion of the midcarpal joint consists of the proximal portion of the scaphoid, the lunate, the hamate and the triquetrum, which function as a diarthrodial joint about the distal ulnar aspect of the capitate.

The ligamentous apparatus of the carpal bones is such that the proximal portion of the scaphoid and the lunate work as a separate unit and intimately relate to the radius, while the trapezoid, the distal portion of the scaphoid, the capitate, the hamate and the triquetrum function as a unit and relate to the metacarpals.

In addition, the scaphoid has some independent rotatory motion; also it is the only carpal bone which spans both rows so that its normal relationship to both the proximal and distal row is essential to the performance of smooth painless motion of the wrist joint.

Radial Deviation of the Wrist

1. The proximal row glides toward the ulna.
2. The distal row with the metacarpals moves toward the radius.

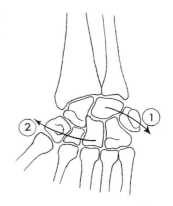

Ulnar Deviation of the Wrist

1. The proximal row glides toward the radius.
2. The distal row and the metacarpals move toward the ulna.

Extension of the Wrist

1. Proximal row moves forward against anterior lip of the radius.
2. The distal row moves dorsally.

Flexion of the Wrist

1. Proximal row moves backward against dorsal lip of the radius.
2. Distal row moves forward.

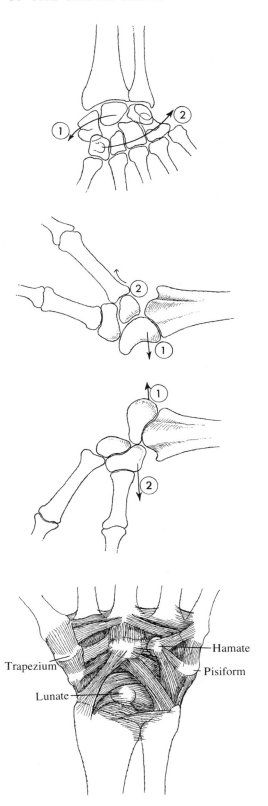

The strength of the wrist depends upon the numerous strong bands which encircle it and also upon a tough intricate complex of ligaments of which the volar component is the strongest. The strong ligaments anchor the bones in place and to each other, to the radius and to the metacarpal bones; this is especially true on the volar surface of the bones. The pisiform bone actually lies within the tendon of the flexor carpi ulnaris, which in turn continues onto the carpus and metacarpals and hamate through strong ligaments extending from the pisiform to these bones.

Page 955

Flexion of the Wrist (Continued)

The volar carpal ligament is a strong broad fibrous band which extends from the trapezium to the hook of the hamate. It forms the anterior surface or roof of an osseous fibrous tunnel; the remaining surfaces of the tunnel are formed by the carpal bones. Within the tunnel lies the median nerve and the flexor tendons of the fingers. Any encroachment of the space in the tunnel predisposes the median nerve to compression.

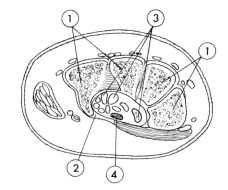

1. Bony sides of the tunnel.
2. Volar carpal ligament.
3. Flexor tendons of the fingers.
4. Median nerve.

Fractures of the Scaphoid

REMARKS

Of all the carpal bones the scaphoid is most frequently fractured. Its size, position and relationship to the radius and the surrounding carpal bones render it vulnerable to injury. During radial deviation and dorsiflexion of the wrist it is impinged upon by the radius; its midportion is narrow and its vertical axis lies in both the proximal and distal row of the carpal bones; these features predispose it to injury.

The healing process following fracture depends much on the integrity of the blood supply, which, because of its manner of distribution, may be interrupted by certain types of fractures.

The arteries enter the bone on the dorsal surface in the region of the tubercle and in the midposition (the waist); the proximal portion has no vessels entering it and depends for its blood supply on the vessels piercing the midportion.

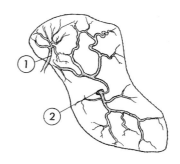

1. Vessels entering the tubercle of the scaphoid.

2. Vessels entering the waist of the scaphoid.

Mechanism of Injury

The scaphoid is fractured during forceful hyperextension of the wrist such as a fall on the outstretched hand. It becomes wedged between the radius and the surrounding carpal bones, especially the capitate. The type of fracture sustained depends upon the direction of the arm at the time of impact. The resulting fractures can be placed into four groups:

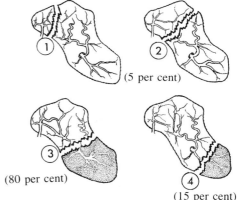

1. Fracture of the tuberosity.
2. Fracture of the distal one-third.
3. Fracture of the middle one-third (waist).
4. Fracture of the proximal one-third.

Note: There may be any combination of these and occasionally a segmental fracture of the scaphoid occurs.

Approximately 80 per cent of all fractures of the scaphoid occur through the middle third, 15 per cent through the proximal third and 5 per cent through the distal third; 85 per cent occur as isolated lesions.

Some of the associated injuries are:

Dislocation of the radiocarpal joint.

Dislocation between the two rows of carpal bones.

Fracture-dislocation of the distal end of the radius.

Fracture of the base of the thumb metacarpal (Bennett's fracture).

Dislocation of the lunate.

Page 957

Epidemiology

The lesion occurs in all age groups, the highest incidence being in young adult males (approximately 50 per cent before the age of 25 years).

It occurs in children more often than is generally appreciated.

Approximately 95 per cent occur in men.

The right hand is involved more frequently than the left (70 per cent).

Bilateral involvement occurs in 2 to 3 per cent.

Recent Fractures of the Scaphoid (Under Four Weeks from Time of Injury)

REMARKS

These lesions continue to be underdiagnosed or completely overlooked. Suspect a fracture of the scaphoid in every case of an acutely sprained wrist.

X-ray examination should always include:

Anteroposterior view.

Lateral view.

Right oblique view.

Left oblique view.

In fresh lesions the x-ray may fail to show a fracture. If so, treat the patient with adequate plaster fixation of the wrist and repeat the x-rays in two weeks. If at this time pain and marked limitation of motion are still present but the x-rays are still negative one must assume that a fracture of the scaphoid exists. Fissure fracture of the scaphoid may not be demonstrable by x-ray for three or four weeks.

A bipartite scaphoid may be mistaken for a fracture through the waist. In the former, the anomaly is frequently bilateral and both bones have normal bone texture with smooth margins; in the latter the line of demarcation is irregular and the bone fragments show evidence of demineralization.

PROGNOSIS

Ninety-five per cent of recent fractures of the scaphoid (this includes fractures not diagnosed or treated for three or four weeks) heal if they are adequately fixed in plaster for a sufficient period of time. In fact 70 to 75 per cent of the fractures in which a diagnosis is not established and treatment is not instituted for several months (up to six months) will heal with adequate and prolonged immobilization.

Some fractures are more likely to go on to delayed union or nonunion regardless of the type of treatment instituted; these include:

Fractures through the proximal third.

Comminuted fractures.

Lesions in which the line of fracture approaches the long axis of the arm as opposed to those which approach the horizontal axis.

Displaced fractures.

Failure to adequately immobilize the limb for a sufficient period of time definitely increases the chance for the development of nonunion.

Failure to immobilize the hand, wrist and forearm in the position which provides the greatest stability possible for displaced and unstable fragments favors delayed union and nonunion.

TYPE OF IMMOBILIZATION

FOR UNDISPLACED FRACTURES

Apply a skin-tight cast (except for a layer of stockinet) extending from just below the elbow to just proximal to the metacarpophalàngeal joints; the wrist is slightly dorsiflexed; the thumb, in the grasp position, is included up to the base of the thumbnail. The wrist is in the neutral position as regards radial and ulnar deviation. At one time I was of the impression that slight radial deviation helped to reduce and fix displaced and unstable fractures; I no longer believe this to be true.

There is evidence indicating that in a stable fracture there is still some continuity between the fragments, particularly at the level of the articular cartilage, which permits the fragments to move in unison and prevents gross motion or displacement at the fracture site. On the other hand, in unstable and displaced fractures there is complete loss of continuity between the fragments, which now are permitted to move as independent bodies. No single position will approximate the fragments and no position will completely prevent motion at the fracture site. In these instances the most favorable position must be determined by x-rays.

LENGTH OF IMMOBILIZATION

There is agreement that longer periods of adequate, continuous immobilization are required for certain fractures such as fractures of the proximal third of the bone, comminuted fracture, fractures with planes approaching the vertical axis of the forearm and for older fractures. In general, fractures of the distal and middle third heal in six to eight weeks; fractures through the proximal third heal in ten to 12 weeks; fractures approaching the horizontal axis of the forearm heal in six to eight weeks while those approaching the vertical axis require ten to 12 weeks.

I no longer believe that prolonged immobilization is justified until there is x-ray evidence of union or x-ray evidence of an established nonunion. Long and indefinite periods of immobilization require great forebearance on the part of the patient, his employer and the insurance carrier; not to mention the strain on the waiting and hopeful surgeon.

There is evidence to affirm that periods of immobilization beyond three or at the most four months are not justifiable, because 95 per cent of the fractures will attain bony union regardless of the appearance of the x-ray at the end of this period. Also, most patients with established nonunions are free of pain and have little if any restriction of motion; however, these wrists are vulnerable to excessive strains which may give rise to temporary symptoms.

Only a few cases of nonunion present symptoms of such severity as to require surgical intervention.

TYPE OF IMMOBILIZATION

FOR DISPLACED FRACTURES

REMARKS

Displacement of fragments is determined by their relationship to the surrounding carpal bones as noted on x-ray.

When displacement is apparent it is essential to determine which position of the wrist will restore anatomic alignment or at least reduce the displacement of the fragments. This is best determined by viewing the position of the fragments when different positions of the wrist are assumed. Cineradiography shows this best; if this modality is not available, take x-rays with the hand extended, flexed, deviated toward the radius and deviated toward the ulna.

Immobilize the hand and wrist in the position found to be the most stable for the fragments. The cast extends from just below the elbow to just proximal to the metacarpophalangeal joints. Place the thumb in the grasp position and extend the cast to the base of the thumbnail.

From this point on the treatment is the same as for undisplaced fractures.

MANAGEMENT OF RECENT FRACTURES OF THE SCAPHOID

REMARKS

Management of undisplaced and displaced fractures of the scaphoid differ only in the position of immobilization of the hand and wrist.

In undisplaced fractures the plaster cast is applied with the wrist slightly dorsiflexed and in a neutral position with regard to radial or ulnar deviation.

For displaced fractures the position of stability for the fragments must first be determined by cineradiography or x-ray studies; and the hand and wrist must be immobilized in this position.

Types of Undisplaced Fractures Usually Encountered

Fracture through the waist (middle third).

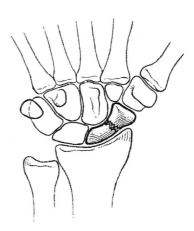

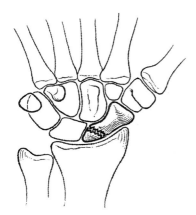

Fracture through the proximal third.

Fracture through the distal third.

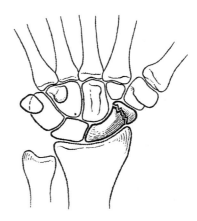

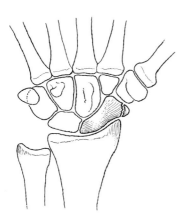

Fracture through the tubercle.

Types of Displaced Fractures

Fracture of the middle third — the normal relationship of the fragments of the scaphoid to the surrounding carpal bones is disturbed.

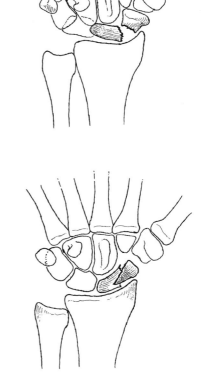

Displaced fracture of the body of the scaphoid; this is really a compression fracture.

Immobilization for Undisplaced Fractures

If the patient is seen immediately after the injury and exhibits considerable swelling of the hand and wrist, apply anterior and posterior plaster splints.

1. The splints extend from below the elbow to the metacarpophalangeal joints.

2. The thumb is in the grasp position and included in the plaster as far as the base of the thumbnail.

3. The wrist is in the neutral position except for slight dorsiflexion.

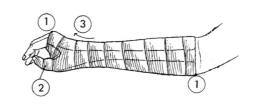

Immobilization for Undisplaced Fractures (Continued)

After all swelling has subsided, usually in ten to 14 days, apply a circular cast over stockinet without padding.

1. The cast extends from just below the elbow to the metacarpophalangeal joints.

2. The wrist is slightly dorsiflexed and in a neutral position.

3. The thumb is in the grasp position and the thumb is

4. Included in the cast as far as the base of the thumbnail.

5. The plaster is well molded in the palm.

6. The cast extends to the distal palmar crease.

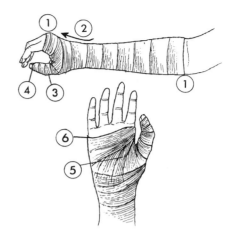

Immobilization for Displaced and Unstable Fractures

After determining the optimum position for the wrist, the hand, wrist and forearm are encased in plaster holding this position.

A. AN EXAMPLE OF A FRACTURE WITH DISPLACEMENT OF THE FRAGMENTS

Prereduction x-ray:

1. Fracture of the middle third of the scaphoid.

2. The normal relationship of the fragments to the surrounding carpal bones is disturbed.

3. The fragments are angulated.

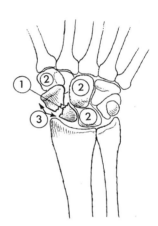

X-ray study revealed that a position of moderate radial deviation of the hand realigned the fragments.

1. The hand is deviated toward the radius.

2. The fragments are in normal alignment.

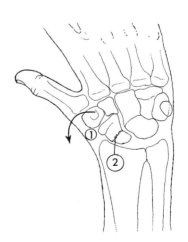

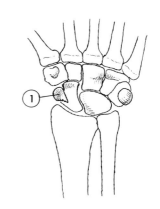

Immobilization for Displaced and Unstable Fractures *(Continued)*

B. ANOTHER EXAMPLE OF A DISPLACED FRACTURE

Prereduction x-ray:

1. Fracture of the tuberosity of the scaphoid.

2. X-ray revealed that ulnar deviation of the hand without dorsiflexion or palmar flexion corrected the displacement.

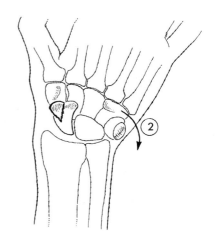

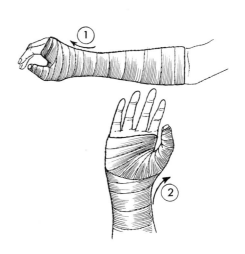

Immobilization for Example A

Apply a circular cast over stockinet without padding.

1. Hold the wrist slightly dorsiflexed and

2. In moderate radial deviation.

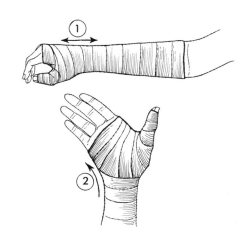

Immobilization for Example B

Apply a circular cast over stockinet without padding.

1. Hold the wrist in line with the forearm.

2. The wrist and hand are deviated toward the ulna.

Management

Immobilization of the wrist must be rigid and complete.

Inspect the cast every two weeks; if it becomes loose apply a new cast.

Maintain immobilization for eight weeks, then take the cast off and x-ray the wrist. If there is evidence of solid bony union and there is no pain and a reasonable amount of painless motion, take the cast off.

If there is evidence of bony union but the union is still not adequate and motion of the wrist is painful, reapply the plaster cast for four more weeks, or even for six or eight more weeks, until union is solid.

If there is no evidence of bony union at the end of eight weeks, reapply the plaster cast.

Remove the cast at the end of four months regardless of the state of union.

Check the status of healing every four weeks; if healing occurs before four months remove the cast; if union is still not demonstrable by x-ray at the end of four months remove the cast and permit free use of the hand.

Note: It was previously stated that 95 per cent of fresh fractures heal by solid bony union if early treatment is adequate.

In some instances bony union is incomplete at the end of four months but, nevertheless, healing progresses until solid union is achieved without plaster immobilization of the limb within six to 12 months after discarding the cast.

Should fibrous union develop, the condition may produce no symptoms; and in many instances it is not recognized until the arm is subjected to some form of trauma.

MANAGEMENT OF FRACTURE OF THE SCAPHOID WITH DISPLACED FRAGMENTS

REMARKS

Displaced fragments of a fractured scaphoid indicate that a perilunar dislocation has occurred and reduced spontaneously.

Page 965

These lesions are associated with severe soft tissue damage, carrying a very unfavorable prognosis insofar as the viability of the proximal fragment and the chances of a bony union are concerned.

In undisplaced fractures the incidence of avascular necrosis of the proximal fragment approaches 50 per cent; in displaced fractures it is almost 100 per cent.

When closed methods fail to approximate the fragments anatomically, I recommend the following course of management:

1. If the proximal fragment is small or comminuted, remove it.

2. If the proximal fragment is one-third or more, perform an open reduction and fix the fragments with a bone peg or a threaded wire (see page 968).

Subacute Fractures of the Scaphoid (Under Six Months)

REMARKS

Many of these lesions go unrecognized and frequently are treated as sprains of the wrists.

During this period certain alterations occur at the fracture site that may delay union but do not preclude it, provided correct and prolonged immobilization of the wrist is instituted.

Seventy to 75 per cent of these lesions will heal eventually.

The changes that may be presented at the site of the fracture are:

Absorption of bone at the fracture site.

Formation of vacuoles or cysts in the fragments.

Avascular necrosis.

In late cases, sclerosis of the fragments.

These abnormalities do not preclude bony union when the wrist is adequately protected for a long period of time; nor does the appearance of these changes during the course of treatment indicate a hopeless situation prompting discontinuance of the immobilization.

Factors which favor union in old cases are:

Absence of arthritis.

Absence of sclerosis of the fragment.

No displacement or very little displacement of the fragments.

MANAGEMENT

Treat these fractures by continuous plaster immobilization as described for recent fractures of the scaphoid (see page 960).

Remove the cast at the end of four months regardless of the state of repair or the absence of repair at the fracture site. If union occurs earlier than in four months discard the cast at this time.

The management of those patients who develop an established nonunion is governed by the intensity of the symptoms (if present) and the degree of functional impairment of the wrist.

Nonunion of the Scaphoid

REMARKS

Established nonunion of the scaphoid may exist without symptoms or impairment of function. This is true in the great majority of cases; the wrist becomes symptomatic only when subjected to abusive stresses or when traumatized.

The pathologic conditions at the site of fracture vary considerably.

1. The fragments may be viable with an actual joint space between them with no change in the trabecular pattern of the bone. There may be no reactive changes such as osteoarthritis.
2. There may be avascular necrosis of one or both fragments with cyst formation. These alterations are usually associated with varying degrees of osteoarthritis but not necessarily so.
3. There may be dense sclerosis of one fragment with cyst formation in the other.
4. The affected fragment may be comminuted and fragmented with changes in the intercarpal and radiocarpal joints.
5. There may be severe disintegration of the radiocarpal and intercarpal joints (particularly the proximal joints).

The preceding alterations may not be associated with disabling symptoms. The incidence of avascular necrosis of a fragment in nonunion is approximately 40 per cent; osteoarthritis is encountered in 35 per cent of the cases. In general, the older the nonunion the greater the likelihood of osteoarthritis, but this is not necessarily so.

Fibrous union may stabilize the fragments sufficiently to eliminate symptoms or impairment of function unless there is a superimposed injury.

Surgery is not indicated unless the lesion fails to respond to a period of rest (four weeks) and produces marked impairment of function.

Many elderly patients and patients with sedentary occupations are capable of adjusting their activities to the tolerance of the wrist and need no other treatment.

CONSERVATIVE MANAGEMENT OF NONUNION OF THE SCAPHOID (OVER SIX MONTHS SINCE INJURY)

All cases of established nonunion, especially if the symptoms were heralded by overuse of the wrist or by an injury, should be treated by a period of rest for four weeks.

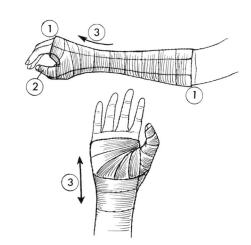

Apply anterior and posterior plaster slabs.

1. The plaster slabs extend from just below the elbow to the metacarpophalangeal joints.

2. The thumb is in the grasp position and is included in the splints as far as the interphalangeal joint.

3. The wrist is slightly dorsiflexed and in the neutral position in regard to ulnar and radial deviation.

Allow free use of the fingers and elbow.

Remove the splint after four weeks.

Institute a program of gentle exercises to restore normal motion at the wrist.

Apply radiant heat and gentle massage.

Refrain from strenuous use of of the wrist for four to six weeks.

SURGICAL PROCEDURES FOR NONUNION OF THE SCAPHOID

REMARKS

Most patients will respond to the conservative form of treatment just outlined and they will be capable of performing normal activities without pain or serious disability.

Those that fail to respond, if they are young or middle-aged persons leading an active life, should be subjected to that surgical procedure most likely to relieve pain and improve the function of the wrist.

Do not "fit" the patient to any particular operation.

Study the patient as a whole as to his age, activities, occupation and other functional demands made on the wrist. Study the nature of the local pathologic conditions carefully and choose the operation that is best suited for the individual case.

I do not believe that any nonunion of over six months duration should be treated by continuous, prolonged immobilization; this period may extend into many, many months and then terminate in failure.

If symptoms and serious impairment persist after a period of rest (four weeks) then choose the operation best fitted for the patient.

Bone Grafting and Radial Styloidectomy

REMARKS

This procedure is best suited:

When both fragments are viable and the smaller fragment is not less than one-third of the scaphoid.

When no arthritic changes are demonstrable in the radiocarpal or intercarpal joints. However, mild arthritic changes on the radial side of the joint, indicated by some narrowing of the joint space and spurring, do not preclude this procedure.

When cysts are demonstrable in one or both fragments.

Note: Do not perform the operation when there is extensive arthritis implicating the radiocarpal and intercarpal joints or when one fragment is dense and sclerotic.

Appearance on X-Ray

1. Old ununited fracture through the body.

2. Fractured surfaces are smooth and sclerotic.

3. Bone texture is indicative that both fragments are viable.

Note: X-ray evidence of arthritis is absent.

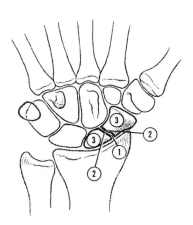

Operative Procedure

BONE GRAFTING

1. Make a 2½ inch incision centered over the anatomic snuffbox; it begins at the base of the first metacarpal and is directed upward and proximally.

2. Divide the fascia between the extensor pollicis longus dorsally and the extensor pollicis brevis ventrally. Identify and protect the sensory branch of the radial nerve and the radial artery.

3. Expose the dorsal carpal ligament proximally.

4. Mobilize the tendons of the extensor pollicis longus and the extensor carpi radialis from the joint capsule and retract them dorsally.

5. Make a linear incision in the joint capsule and divide the dorsal carpal ligament.

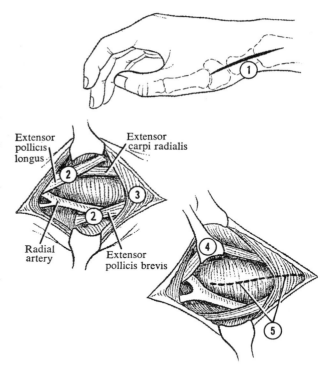

Extensor pollicis longus

Extensor carpi radialis

Radial artery

Extensor pollicis brevis

1. Retract the margins of the capsule.

2. Strip the periosteum and capsule from the radius for ¾ inch.

3. Deviate the wrist toward the ulna; the scaphoid is now clearly visualized.

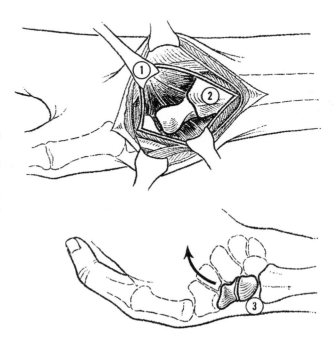

Operative Procedure (Continued)

4. With a fine osteotome resect the styloid process just proximal to the fracture line and perpendicular to the long axis of the bones.

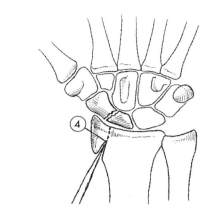

1. Make a channel through both fragments with a ⁵/₁₆ inch drill. The drill channel extends from the distal into the proximal fragment.

CAUTION

a. Do not damage the articular surfaces of the scaphoid or the other adjacent carpal bones with the drill.

b. Avoid excessive stripping of soft tissues.

c. Do not perforate the proximal surface of the proximal fragment.

d. It is not necessary to curette fibrous tissue from between the fragments.

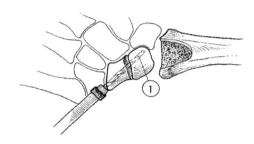

2. Insert a graft, previously obtained from the resected styloid process through the drill channel. The fragments must be impacted by the tightly fitting graft.

3. Cut the protruding end of the graft flush with the surface of the tuberosity.

Note: The graft should be slightly larger in diameter than the drill hole.

Postoperative X-Ray

1. A cortical bone graft traverses the fracture line and stabilizes both fragments.

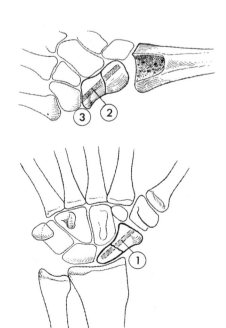

Immobilization

Apply a circular cast over a stockinet without padding.

1. The cast extends from just below the elbow to the metacarpophalangeal joints.

2. The wrist is slightly dorsiflexed and in the neutral position.

3. The base of the thumb is in a position of abduction and its metacarpophalangeal and interphalangeal joints are slightly flexed.

4. The cast incorporates the thumb to the middle of the nail.

5. The plaster is well molded in the palm of the hand.

6. The cast extends to the distal palmar crease of the hand.

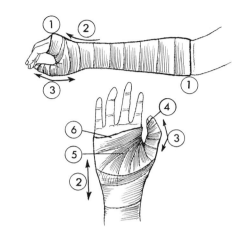

Postoperative Management

As with fresh fractures, immobilization must be rigid and complete.

Reapply the plaster cast if the original cast becomes loose.

Maintain immobilization until bony union is demonstrable by x-ray (three to six months).

If union is not completed at the end of six months, the cast is removed and the patient is allowed free use of the limb.

Some residual stiffness must be anticipated in all cases.

The incidence of success is high in carefully selected cases and when the operation is executed skillfully; it is low in ill-selected cases and when the operation is poorly done.

Excision of the Ulnar Fragment of the Scaphoid

REMARKS

This procedure is indicated:

When the fragment is one-third or less of the scaphoid and is comminuted or sclerotic.

When the fragment is less than one-third of the scaphoid regardless of its viability.

When bone grafting of a fragment one-third or less of the scaphoid has failed.

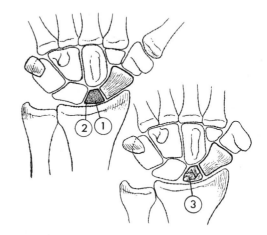

Appearance on X-Ray

1. The proximal fragment is one-third of the scaphoid.
2. The fragment is dense.
3. The fragment is comminuted.

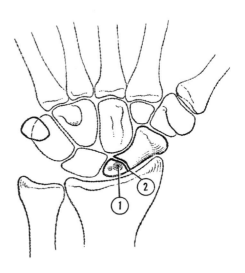

Appearance on X-Ray

1. The fragment shows some cyst formation but is viable.
2. The proximal fragment is less than one-third of the scaphoid.

Excision of the Ulnar Fragment

1. Make a 2½ inch incision centered over the anatomic snuffbox; it begins at the base of the first metacarpal and extends upward and proximally.

2. Divide the fascia between the extensor pollicis longus dorsally and the extensor pollicis brevis ventrally.

3. Expose the dorsal carpal ligament proximally.

4. Retract the tendons of the extensor pollicis longus and the extensor carpi radialis upward.

5. Make a linear incision in the joint capsule and divide the dorsal carpal ligament.

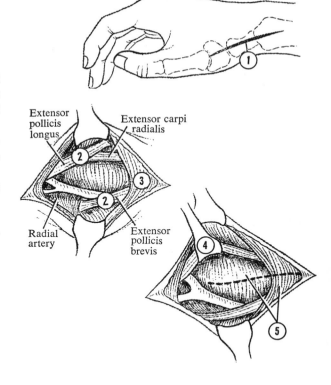

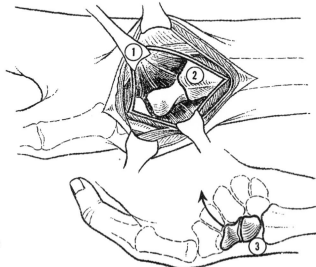

1. Retract the margins of the capsule.

2. Strip the periosteum and the capsule from the radius for ¾ inch.

3. Turn the wrist toward the ulna.

Excision of the Ulnar Fragment
(Continued)

1. Grasp the proximal fragment with a towel clip and by sharp dissection, using a tenotome, sever all soft tissue attachments and remove the bone.

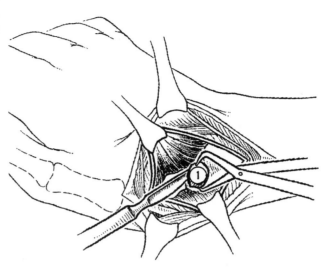

Postoperative X-Ray

1. The ulnar fragment has been removed.

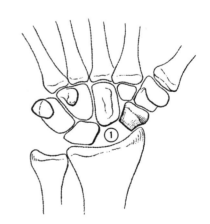

Immobilization

Apply an anterior plaster slab.
1. The plaster slab extends to the distal palmar crease.
2. The wrist is slightly dorsiflexed.

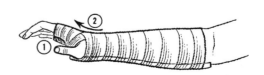

Page 975

Postoperative Management

Remove the plaster slab after ten days.
Institute active motion of the wrist and fingers.
Institute physical therapy (heat and underwater massage).

Note: In all instances, some restriction of dorsiflexion and palmar flexion must be anticipated.

Styloidectomy

REMARKS

This procedure is of significant value when performed in conjunction with bone grafting for nonunion of the scaphoid, especially if there are mild arthritic changes implicating the radial aspects of the radiocarpal joint.

It may be performed as a single procedure when mild or moderate arthritic changes of the radial aspect of the radiocarpal joint are present and bone grafting of an ununited scaphoid is contraindicated.

It may be performed in conjunction with excision of the proximal fragment of an ununited scaphoid. Finally, in severe instances of arthritis associated with an ununited scaphoid, when the only alternative is fusion of the wrist which is contraindicated for some reason, styloidectomy may provide sufficient relief of pain to make the situation tolerable.

Styloidectomy has no effect on the state of union of an ununited scaphoid.

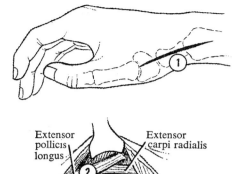

Operative Procedure

1. Make a 2½ inch incision centered over the anatomic snuffbox; it begins at the base of the first metacarpal and is directed upward and proximally.

2. Divide the fascia between the extensor pollicis longus dorsally and the extensor pollicis brevis ventrally. Identify and protect the sensory branches of the radial nerve and the radial artery.

3. Expose the dorsal carpal ligament proximally.

4. Mobilize the tendons of the extensor pollicis longus and extensor carpi radialis from the joint capsule and retract them dorsally.

5. Make a linear incision in the joint capsule and divide the dorsal carpal ligament.

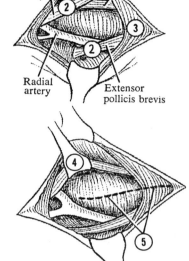

Extensor pollicis longus · Extensor carpi radialis · Radial artery · Extensor pollicis brevis

1. Retract the margins of the capsule.

2. Expose the radial styloid by sharp subperiosteal dissection.

3. Locate the ridge in the radius which separates the articular surface of the lunate from that of the scaphoid.

4. With a fine osteotome, osteotomize the styloid process perpendicular to the long axis of the radius, the ulnar margin being at the level of the bony ridge previously identified. The line of the osteotomy should be proximal to the fracture line of the radius.

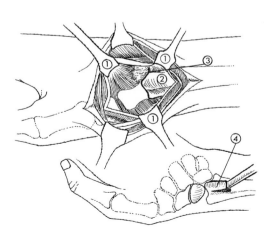

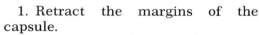

Postoperative Management (If Performed as an Isolated Procedure)

Apply an anterior plaster slab.

1. The plaster slab extends from below the elbow to the distal palmar crease.

2. The wrist is slightly dorsiflexed.

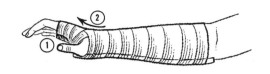

Remove the plaster splints after ten days.

Institute active motion of the wrist and fingers.

Institute physical therapy (heat and underwater massage).

Note: In most instances, some restriction of motion at the wrist must be anticipated.

Arthrodesis of the Wrist Joint

REMARKS

Arthrodesis is indicated when one fragment is greater than one-third of the scaphoid and is densely sclerotic. (Never excise a fragment such as this; the results are poor. The capitate migrates into the defect; the anatomy of the intercarpal joints is severely disturbed.)

Also, arthrodesis is indicated when there is advanced osteoarthritis implicating the radiocarpal and intercarpal joints.

Many patients are able to carry on their work with minimal distress in spite of the x-ray evidence of advanced arthritic changes. Such patients need no surgical intervention.

Occasionally such patients have acute exacerbations of symptoms following excessive use of the wrist; rest, restricted activity or a change of the patient's work may suffice to obtain the desired relief.

In some cases, pain is severe and constant and there is marked dysfunction of the wrist, particularly if strenuous activity is demanded of this joint; in such cases, the treatment of choice is arthrodesis of the wrist joint.

Appearance on X-Ray

1. Nonunion of the fracture of the scaphoid.

2. The ulnar fragment is dense and sclerotic.

3. The radial fragment shows cystic changes.

4. The joint space is narrowed, indicative of degeneration of articular cartilage.

5. Bony spurs are consistent with osteoarthritis.

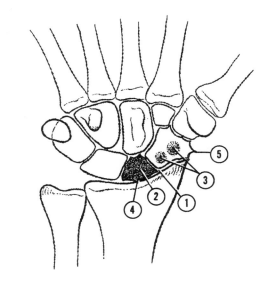

Arthrodesis of the Wrist Joint

1. Make an S incision centered on the radius; it begins just distal to the proximal end of the third metacarpal and ends approximately 3 inches above the wrist joint.

2. Incise the dorsal carpal ligament and the deep fascia proximally and distally.

3. Develop the interval between the extensor pollicis longus and the extensor digitorum communis tendon of the index finger and expose the radius.

4. Incise the periosteum and by subperiosteal dissection expose the dorsal surface of the radius.

5. Retract the extensor pollicis longus and its fascial canal together with the tendons of the extensor carpi radialis longus and brevis to the radial side of the wound.

6. Extend the radial incision into the capsule as far as the base of the third metacarpal bone and reflect the capsule from the margin of the radius and from the adjacent carpal bones and from the base of the third metacarpal bone.

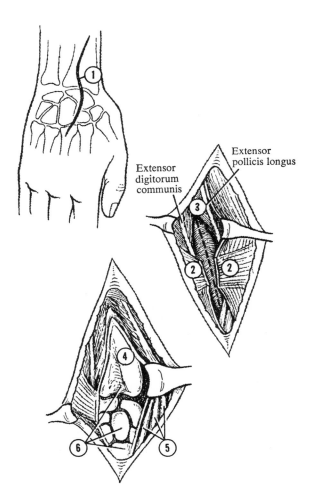

Arthrodesis of the Wrist Joint (Continued)

1. With a sharp, thin osteotome, cut a trough ½ inch wide in the dorsum of the carpus connecting the distal end of the radius with the base of the third metacarpal bone.

2. With sharp curettes, open the medullary canal in the radius and the base of the third metacarpal.

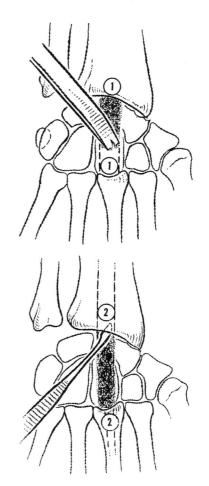

A cortical graft, ½ inch wide and 2 inches longer than the prepared bed, is obtained from the tibia.

1. One end of the graft is shaped to fit tightly in the medullary canal of the third metacarpal.

2. The other end is driven into the medullary canal of the radius.

3. While traction is made on the hand, the distal end of the graft is tapped into the medullary canal of the third metacarpal bone.

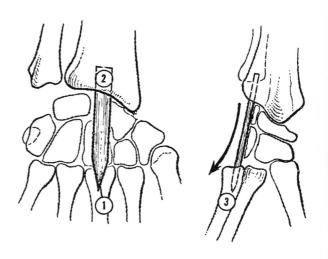

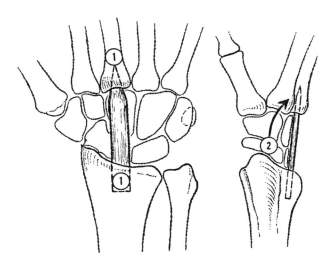

Postoperative X-Ray

1. The tibial graft is well seated in the medullary canal of the radius and third metacarpal bone.

2. The wrist is dorsiflexed 15 to 20 degrees.

Immobilization

Apply a circular cast from the upper arm to the metacarpophalangeal joints; include the base of the thumb.

1. The elbow is at a right angle.

2. The forearm is in midposition.

3. The wrist is dorsiflexed 15 to 20 degrees.

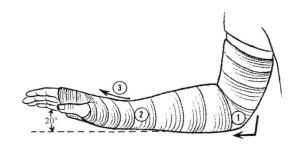

Postoperative Management

Watch for swelling and evidence of circulatory embarrassment.

Elevate the arm and apply ice bags.

If the swelling is excessive, split the dorsum of the cast throughout its entire length and cut all padding beneath the cast.

After three weeks, remove the long arm cast and apply a short cast extending from below the elbow to the metacarpophalangeal joints.

Continue immobilization until union is firm (ten to 14 weeks).

Lunate and Perilunar Dislocations

REMARKS

These lesions are rare — dislocation of the lunate is more common than perilunar dislocation.

The lesions may occur in any age group but the greatest incidence is between 25 and 50 years of age.

Females are rarely affected, the incidence among them being about 3 per cent.

Dislocations may be either anterior or posterior; the former is by far more common.

Dislocations of the carpal bones are frequently not recognized and often the seriousness of the lesion is underestimated. Delay in the reduction of the lesion is directly reflected in the prognosis: the greater the delay the worse the prognosis.

The lesions are listed here in the order of greatest frequency:

    Anterior dislocation of the scaphoid.

    Trans-scaphoid perilunar dislocation.

    Perilunar dislocation without fracture of the scaphoid.

    Dislocation of the proximal row of carpal bones.

The exact diagnosis may be difficult to establish by x-rays.

Always take the following four projections; also, take x-rays of the uninjured wrist for comparison:

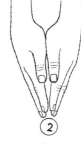

AP.

1. Anteroposterior.
2. Lateral.
3. Pronation (45 degrees).
4. Supination (45 degrees).

Lat.

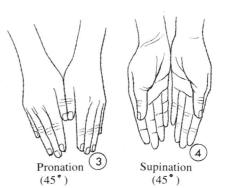

Pronation (45°)   Supination (45°)

POSITION OF HAND AND WRIST FOR LESIONS OF THE CARPAL BONES

MECHANISM

Dislocations of the carpal bones are the result of extension or flexion injuries of the wrist. The type of dislocation or fracture-dislocation produced by these mechanisms depends upon the direction and intensity of the acting force and the position of the hand in relation to the forearm at the moment of impact. The most crucial factor in all dislocations is the integrity of the lunate-capitate relationship. The resulting lesions are directly related to the disruption or the preservation of this articulation.

EXTENSION LESIONS

When the hand is forced into extension, such as in a fall on the out-stretched hand, either dislocation of the lunate or a dorsal perilunar dislocation ensues. The type of lesion produced is governed by the degree of hyperextension and the intensity and direction of the acting force.

Volar Dislocation of the Lunate

This lesion occurs when the hand and carpus are severely hyperextended, such as occurs in a fall on the outstretched hand close to the body.

The fingers and metacarpal heads, which are the point of contact with the ground, together with the downward force acting through the radius, force the hand and carpus into severe hyperextension. The capitate rolls dorsally on the lunate and, as the forces continue, the lunate is driven forward out of the joint.

The hand and carpus are severely hyperextended by:

1. The force acting upward on the fingers and metacarpal heads and

2. The force acting downward in the line of the radius.

3. The capitate rotates dorsally on the lunate.

4. The lunate is squeezed out of the wrist joint.

5. The rotated lunate lies anterior to the wrist joint.

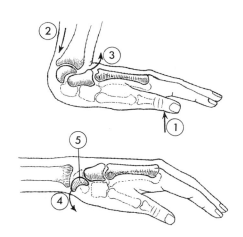

Dorsal Perilunar Dislocation

This lesion occurs when the hand is only moderately hyperextended, such as in a fall on the outstretched hand away from the body.

The main point of impact is on the palm of the hand. The force thus generated together with the oblique downward force traveling along the radius disrupts the lunate-capitate articulation and drives the carpal bones dorsally behind the lunate.

The hand and carpus are not severely extended.

1. The force acting upward on the palm of the hand.

2. The force acting obliquely downward along the shaft of the radius.

3. The lunate-capitate articulation is disrupted.

4. The carpal bones (except the lunate) are driven dorsally and behind the lunate.

5. Perilunar dislocation.

6. The radiolunate relationship is preserved.

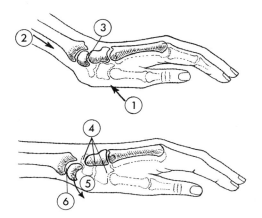

Dorsal perilunar dislocation may be complicated by a fracture or fracture-dislocation of the scaphoid. Depending on the direction of the forces acting, the following lesions involving the scaphoid may follow:

The scaphoid may fracture but its fragments may maintain their normal position to the rest of the carpus.

The scaphoid fragments may separate, the proximal part remaining with the lunate while the distal fragment maintains its normal relationship with the rest of the carpus and with it is displaced dorsally. Should spontaneous reduction occur following the injury, the only evidence that a perilunar dislocation has occurred is the disalignment of the scaphoid fragments. The prognosis in this lesion is poor; the incidence of avascular necrosis of the proximal fragment is almost 100 per cent.

These lesions may be further complicated by a fracture of the styloid process of the radius and ulna.

Also dorsal perilunar dislocation may be complicated by a fracture of the capitate which may be associated with a fracture of the scaphoid. Upon reduction of the dislocation, the proximal fragment of the capitate may remain behind. Closed reduction of this lesion rarely is successful. As a rule, an open reduction must be performed.

FLEXION LESIONS

REMARKS

These lesions are very rare, especially volar perilunar dislocation.

Dorsal Dislocation of the Lunate

This lesion occurs when the hand and carpus are severely hyperflexed, as occurs in a fall on the back of the hand with the hand close to the body.

The upward force generated when the hand makes contact with the ground together with the downward force acting through the radius forces the capitate to rotate anteriorly and drives the lunate backward into a dorsal position.

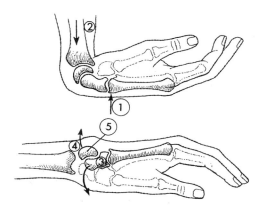

The hand and carpus are severely flexed.

1. The upward force acting on the dorsum of the hand and
2. The force traveling along the radius
3. Rotate the capitate anteriorly and
4. Force the lunate out of the joint posteriorly.
5. The rotated lunate is in a dorsal position.

Volar Perilunar Dislocation

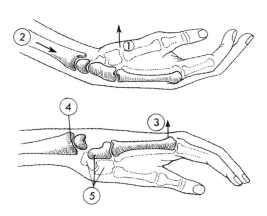

The hand and carpus are not hyperflexed.

1. The upward and backward forces acting on the back of the hand together with
2. The oblique downward force acting along the radius
3. Drive the carpus anterior to the lunate.
4. The lunate retains its normal position with the radius.
5. The rest of the carpus is anterior to the lunate.

Note: Fracture of the scaphoid may also occur with this mechanism.

Page 985

MANAGEMENT OF VOLAR DISLOCATION OF THE LUNATE BONE

REMARKS

Replacement of the lunate by closed methods is generally achieved if the reduction is performed early; in rare instances closed methods fail even in fresh lesions, making open reduction necessary.

After two weeks, closed methods rarely achieve a reduction; therefore, when the dislocation is more than two weeks old, perform an open reduction through the posterior approach.

Excision of the lunate in patients seen many weeks after injury should not be performed; replacement of the bone should be achieved by an open reduction using the posterior incision.

A volar dislocation of the lunate may be secondary to an initial dorsal perilunar dislocation. Reduction of the dislocation may be spontaneous or voluntary; in these instances, during reduction, the lunate is displaced forward as the capitate and hand are brought into alignment with the radius. The scaphoid, which had dislocated with the rest of the carpus, may not be rotated.

Following reduction of the lunate, the scaphoid may still remain rotated requiring realignment to the lunate and the capitate; this must be done by open reduction.

Prereduction X-Ray

1. The lunate lies in front of the wrist and its articular surface tilts forward.

2. The capitate articulates with the articular surface of the radius.

3. In the anteroposterior view, the lunate appears to be triangular instead of quadrilateral.

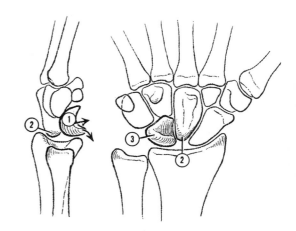

Reduction by Traction and Manipulation

1. Apply finger traction (Weinberg finger traction apparatus is preferred).
2. The elbow is flexed at a right angle.
3. The forearm is fully supinated.
4. Counter traction is made by muslin bandage secured to the bottom of the table.
5. Make strong traction directly upward.

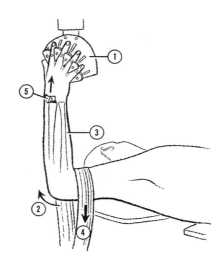

While traction is maintained:
1. Place both thumbs against the front of the lunate and make strong pressure directly backward, while
2. The wrist is dorsiflexed.

Note: Check the position of the lunate by x-ray before application of the plaster slabs.

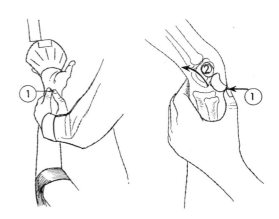

Postreduction X-Ray

1. The lunate is in its normal anatomic position and articulates with the radius.
2. Its concave articular surface articulates with the capitate.
3. In the anteroposterior view, its profile is quadrilateral.

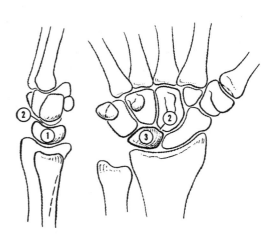

Immobilization

1. Apply anterior and posterior plaster slabs from just below the elbow to just proximal to the metacarpophalangeal joints.
2. The wrist is flexed 45 degrees.

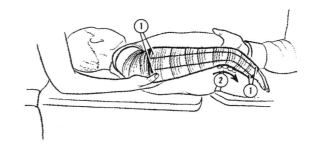

Postreduction Management

After one week, remove the plaster slabs, bring the wrist to a neutral position and again immobilize with anterior and posterior plaster slabs.

Continue immobilization for two more weeks and then remove the plaster slabs.

During the period of immobilization, insist on a program of active finger exercises.

After removal of the plaster slabs, institute a program of active finger exercises.

The prognosis is good in recent cases; recovery should be complete in eight to 12 weeks.

Note: Rarely the lunate is dislocated posteriorly; the treatment is the same as for forward dislocation, except that the wrist is immobilized in slight dorsiflexion.

OPEN REDUCTION OF VOLAR DISLOCATION OF THE LUNATE BONE

REMARKS

Do an open reduction if closed reduction fails in fresh lesions and when the dislocation is over two weeks old.

This same approach may be utilized to realign a rotated scaphoid bone or to stabilize displaced fragments of a fractured scaphoid complicating a perilunar dislocation which, upon reduction, was converted to a volar dislocation of the lunate with some residual dorsal displacement of the scaphoid and capitate.

1. Make a transverse incision across the dorsum of the wrist from just proximal to the tip of the styloid process of the radius and the tip of the styloid process of the ulna.

2. Incise the dorsal carpal ligament and deep fascia longitudinally between the extensor pollicis longus and the extensor digitorum communis tendon to the index finger.

3. Apply traction to the hand.

4. Locate the defects in the dorsum of the carpus.

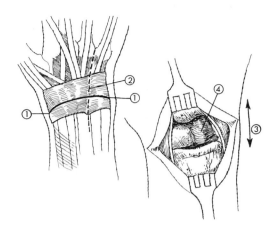

1. By sharp dissection clean out the scar tissue occupying the space of the lunate bone.

2. Identify the capitate distally and the articular surface of the radius proximally.

3. While traction and slight dorsiflexion is maintained lever the lunate into its normal position.

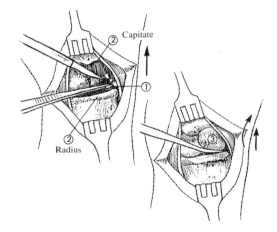

Postoperative Management

If this is an uncomplicated volar dislocation, an attempt is made to approximate the edges of the dorsal radiocarpal ligament, and the forearm, wrist and hand are immobilized by:

1. Anterior and posterior splints.
2. The wrist is flexed slightly.

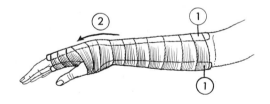

Encourage full use of the fingers and elbow.

After three weeks remove the plaster splints.

Institute a program of physical therapy and active exercises to restore finger and wrist motion.

Check by x-ray the state of the lunate bone for at least 18 months because it may develop avascular necrosis.

CORRECTION OF ROTATORY DISPLACEMENT OF THE SCAPHOID ASSOCIATED WITH VOLAR DISLOCATION OF THE LUNATE

REMARKS

After closed or open reduction of the lunate there may still be some rotation of the scaphoid.

The displacement is corrected and fixed by open reduction.

Failure to recognize this lesion results in poor function of the wrist.

1. The lunate is in normal alignment with the capitate and radius.

2. The scaphoid is rotated posteriorly and is not in alignment with the lunate, the capitate or the radius.

While traction is made with the wrist slightly dorsiflexed:

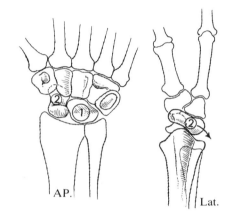

1. Lever the scaphoid into its normal anatomic position with a blunt dissector or periosteal elevator.

2. Transfix the lunate and the scaphoid with a threaded Kirschner wire (⁵/₆₄ inch) which enters the scaphoid on the radial side of the tendon of the extensor pollicis longus. Cut the wire below the level of the skin.

Note: While the wire is being inserted, take care in maintaining at all times the normal relationship between the lunate and scaphoid. The wire should be removed at the end of three weeks.

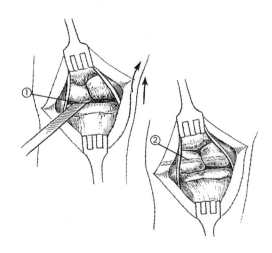

STABILIZATION OF DISPLACED FRAGMENTS OF THE SCAPHOID ASSOCIATED WITH VOLAR DISLOCATION OF THE LUNATE

REMARKS

After closed or open reduction of the lunate, the fragments of the fractured scaphoid may exhibit some displacement.

If the proximal fragment is very small (less than a third of the scaphoid), remove it.

If the fragments are large, reduce the displacement and transfix them with a threaded Kirschner wire ($^5/_{64}$ inch).

1. The lunate is in normal alignment with the capitate and radius.

2. Displaced fragments of the scaphoid.

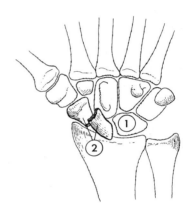

1. Realign the fragments into normal position.

2. Hold the reduced fragments with a towel clip.

3. Transfix the fragments with a threaded wire ($^5/_{64}$ inch) which enters the scaphoid on the radial side of the extensor pollicis longus.

Note: If the stability of the scaphoid is not satisfactory, pass the threaded wire into the lunate. Cut the wire below the level of the skin; it should be removed at the end of six to eight weeks.

The fragments of the scaphoid may be stabilized by a bone peg instead of a wire (see page 968).

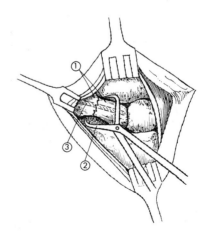

Postoperative Immobilization

1. Apply anterior and posterior plaster splints.
2. The wrist is slightly dorsiflexed.

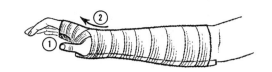

For correction of rotatory displacement of the scaphoid without fracture, remove the wire at the end of three weeks.

Institute a program of physical therapy to restore normal finger and wrist motion.

For Stabilization of Displaced Fragments of the Scaphoid

1. After ten to 14 days, apply a circular cast from below the elbow to the metacarpophalangeal joints.
2. The thumb is in the grasp position and is included in the cast to the base of the thumbnail.
3. The wrist is slightly dorsiflexed; otherwise it is in the neutral position.

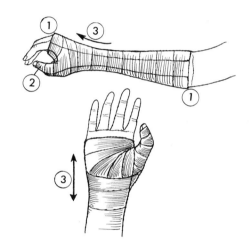

Remove the wire at the end of six to eight weeks depending on the state of healing at the fracture site.

Continue immobilization in a plaster cast until bony union is achieved, usually in three to four months. If bony union is not attained at the end of six months, take the cast off and mobilize the wrist.

OLD UNCOMPLICATED DISLOCATION OF THE LUNATE BONE WITH ASEPTIC NECROSIS

REMARKS

The method of reduction described for recent dislocations of the lunate bone can be employed in dislocations up to two weeks old.

After two weeks this method usually fails; open reduction as described should be performed.

Open reduction of old dislocations through the posterior approach as described for unreducible fresh dislocations should be performed for all old dislocations of the lunate provided the bone is viable.

Excision through the anterior route is performed only when the lunate shows definite evidence of aseptic necrosis.

The results following excision of the lunate are generally not good.

Preoperative X-Ray

Dislocation of the lunate is eight months old.

1. The lunate is in front of the wrist.
2. The capitate is in line with the radius.
3. The lunate is dense and sclerotic, indicative of aseptic necrosis.

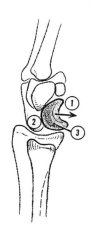

Operative Procedure (Excision of Lunate)

1. Make an S-shaped incision on the volar aspect of the wrist beginning at the base of the thenar eminence.
2. Divide the fascia and the transverse carpal ligament.

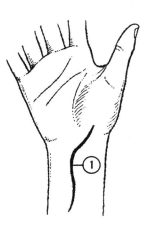
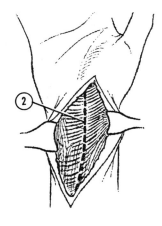

Operative Procedure (Excision of Lunate) (Continued)

1. Retract the median nerve, the palmaris longus and the tendon of the flexor pollicis longus to the radial side.

2. Retract the tendons of the flexor digitorum sublimis and the profundus to the ulnar side.

3. Incise the capsule of the joint if intact.

4. Grasp the lunate with a towel clip and by sharp dissection free it from all soft tissue attachments.

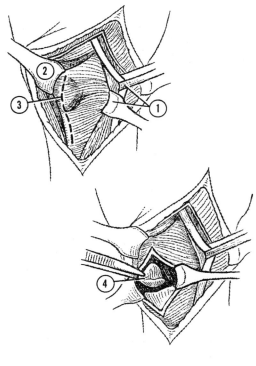

Immobilization

Apply an anterior plaster slab.
1. The wrist is in the neutral position.

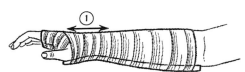

Postoperative Management

Encourage full finger movements at all times.

Remove the plaster splint after one week.

Institute a program of physical therapy and active exercises to restore finger and wrist motions.

Some restriction of flexion and extension of the wrist and some weakness of the wrist must be anticipated in all cases.

MANAGEMENT OF UNCOMPLICATED DORSAL PERILUNAR DISLOCATIONS

REMARKS

This lesion is relatively common.

The lunate is the focal point around which the dislocation of the remaining carpus occurs.

The lunate maintains its normal anatomic position in relation to the radius; the rest of the carpus is displaced upward, backward and outward.

Open reduction is rarely indicated in fresh lesions; it may be necessary in old lesions which cannot be reduced by closed methods.

Postreduction X-Ray

1. The normal relationship of the lunate to the remaining carpal bones is lost; the carpus is displaced to the radial side.

2. The lunate is in normal relation with the radius.

3. The remaining carpus is displaced upward and backward.

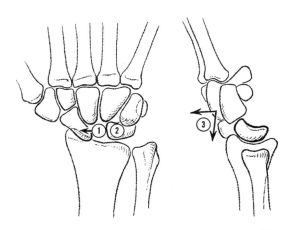

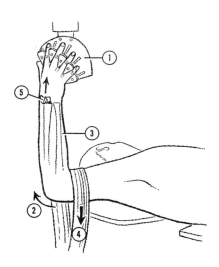

Reduction by Traction and Manipulation

1. Apply finger traction.

2. The elbow is flexed at a right angle.

3. The forearm is fully supinated.

4. Counter traction is made by a muslin bandage secured to the bottom of the table.

5. Make strong traction directly upward.

While traction is maintained:

1. Place both thumbs against the posterior aspect of the carpus and make strong pressure forward and outward, and at the same time flex the wrist.

Note: Check the position of the carpus by x-ray before application of the plaster cast.

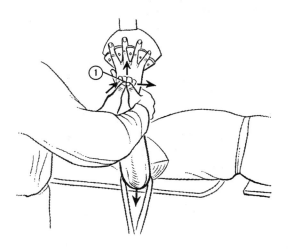

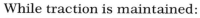

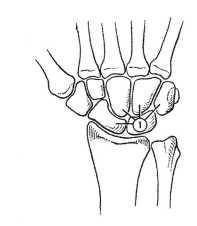

Postreduction X-Ray

1. The carpus is in normal anatomic relationship to the lunate bone.

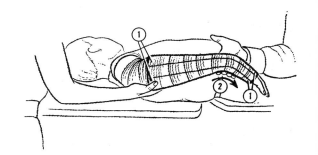

Immobilization

1. Apply anterior and posterior plaster slabs from just below the elbow to just proximal to the metacarpophalangeal joints.
2. The wrist is flexed 45 degrees.

Postreduction Management

Remove the plaster slabs after one week, bring the wrist to a neutral position and again immobilize with anterior and posterior plaster slabs.

Continue immobilization for two more weeks.

During the period of immobilization, insist on a program of active finger exercises.

After removal of the plaster slabs, institute a regimen of physical therapy and active exercises for the wrist and fingers.

The prognosis is good in recent cases; recovery should be complete in eight to 12 weeks.

Note: The aforementioned method may be employed in old unreduced cases of several weeks duration. As a rule, if this method fails, operative reduction is indicated.

DORSAL PERILUNAR DISLOCATIONS COMPLICATED BY FRACTURE OR DISLOCATION OF OTHER CARPAL BONES

Dorsal perilunar dislocations are frequently complicated by lesions of the other carpal bones; the scaphoid is most frequently involved.

Dorsal Perilunar Dislocation with Fracture of the Scaphoid Without Displacement of the Fragments

REMARKS

Lack of displacement of the scaphoid fragments indicates that there is still continuity of the fragments through the articular cartilage. The prognosis is good.

Appearance on X-Ray

1. Normal relationship of the lunate to the remaining carpal bones is lost; the carpus is displaced to the radial side.

2. The lunate is in normal relationship to the radius.

3. The remaining carpus is displaced upward and backward.

4. Fracture of the scaphoid with no displacement of the fragments.

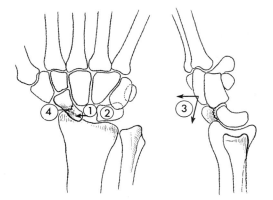

Management

Reduce the perilunar dislocation by traction and manipulation as described on page 994.

Then treat the fracture of the scaphoid by continuous plaster fixation as described on page 962.

DORSAL PERILUNAR DISLOCATION WITH DISPLACEMENT OF THE FRAGMENTS OF THE SCAPHOID

(The proximal fragment remains with the lunate and the distal fragment is displaced dorsally with the rest of the carpus.)

Trans-scaphoid Perilunar Fracture-dislocation

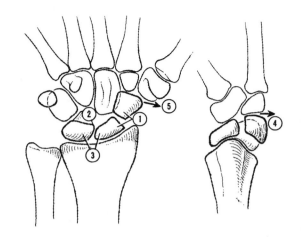

APPEARANCE ON X-RAY

1. Fracture through the waist of the scaphoid.

2. Normal relationship of the carpal bones is disturbed; note the wide gap between the lunate and the capitate.

3. The lunate and the proximal half of the scaphoid are in normal relationship to the radius.

4. The carpus and the distal half of the scaphoid are displaced backward.

5. The carpus distal to the lunate and the proximal half of the scaphoid are displaced radially.

REMARKS

Generally the proximal fragment is large; if the fracture is anatomically reduced and fixed internally, the prognosis is good; however, the incidence of avascular necrosis of the proximal fragment is high. On the other hand, if not reduced, the incidence of avascular necrosis is almost 100 per cent.

Management

Reduce the perilunar dislocation by traction and manipulation as described on page 994.

Then expose the scaphoid through a dorsal approach.

Realign the fragments and fix them with a threaded wire or a bone peg as described on page 968.

Note: If the proximal fragment is very small and comminuted, it is best to excise it.

DORSAL PERILUNAR DISLOCATION WITH FRACTURE OF THE CAPITATE

REMARKS

Following reduction of the dislocation the proximal fragment of the capitate may remain displaced.

Closed reduction usually fails; open operation is usually necessary to replace the fragment.

Results are poor if the fragment remains displaced.

If small, remove it; if large, realign the fragment with the distal fragment of the capitate and fix it with a threaded wire.

This fracture may also be associated with a displaced fracture of the scaphoid.

Appearance on X-Ray

1. Fracture of the capitate.
2. Fracture of the scaphoid with displacement.
3. Dorsal displacement of the carpus distal to the lunate.

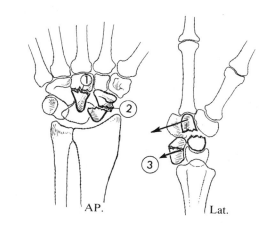

AP.   Lat.

Management

Reduce the perilunar dislocation by traction and manipulation as described on page 994.

Through a dorsal incision expose the capitate, scaphoid and lunate bones.

With a blunt dissector, lever the fragments of the capitate into normal position and transfix them with a threaded wire.

Note: If the proximal fragment of the capitate is small, excise it. If there is a displaced fracture of the scaphoid, realign the fragments and transfix them with a threaded wire or bone peg as described on page 968.

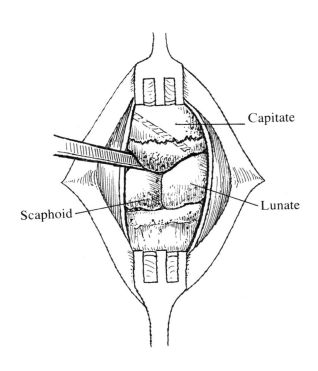

Capitate

Scaphoid

Lunate

Other Dislocations and Fracture-dislocations of the Carpus

DORSAL PERISCAPHOLUNAR DISLOCATION

REMARKS

In this lesion the lunate and scaphoid remain articulated with the radius, and the capitate with the remaining carpus is displaced dorsally. The scaphoid may be forced into a volar position as the carpus is shortened.

After reduction always check for any malposition of the scaphoid. Usually realignment is achieved by closed reduction. Open reduction is rarely indicated except in old cases.

Appearance on X-Ray

1. The scaphoid and lunate articulate with the radius.
2. The remaining carpus is displaced upward and backward.

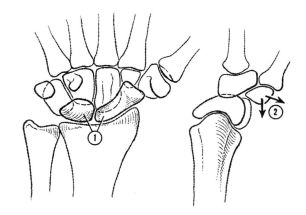

Management

Reduce the dislocation by traction and manipulation as described on page 994.

DISLOCATION OF THE LUNATE AND THE PROXIMAL HALF OF THE SCAPHOID

Appearance on X-Ray

1. The lunate and the proximal half of the scaphoid do not articulate with the radius but are in an anterior position.

2. The capitate articulates with the radius.

Note: After reduction the fragments of the scaphoid may be displaced; if so, open reduction and internal fixation with a threaded wire or bone peg is indicated, as described on page 968.

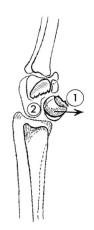

DISLOCATION OF THE LUNATE AND SCAPHOID

Appearance on X-Ray

1. The lunate and the entire scaphoid are displaced anteriorly.

2. The capitate articulates with the radius.

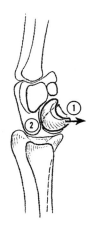

BACKWARD AND ANTERIOR DISLOCATION OF THE METACARPAL BONES ON THE CARPUS

Appearance on X-Ray

1. The metacarpal bones together with

2. The trapezium are displaced anterior to the remaining carpus.

3. The trapezoid is displaced to the dorsum of the wrist on the ulnar side. (In this instance this bone was excised.)

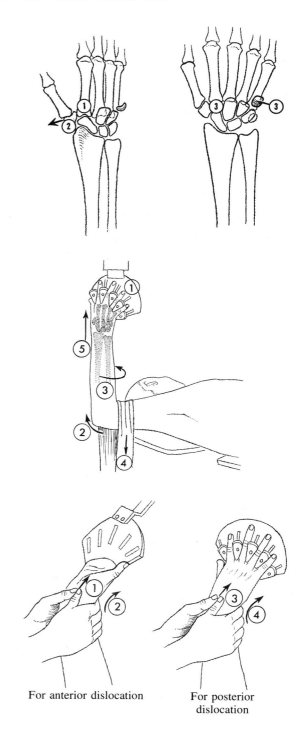

Reduction by Traction and Manipulation

1. Apply finger traction.

2. The elbow is flexed at a right angle.

3. The forearm is fully supinated.

4. Counter traction is made by a muslin bandage secured to the bottom of the table.

5. Make strong traction directly upward.

While traction is maintained, pressure is made on the displaced elements.

1. If one or two metacarpal bones are displaced anteriorly, pressure is made directly backward and at the same time

2. The wrist is dorsiflexed.

3. If these elements are displaced posteriorly, pressure is made directly forward and

4. The wrist is palmar flexed.

Note: If lateral displacement is present, pressure is directed in the opposite direction to correct the disalignment.

For anterior dislocation

For posterior dislocation

Immobilization

1. Apply anterior and posterior plaster slabs; flex the wrist for anterior dislocation.

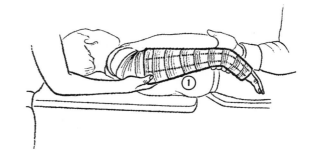

Postreduction Management

Management is the same as described for simple dislocation of the lunate or perilunar dislocation, except that in cases of fracture-dislocation immobilization must continue until bony union of the carpal bone or bones is achieved.

Change the position of flexion of the wrist to a neutral position after ten to 14 days. In uncomplicated dislocations remove the cast after three weeks.

In the event that traction and manipulation fail to obtain an anatomic reduction, open operation is indicated.

DISRUPTION OF THE PROXIMAL ROW OF THE CARPUS

REMARKS

Occasionally as the result of severe violence the proximal row of the carpus may be completely disrupted by fractures and dislocations.

Because of the multiplicity of the injuries and the great likelihood of avascular necrosis developing in the fragments, excision of the proximal row of the carpal bones is justified as a primary procedure.

This means excision of the lunate, scaphoid and triquetrum. Although the end result is not an excellent one, the patient generally attains good functioning and a painless wrist with varying degrees of restriction of motion. This procedure is preferred to arthrodesis of the wrist.

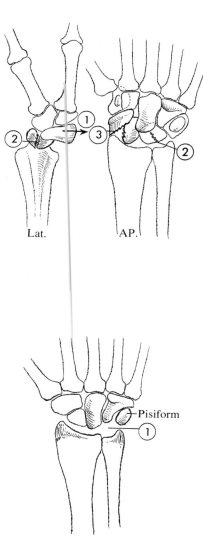

1. Dorsal perilunar dislocation of the carpus.

2. The lunate is fractured.

3. The scaphoid is fractured and its distal fragment is dislocated on the radius.

Postoperative X-Ray

1. The proximal row of carpal bones (except the pisiform) has been excised.

VOLAR PERILUNAR DISLOCATIONS AND FRACTURE-DISLOCATIONS

REMARKS

These are indeed rare lesions. Volar perilunar dislocation may be complicated by fracture or fracture-dislocation of the scaphoid just as the dorsal lesion.

Volar Perilunar Dislocation

1. The lunate is in normal relation to the radius.
2. The remaining carpus is displaced anterior to the lunate.

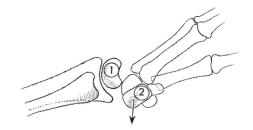

The principles of management are the same as for dorsal dislocation with or without associated fractures of other carpal bones.

FRACTURE OF THE CAPITATE

REMARKS

Fracture of the capitate occurs more frequently than generally realized. Approximately 15 per cent of all fractures of the carpal bones involve the capitate.

Anatomic Considerations

Its size and relationship to the other carpal bones make the capitate vulnerable to injury; it is the largest of all the carpal bones and articulates with seven bones: the scaphoid and the lunate proximally, the lesser multangular on the radial side, the hamate on the ulnar side and the second, third and fourth metacarpals distally.

It receives its blood supply from vessels penetrating the dorsal surface of the neck and waist of the bone, so that trauma may sever a portion of the bone from an adequate blood supply, thus causing aseptic necrosis of the affected segment.

It is firmly anchored to the bases of the second, third and fourth metacarpal bones by an intricate system of tough intercarpal ligaments.

It is intimately related to the axial motion of the third metacarpal bone.

1. The capitate, the largest bone, occupies a central position in the carpus.
2. Distally it articulates with the second, third and fourth metacarpals.
3. Proximally it articulates with the scaphoid and lunate.
4. It is related to the axial movements of the third metacarpal.

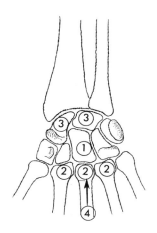

Mechanism of Fracture

Fractures of the capitate are produced either as the result of:

Direct violence, which usually causes injury to other carpal bones or

Indirect violence due to a fall on the outstretched hand; this is by far the most common mechanism. The type of lesion produced depends on the direction of the hand and wrist.

    a. If the hand and wrist are dorsiflexed and are deviated toward the ulna, the lunate is caught between the radius and the capitate and is squeezed volarly out of the wrist joint. This lesion may be associated with a fracture of the distal tip of the radius or the capitate.

    b. If the hand and wrist are dorsiflexed and are deviated toward the radius, the styloid process of the radius digs into the waist of the scaphoid producing a fracture; with continuance of the force the capitate is also fractured through its waist and the proximal fragments may rotate as much as 180 degrees.

Also, trauma to the radial side of the dorsum of the hand with the wrist palmar flexed may result in a fracture of the capitate.

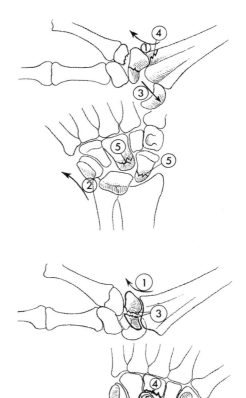

1. Wrist is in extreme dorsiflexion.

2. The wrist and the hand are deviated toward the ulna.

3. Lunate is forced volarly out of the wrist joint.

4. The distal tip of the radius may fracture.

5. The capitate may fracture; also a fracture may occur through the proximal head of the scaphoid.

1. The wrist is in extreme dorsiflexion.

2. The wrist and the hand are deviated toward the radius.

3. The styloid process of the radius digs into the waist of the scaphoid producing a fracture. With continuance of the force

4. The capitate fractures through the waist and

5. Its proximal fragment rotates (almost 180 degrees).

Many fractures of the capitate are missed; take oblique x-rays and laminograms to establish the diagnosis, especially if symptoms localized to the region of the capitate persist.

The fractures may be transverse (the most common), oblique, vertical and incomplete.

Most of the fractures are isolated lesions, although many are associated with other carpal injuries.

When the scaphoid and capitate bones alone are involved, the combination is referred to as the "scaphoid-capitate fracture syndrome."

MANAGEMENT OF ISOLATED FRACTURE OF THE CAPITATE

REMARKS

Most of these lesions are the result of a fall on the palm of the hand.

Most fractures are transverse and show little or no displacement.

Simple plaster fixation for eight weeks is adequate treatment.

Bony union is the rule.

If fibrous union or avascular necrosis of a fragment should occur and it produces painful disability, the fragment should be excised.

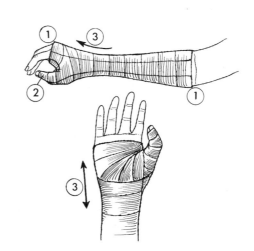

1. Apply a plaster cast from below the elbow to the metacarpophalangeal joints.

2. The thumb is in the grasp position and included in the cast up to the base of the thumbnail.

3. The wrist is only slightly dorsiflexed; otherwise it is in the neutral position.

Maintain immobilization for eight weeks.

Reapply the cast every two or three weeks if it should get loose.

After eight weeks remove the cast and

Institute a program of physical therapy to restore finger and wrist motion.

Note: If fibrous union or aseptic necrosis of the proximal fragment occurs and produces a painful wrist, excise the fragment through a dorsal incision.

MANAGEMENT OF "SCAPHOID-CAPITATE FRACTURE"

REMARKS

As a rule, the fracture of the capitate is transverse and the proximal fracture is rotated up to 180 degrees.

This lesion may have been produced in association with a dorsal perilunar dislocation which reduced spontaneously. In these instances the proximal capitate fragment may remain in a displaced position on the dorsum of the wrist.

If the fragment is small excise it; if it is large replace it and fix it to the other fragment with a threaded wire.

The incidence of aseptic necrosis when the fragments are unreduced, and particularly if the proximal fragment is rotated, is very high; hence, operative reduction or excision gives the best chance for a satisfactory result.

Operative Procedure

1. Make a transverse incision on the dorsum of the wrist at a level just proximal to the base of the third metacarpal.

2. Divide the deep fascia longitudinally in line with the shaft of the third metacarpal.

3. Deepen the incision between the extensor tendons of the fourth and fifth fingers.

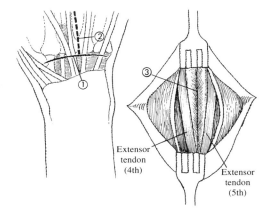

Extensor tendon (4th)

Extensor tendon (5th)

1. By sharp dissection, expose the fragments of the capitate. (Don't strip them of soft tissue attachment any more than is necessary.)

2. With a blunt dissector pry the proximal fragment into its normal position and transfix the fragments with a threaded wire ($^5/_{64}$ inch). Cut the wire below the level of the skin.

Note: If the proximal fragment is small or severely comminuted excise it.

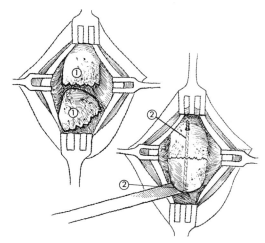

Operative Procedure (Continued)

If there is an unstable fracture of the scaphoid:

1. Expose the styloid process of the radius.

2. Divide the dorsal carpal ligament and deep fascia longitudinally between the extensor pollicis longus and the extensor tendon of the index finger; open the capsule to expose the scaphoid.

3. Make traction on the hand toward the ulna to bring into view both fragments of the scaphoid.

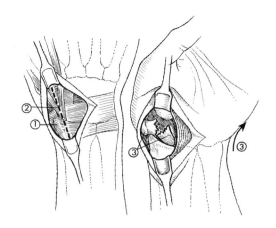

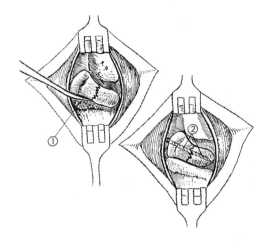

1. Lever the fragments into normal position.

2. Transfix them with a threaded wire (⁵/₆₄ inch).

Note: If necessary, run the wire through the lunate for further stability.

Postoperative Immobilization

Apply anterior and posterior plaster splints holding the wrist slightly dorsiflexed and otherwise in the neutral position. After ten to 14 days apply a circular cast.

1. The cast extends from below the elbow to the metacarpophalangeal joints.

2. The thumb is in the grasp position and is included in the cast to the base of the thumbnail.

3. The wrist is slightly dorsiflexed; otherwise it is in the neutral position.

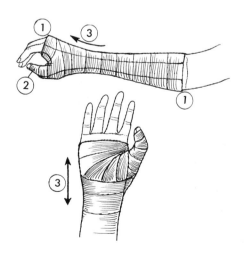

Postoperative Immobilization (Continued)

Remove the wires at the end of six to eight weeks.

Continue immobilization in plaster until bony union is achieved (usually three to four months).

If bony union is not obtained in six months take the cast off and mobilize the wrist.

Note: Some cases of apparent nonunion, as seen by x-ray, will eventually achieve bony union after the cast is removed. Also avascular necrosis of the proximal fragments of the capitate or of the scaphoid does not preclude a painless wrist with good function.

MANAGEMENT OF FRACTURES OF THE CAPITATE WHEN ASSOCIATED WITH OTHER CARPAL INJURIES

In general, treatment of these injuries is the same as that described for isolated and scaphoid-capitate fractures, except that the treatment is also directed to the other associated injuries, which in some instances may be more severe than the fracture of the capitate; for example, a fracture of the distal end of the radius.

If the principles of the treatment of capitate fractures just described are adhered to in conjunction with other carpal injuries, a plan of adequate management should readily evolve.

FRACTURES OF THE TRIQUETRUM

REMARKS

Fractures of the triquetrum rank second in frequency of all fractures of the carpal bones.

These fractures are frequently missed, even by x-ray examination.

In order to establish the diagnosis by x-ray, it is essential to take oblique projections.

Mechanism of Fracture

By direct violence to the dorsum of the hand.

Extreme dorsiflexion, as in a fall on the outstretched hand (this is the commonest mechanism) or extreme palmar flexion due to a fall on the flexed hand.

Twisting movements against resistance.

The type of fracture may be a chip fracture, varying in size, of the dorsum of the bone with some separation of the fragments or a fracture of the body which may be comminuted.

Separation of fragments is never marked; bony union is the rule; fibrous union occurs rarely. Aseptic necrosis does not occur.

The lesions may be isolated or associated with other injuries, such as fractures of the scaphoid or of the distal end of the radius.

Untreated cases frequently parade as chronic sprains of the wrist.

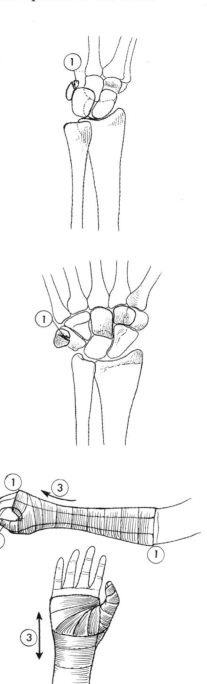

Appearance on X-Ray (Lateral View)

1. Chip fracture from dorsum of the bone.

Appearance on X-Ray (Oblique View)

1. Fracture through the body of the bone.

Management of Isolated Fractures

1. Apply a plaster cast from below the elbow to the metacarpophalangeal joints and including the thumb to the base of the thumbnail.

2. Thumb is in the grasp position.

3. Wrist is slightly dorsiflexed; otherwise it is in the neutral position.

Management of Isolated
Fractures (Continued)

Remove the cast after six to eight weeks, regardless of what the status of union may be as interpreted by x-ray.

The wearing of a wrist support for several weeks after the cast is removed may be helpful in some instances.

Institute a program of physical therapy and exercises to restore normal motion of the fingers and wrist.

Note: Union may be delayed, especially in fractures with separation of the fragments. Bony union may not occur for many weeks after the cast is removed; fibrous union or delayed union does not preclude a wrist with good function and without pain.

MANAGEMENT OF FRACTURES OF THE TRIQUETRUM ASSOCIATED WITH OTHER INJURIES

When associated with other injuries, direct your attention to the treatment of the associated injuries, which usually are more serious than fracture of the triquetrum.

The most common associated injuries are:

Fracture of the scaphoid.

Fracture of the distal end of the radius.

FRACTURES OF THE PISIFORM

REMARKS

The anatomic features of this bone render it vulnerable to injury.

Its volar surface is attached to the volar ligament and the tendon of the flexor carpi ulnaris which sends fibrous strands to the hamate and metacarpal bones forming the pisohamate and pisometacarpal ligaments.

The dorsal surface of the bone articulates with the triquetrum forming the pisotriquetrum joint which is enclosed in a tough fibrous capsule.

Mechanism of Injury

The bone may be fractured by direct trauma (the most common mechanism) or by

Forceful hyper-dorsiflexion as produced by a fall on the outstretched hand or when the wrist is forcefully dorsiflexed against resistance.

The types of fracture produced are:

Avulsion fracture by the action of the flexor carpi ulnaris.

Transverse or linear fracture of the body of the pisiform.

Comminuted fracture.

Mechanism of Injury
(Continued)

Because the capsule and ligaments are attached to the bone, separation of the fragments is never marked.

The fractures may be isolated lesions or associated with other carpal injuries.

The diagnosis is often missed; oblique x-ray projections are necessary to show the lesions.

Appearance on X-Ray (Anteroposterior and Oblique Views)

1. Fracture of pisiform involving the articular surface.

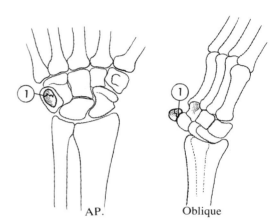

AP.   Oblique

Appearance on X-Ray (Oblique View)

1. Comminuted fracture of pisiform.

Nonunion is rare but may occur; bony union is nearly always achieved and recovery is usually complete.

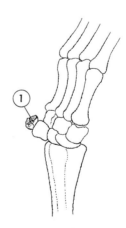

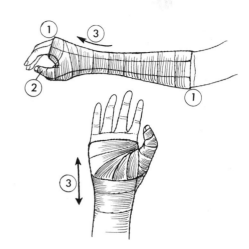

Management of Isolated Lesion

1. Apply a plaster cast from below the elbow to the metacarpophalangeal joints.

2. The thumb is in the grasp position; the plaster extends to the base of the thumbnail.

3. The wrist is slightly dorsiflexed; otherwise it is in a neutral position.

Remove the cast after six weeks.

Institute a program of physical therapy and exercises to restore normal finger and wrist motion.

Management of Fractures of the Pisiform when Associated with Other Carpal Injuries

Usually the associated lesions are more serious; direct your attention primarily to the treatment of the associated injuries.

These are:

Fracture of the triquetrum.

Fracture of the hamate.

Fracture of the distal end of the radius.

CHRONIC SPRAIN OF THE PISOTRIQUETRAL JOINT

Persistent pain localized over the pisiform and aggravated by radial deviation of the wrist may be caused by a chronic sprain of the pisotriquetral joint, usually seen in women. Pain may be referred to the fourth and fifth fingers.

Treat this lesion as a strain.

Injection of a steroid into the joint may be effective.

If symptoms persist, excise the pisiform bone.

Don't traumatize the ulnar nerve.

Calcification, such as is seen in the supraspinatus tendon, may occur in the tendon of the flexor carpi ulnaris producing an acute or chronic syndrome. Treat this lesion as you would a calcific deposit causing pain in the supraspinatus tendon.

FRACTURE OF THE TRAPEZIUM (GREATER MULTANGULAR)

REMARKS

This lesion occurs in approximately 5 per cent of all carpal fractures. Closed reduction usually fails. Anatomic reduction of the fracture is essential in order to assure normal thumb motion.

Mechanism of Injury

Fracture of the trapezium is produced by direct trauma to the radio-dorsal aspect of the joint or by extreme dorsiflexion of the wrist, as occurs in a fall on the outstretched hand. The bone is caught between the styloid process of the radius and the base of the first metacarpal bone.

The fracture may be an isolated lesion or associated with other carpal lesions, the most frequent being fracture of the first metacarpal and fracture of the distal end of the radius.

Anatomic Features

The trapezium (greater multangular) is trapezoid in shape and articulates with the first and second metacarpals, the scaphoid and the trapezoid (lesser multangular).

The articulation with the first metacarpal is saddle-shaped and enveloped in a loose capsule, permitting a wide range of motion.

Fractures may be of various types; they may be vertical, comminuted or avulsion fractures. The vertical type is by far the most common and is invariably associated with dislocation of the first metacarpal bone.

Management

Accurate restoration of the fragments is most essential for normal function of the thumb; therefore, open reduction and internal fixation, unless contraindicated, are the treatment of choice.

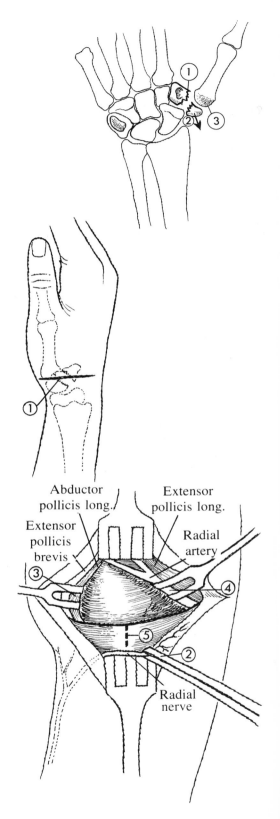

Appearance on X-Ray

1. Fracture of the trapezium.
2. The outer fragment is displaced proximally.
3. The articular surface of the first metacarpal is subluxated.

Operative Procedure

1. Make a transverse incision 2 inches long proximal to the base of the first metacarpal.
2. Identify the cutaneous branch of the radial nerve and retract it ulnarward.
3. Retract the abductor pollicis longus and the extensor pollicis brevis volarward and
4. The extensor pollicis longus together with the radial artery dorsally.
5. Divide longitudinally for ½ inch the dorsal carpal ligament.

Operative Procedure (Continued)

1. Open the capsule with a transverse incision.

2. Make traction on the thumb and bring the fracture into view.

3. Approximate the fragments and hold them with a towel clip.

4. Transfix the fragments with a threaded wire (5/64 inch).

5. Cut the wire below the level of the skin.

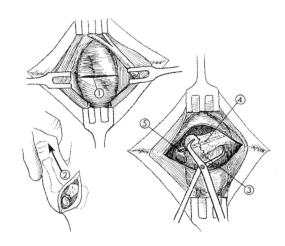

Postoperative Immobilization and Management

1. Apply a plaster cast from below the elbow to the metacarpophalangeal joints including the thumb to the base of the thumbnail.

2. The thumb is in the grasp position.

3. The wrist is slightly dorsiflexed; otherwise it is in the neutral position.

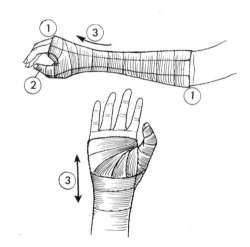

Remove the cast after six weeks.

Institute a program of physical therapy and exercises to restore motion of the fingers, thumb and wrist.

Management of Severe Comminuted Fractures of the Trapezium

REMARKS

Comminution may be so severe that it is impossible to reassemble the fragments of the bone to their anatomic position by internal fixation.

In these instances treat the fracture by skeletal traction in the same manner that comminuted fractures of the base of the first metacarpal are treated (see page 1048).

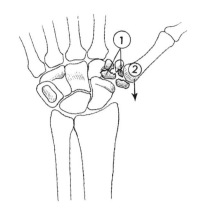

1. Severe comminution of the trapezium.

2. Proximal displacement of the first metacarpal.

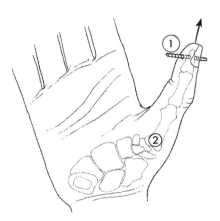

1. Wire through distal phalanx for traction.

2. Proximal displacement of the first metacarpal is corrected.

DISLOCATION OF THE TRAPEZOID (LESSER MULTANGULAR)

REMARKS

This is a rare lesion. It may occur as an isolated injury or with other lesions of the carpal bones.

The dislocation is usually dorsal but in rare instances it is volar.

Aseptic necrosis of the bone is a common sequela.

Management

Closed reduction rarely is successful.

Excision of the bone is the procedure of choice whether it occurs as an isolated lesion or with other carpal injuries.

Nerve Complications with Carpal Injuries

ULNAR NERVE INVOLVEMENT

In closed fractures of the pisiform, hamate, triquetrum and the fourth and fifth metacarpals the motor branch of the ulnar nerve, which is the chief motor nerve of the hand, may be injured; the sensory branch is rarely affected.

Blunt trauma to the hypothenar eminence of the hand may also contuse the ulnar nerve.

Following fracture or soft tissue injuries, the nerve may be compressed by edema or hemorrhage. Intraneural fibrosis may result, as indicated by delayed or progressive paralysis of the intrinsic muscles of the hand.

Management

If there is a large hematoma it should be evacuated. Generally, spontaneous recovery occurs; however, if there is no recovery after six or eight weeks the ulnar nerve should be explored.

If compressed, incise the tight ligament.

If a neuroma is present, excise it.

Neurolysis of the nerve may be necessary. This is best performed by injection of a saline solution into the sheath above the level of constriction.

MEDIAN NERVE INVOLVEMENT

CARPAL TUNNEL SYNDROME

REMARKS

This disorder is characterized by sensory disturbances in the index and middle fingers such as tingling. Pressure over the volar ligament accentuates pain and paresthesia along the course of the median nerve.

Late in the disorder the thenar eminence exhibits muscular atrophy.

Implication of the median nerve is the result of compression due to either constriction of the osseofibrous tunnel containing the flexor tendons of the fingers and the median nerve or as the result of the swelling of the structures within the tunnel, as in tenosynovitis of the flexor tendons. Direct trauma to the volar aspect of the wrist may cause swelling of the volar ligament.

Occasionally the syndrome is associated with Colles' fracture, fracture of one of the carpal bones, or perilunar dislocation.

During the early stages of the disorder, simple rest of the limb in a plaster splint for several weeks will permit subsidence of any reactive process of the structure within the tunnel or of the walls of the tunnel, and hence decompression of the median nerve ensues. If conservative measures fail, either in recent lesions or in old established syndromes, resection of a portion of the volar ligament is the treatment of choice.

Appearance on X-Ray

RECENT LESIONS

1. Perilunar dislocation.
2. Fracture of the scaphoid.
This patient had an acute compression of the median nerve.

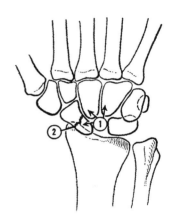

Appearance on X-Ray

LATE LESION

1. Old nonunion of fractured scaphoid.
2. The ulnar fragment is dense and sclerotic.
3. The radiocarpal joint is thin.
4. Osteophytes indicative of advanced osteoarthritis.

Note: This lesion was six years old and was complicated by compression of the median nerve.

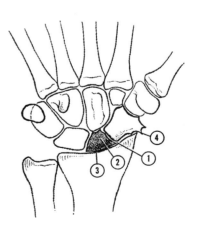

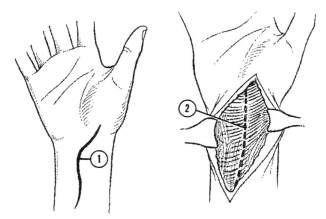

Operative Procedure

1. Make an S-shaped incision on the volar aspect of the wrist, beginning at the base of the thenar eminence.

2. Make a longitudinal incision in the transverse carpal ligament; retract its margins.

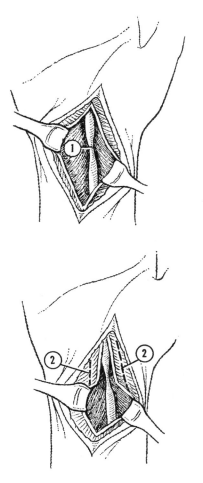

1. Expose the median nerve; it is compressed.

2. Excise a portion of the transverse carpal ligament from each margin.

Note: If the contracture of the median nerve is severe, perform a neurolysis by injecting saline with a fine needle into the nerve sheath to stretch the sheath and decompress the nerve.

Immobilization

1. Apply an anterior plaster slab holding the wrist in the neutral position.

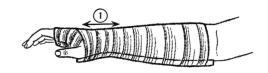

Postoperative Management

Remove the plaster slab after seven days.

Institute physical therapy and active exercises to restore function in the wrist and fingers.

FRACTURES AND DISLOCATIONS OF THE HAND

ANATOMIC FEATURES

The entire upper extremity is designed in such a fashion that the hand can function as an efficient prehensile organ.

Comprehension of the anatomic and functional characteristics of this organ are essential in order to plan an adequate regimen of therapy for the many and varied injuries which affect the hand.

Lack of this comprehension invariably ends in catastrophic consequences.

Some of the most pertinent anatomic and functional features of the hand which relate to the proper management of fractures and dislocations are described in this section. However, one who aspires to treat the many disorders which can affect the hand should delve deeper into the intrinsic and functional characteristics of this organ.

OSSEOUS COMPONENTS OF THE HAND

REMARKS

The distal row of the carpus, comprising the trapezium, the trapezoid, the capitate and the hamate, collectively articulates with the five metacarpals of the hand. The articular surfaces of the metacarpals and the carpal bones vary in size and shape and are designed to meet the demands of the individual rays and the hand as a whole.

The capitate articulates with the second, third and fourth metacarpals whereas the second metacarpal articulates with the trapezium, the trapezoid and the capitate. The second and third metacarpals have the largest articular surfaces of all the carpal bones.

The metacarpals of the fingers are roughly parallel to one another and their bases articulate with each other. On the other hand the metacarpal of the thumb is at a distance from the other metacarpals and articulates with the trapezium at an angle of approximately 45 degrees to the metacarpals of the index finger.

The thumb carpometacarpal articulation is saddle-shaped; the fourth and fifth articulations are hinge-shaped. All three of these joints are very mobile, especially the thumb and the fifth articulation; however, the second and the third carpometacarpal articulations are practically immobile.

The thumb carpometacarpal joint has a separate capsule and is in no way related to the remaining carpometacarpal joints.

The volar aspect of each metacarpal from the base to the head is concave so that collectively they are responsible for the concavity of the palm.

Volar Aspect of the Wrist and Hand

1. Capitate articulates with second, third and fourth metacarpals.

2. Second metacarpal articulates with the trapezium, trapezoid and capitate.

3. The metacarpals of the fingers are parallel to one another.

4. The metacarpal of the thumb is 45 degrees to the metacarpal of the index finger.

5. The carpometacarpal articulation of the thumb is saddle-shaped.

6. The carpometacarpal articulations of the fourth and fifth carpometacarpal joints are hinge-shaped.

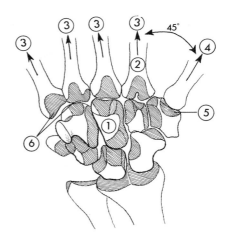

VOLAR LIGAMENTS OF THE WRIST AND HAND

REMARKS

On the volar aspect of the wrist and hand from the radius to the metacarpals is an intricate system of tough fibrous ligaments, the palmar ligaments, which firmly bind together the radius, the carpus and the proximal ends of the metacarpals. The fibers of these ligaments are directed in such a manner that the hand follows the radius in supination.

On the dorsal aspect the ligamentous apparatus is not as strong as the volar but its fibers take the same direction so that the hand follows the radius in pronation.

Palmar Ligaments of the Wrist and Radiocarpal Joint

1. The ligaments are tough and fibrous particularly those to the scaphoid, capitate and lunate.

2. The general direction of the large ligaments is from the radial to the ulnar aspects of the carpus.

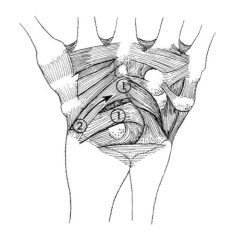

The metacarpals of the fingers are bound together by the intermetacarpal ligaments which span the intervals between them.

At the distal end of the metacarpal region the intermetacarpal ligaments thicken to form the deep transverse carpal ligaments (the transverse capsular ligaments) which loosely bind together the heads of the metacarpal bones.

This arrangement permits considerable volar and dorsal mobility of the distal ends of the metacarpal bones but very little lateral mobility.

The deep transverse ligaments are intimately related to the capsular ligaments and the palmar ligaments or the fibrocartilaginous plate on the volar aspects of the metacarpophalangeal joints.

The lumbricalis muscles pass in front of these ligaments while the interossei pass behind.

Relationship of Deep Transverse Ligaments

1. Palmar ligaments (fibrocartilaginous portion of the anterior capsule).

2. Deep transverse metacarpal ligaments.

3. Attachment of palmar aponeurosis to the palmar ligament.

4. Lumbrical muscles are in front of the ligament.

5. Interossei are behind the ligament.

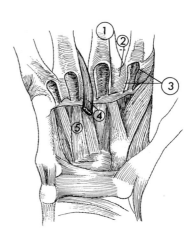

METACARPOPHALANGEAL JOINTS OF THE FINGERS

REMARKS

The configuration of the head of each metacarpal is that of a large single condyle directed slightly volarly which articulates with the shallow concave articular surface of the corresponding proximal phalanx.

Each articulation is so fashioned that upon flexion of the corresponding digit the distal phalanx points to the tubercle of the scaphoid and the fingers do not overlap. This is a very important anatomic arrangement and must always be borne in mind when treating fractures of the phalanges of the fingers.

Malunion with rotation of a phalanx produces overlapping of the finger when the hand makes a fist.

Normal position of finger on flexion:
1. The distal phalanges all point to the tubercle of the scaphoid.
2. The fingers do not overlap.

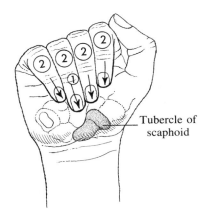

Tubercle of scaphoid

The spherical head also permits the corresponding proximal phalanx to move away from and toward the midline of the hand, and also permits some circumduction, a motion greater in the index and little finger than in the third and fourth fingers.

The stability of the metacarpophalangeal joints depends largely on the capsular ligaments and the lateral collateral ligaments.

The collateral ligaments are strong fibrous cords attached eccentrically to the head of the metacarpal. This arrangement makes the ligaments slack in extension and taut in flexion.

Fixation of this articulation in extension causes shortening of the collateral ligaments.

On the volar side, the capsule is reinforced by a rectangular fibrocartilaginous plate.

The palmar ligament is loosely attached to the metacarpal head but firmly anchored to the base of the proximal phalanx.

In dislocation of the metacarpophalangeal joint this fibrocartilaginous structure may be entrapped between the bones, thereby preventing reduction.

Page 1027

METACARPOPHALANGEAL JOINT OF THE THUMB

REMARKS

The shape of the metacarpal head of the thumb differs from that of the metacarpals of the fingers.

It has more the characteristics of a ginglymoid or hinge joint and therefore resembles very much in structure and function the interphalangeal joints of the fingers.

Its capsular and ligamentous reinforcements are the same as those found in the metacarpophalangeal joints of the fingers.

INTERPHALANGEAL JOINTS

REMARKS

The head of each metacarpal except that of the thumb is a single spherical condyle permitting flexion, extension, abduction and adduction of the corresponding proximal phalanx; however, the distal ends of the first and second phalanges of the fingers are flattened anteroposteriorly and comprise two small condyles which permit motion only in one plane, flexion and extension.

As noted previously, the metacarpophalangeal joint of the thumb functions like the interphalangeal joints of the fingers.

The interphalangeal joints have the same capsular structure, collateral ligaments and volar plates as the metacarpophalangeal joints.

Capsule and Collateral Ligaments of Metacarpophalangeal and Interphalangeal Joints

1. Capsule.
2. Collateral ligaments.
3. Palmar ligament (volar plate).
4. Deep transverse metacarpal ligaments.

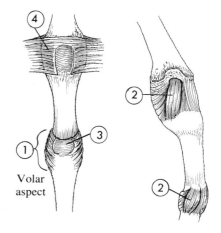

Volar aspect

Capsule and Collateral Ligaments of Metacarpophalangeal and Interphalangeal Joints (Continued)

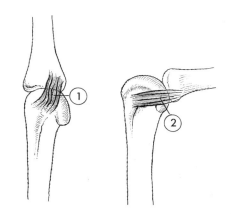

1. Cord component of the collateral ligament is slack in extension, but
  2. Taut in flexion.

MUSCLES OF THE HAND

REMARKS

The hand is capable of a multitude of intricate, delicate and refined movements.

This is made possible by the complex arrangements of the long and intrinsic muscles which motorize the hand.

The long flexor muscles originate in the forearm.

They proceed distally toward the wrist where their tendons are grouped into a compact mass as they pass under the volar and transverse carpal ligaments and then diverge in the hand to reach their respective sites of insertion.

In the hand the long muscles are intimately related to the intrinsic muscles and with them form ingenious mechanisms designed to fulfill the many and diversified functions of the individual rays and of the hand as a whole.

LUMBRICAL AND INTEROSSEI MUSCLES

REMARKS

The important intrinsic muscles of the fingers are the lumbrical and interossei muscles.

The lumbricals are four in number; they arise from the tendons of the flexor digitorum profundus.

The first and second take origin from the volar and radial aspects of the tendons of the index and middle fingers; the third arises from the contiguous surface of the middle and ring finger and the fourth from the contiguous sides of the tendon of the ring and little finger.

The tendons proceed distally on the radial side of the corresponding finger and opposite the metacarpophalangeal joint blend with the dorsal fibrous expansion of the extensor digitorum communis.

Their prime function is to flex the metacarpophalangeal joint and to extend the middle and distal phalanx.

There are seven interossei muscles, four dorsal and three volar; they arise from and occupy the interval between the metacarpal bones. The four dorsal interossei insert into the bases of the proximal phalanges and, with the exception of the first dorsal which has no tendinous insertion, into the dorsal expansion of the extensor digitorum communis.

The first dorsal interosseus is larger than the rest and inserts into the radial side of the base of the proximal phalanx of the index finger; the second and third insert into the base of the proximal phalanx of the middle finger, the second into its radial side and the third into its ulnar side; the fourth inserts into the ulnar side of the ring finger.

The three volar interossei are smaller than the dorsal and arise from the volar surfaces of the metacarpal bones.

The tendon of each muscle inserts into the side of the dorsal expansion of the extensor digitorum communis of the corresponding finger; they do not insert into bone.

With the exception of the fifth, each finger has two interossei muscles.

The action of the lumbrical and interossei muscles is to flex the metacarpophalangeal joint and, except for the first dorsal interosseus, to extend the middle and distal joints of the fingers.

When the metacarpophalangeal joint is stabilized in extension by the long extensor muscles of the fingers, the fingers are capable also of lateral motion.

DORSAL EXPANSION OF THE EXTENSOR COMMUNIS (EXTENSOR APPARATUS)

REMARKS

Essentially this gliding mechanism is an extension of the long extensor tendon consisting of transverse, oblique and longitudinal fibers located over the dorsum of the metacarpophalangeal joint and proximal phalanx.

The tendons of the interossei and, on the radial side, the lumbrical muscles blend with the fibers of this extensor expansion; the former are located more proximal than the latter.

Upon reaching the level of the metacarpophalangeal joint the long extensor divides into a middle and two lateral slips.

The lateral slips are joined by lateral bands from the lumbrical and interossei muscles and then proceed distally across the proximal interphalangeal joint and blend to form the terminal tendon.

A concentration of the transverse fibers of the expansion of the extensor tendon (the hood) is found at the level of the metacarpophalangeal joint; this loosely envelops the joint but is firmly fixed to the palmar ligament on the volar aspect of the joint.

The loose dorsal arrangement of the hood permits the extensor tendon to pull the hood proximally upon contraction and allows the middle slip of the extensor tendon to pull it distally upon flexion of the proximal interphalangeal joint.

Lumbrical Muscles

Observe:

1. Lumbricals arise from the tendons of the flexor digitorum profundus.

2. They insert on the radial side of the fibrous expansion of the extensor digitorum communis.

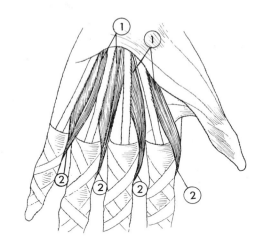

Interossei Muscles

Observe:

1. There are four dorsal and

2. Three volar interossei.

3. The first dorsal is the largest (it has no bony insertion).

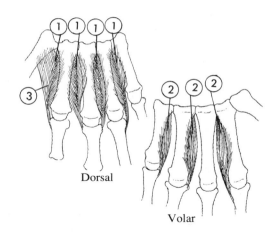

Dorsal

Volar

1. The dorsal inserts into the proximal phalanx and the fibrous dorsal expansion.

2. The interossei and the lumbrical tendons are separated by the deep transverse carpal ligament.

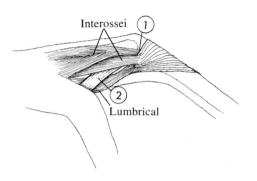

Interossei

Lumbrical

Dorsal Expansion of the Digitorum Communis

Observe:

1. Expansion of the extensor tendon to form a sleeve over the metacarpophalangeal joint.

2. Concentration of the transverse fibers form the mobile hood (this is anchored volarly to the fibrocartilaginous palmar ligament).

3. Two heads of the dorsal interossei; one inserts into the proximal phalanx, the other in the fibrous dorsal expansion.

4. Lumbrical muscle inserts into the fibrous expansion distal to the insertion of the interossei.

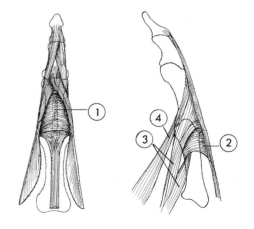

SHIFT OF THE DORSAL EXPANSION

On flexion the middle slip of the extensor tendon pulls the dorsal expansion distally in front of the proximal phalanx.

On extension the extensor tendon pulls the dorsal expansion over the joint and stabilizes it; the lumbrical and interossei muscles extend the distal joint by pulling on the lateral band.

THENAR AND HYPOTHENAR MUSCLES

REMARKS

The two most mobile rays of the hand are the first and fifth. Each is controlled by a complex muscular apparatus which performs the intricate movements necessary to a prehensile organ.

The muscles peculiar to the first ray are the thenar muscles which comprise:

The abductor pollicis brevis.
The flexor pollicis brevis.
The opponens pollicis.
The adductor pollicis.

The important muscles identified with the fifth ray are:

The abductor digiti quinti.
The flexor brevis digiti quinti.
The opponens digiti quinti.
The palmaris brevis.

Thenar and Hypothenar Muscles

1. Opponens pollicis.
2. Abductor pollicis brevis.
3. Flexor pollicis brevis.
4. Adductor pollicis.
5. Palmaris brevis.
6. Abductor digiti quinti.
7. Flexor brevis digiti quinti.
8. Opponens digiti quinti.

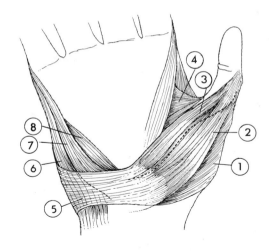

NERVES OF THE HAND

REMARKS

In the hand the ulnar and median nerves contain both motor and sensory components whereas the radial nerve is entirely sensory.

The deep branch of the ulnar nerve innervates the three hypothenar muscles, the two medial lumbrical muscles, all the interossei muscles, of which there are seven, and the adductor pollicis.

The palmaris brevis is supplied by the superficial branch of the ulnar nerve.

The sensory distribution of the ulnar nerve is to the fifth and one-half of the fourth fingers.

The median nerve supplies three thenar muscles (the opponens pollicis, the flexor pollicis brevis and the abductor pollicis brevis), and the two lateral lumbrical muscles.

Its sensory fibers are distributed to the thumb, index, middle, and one-half of the fourth fingers.

Distribution of the Deep Nerves of the Palm

Observe:

1. The median nerve is behind the transverse carpal ligament.

2. The ulnar nerve is in front of the ligament.

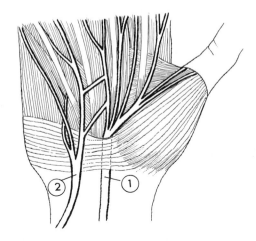

Distribution of the Cutaneous Nerves of the Palm and the Dorsum of the Hand

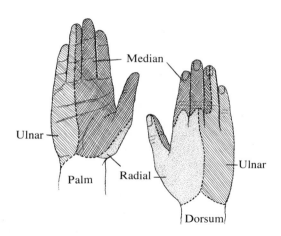

BASIC PRINCIPLES IN THE MANAGEMENT OF INJURIES OF THE HAND

REMARKS

Marked functional impairment is a frequent sequel to injuries of the hand; often this follows what appears to be a trivial injury.

Disastrous results can frequently be traced to inadequate management based on a lack of knowledge of some of the simple basic principles that must be adhered to in the treatment of hand injuries.

The chief causes of functional impairment of the hand are deformities and joint stiffness, both of which in most instances can be avoided.

Deformities are the result of malunion of fractures or fracture-dislocations of the bones of the hand and of chronic subluxation of an interphalangeal joint.

Never immobilize a fractured phalanx in extension; the position causes malunion of the fracture with a deformity of the phalanx in the anteroposterior plane. This deformity restricts flexion and extension of the finger.

Never immobilize or apply traction to a finger in the long axis of its metacarpal; this promotes the development of lateral or rotatory deformities of the fractured phalanx. These deformities cause lateral or rotatory deviations of the finger so that when the hand is closed the fingers overlap.

Always immobilize a fracture of a phalanx with the joint of the finger in the position of flexion.

An immobilized finger, whether in plaster or in a splint or in traction, should always point to the tubercle of the scaphoid.

Do not immobilize uninjured fingers; these must be given free mobility.

The soft tissues of the hand are prone to develop edema and lymphatic stasis after injury; this state lays the basis for development of fibrosis and joint stiffness which may severely cripple a hand.

The best treatment for fibrosis and joint stiffness is prevention which is best achieved by early elevation of the hand, gentle even compression of the soft tissues, early active motion of the uninjured components of the hand, and motion in the injured finger just as soon as healing of the bone and soft tissues permits.

Subluxations and dislocations of the interphalangeal joints that have spontaneously reduced following injury are often underdiagnosed or the diagnosis is never made. These lesions are associated with severe disruption of their ligamentous apparatus, especially one of the collateral ligaments. Inadequate healing of the ruptured ligaments causes a chronic subluxation of the joint; the phalanx distal to the joint deviates to one or the other side. Awareness of these lesions is most important in making the diagnosis. Clinically, lateral instability of the joint can be readily elicited. Adequate splintage of the finger until the ligaments have healed is essential (at least three weeks).

Some lesions may require surgical repair of the ligaments.

CORRECT AND INCORRECT METHODS OF IMMOBILIZATION

Correct

1. The cast extends from below the elbow to the distal flexion crease.
2. The fingers and thumb are free.
3. The wrist is slightly dorsiflexed.
4. The wrist is in the neutral position (no ulnar or radial deviation).

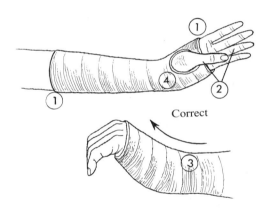

Correct

Incorrect

1. The cast extends beyond the metacarpal heads.
2. The fingers are straight.
3. The thumb is adducted.
4. The wrist and metacarpals are in a straight line.

Note: The metacarpophalangeal joints will stiffen in extension.

5. The hand, including all fingers and the thumb, is bandaged over a roll of gauze.

Note: All finger joints will stiffen; only the injured finger should be immobilized.

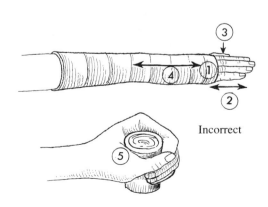

Incorrect

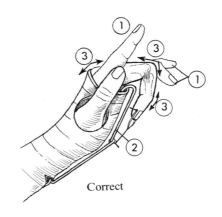

Correct

(For fractures of the metacarpals and phalanges)

1. Properly applied cast—uninjured fingers and thumb are free.

2. Wire extension holding injured finger flexed.

3. The metacarpophalangeal joint is flexed 30 to 45 degrees, the proximal interphalangeal joint 90 degrees and the distal 30 to 45 degrees.

4. The finger points to the tubercle of the scaphoid.

Note: In this position the flexor tendon and the lateral bands are relaxed, and the collateral ligaments are taut.

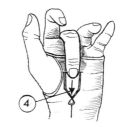

Correct

Incorrect

1. The fingers are pulled straight.

2. The wrist is straight.

3. The fingers diverge.

4. Flexor tendons and lateral bands are tight and displace the fragments.

5. The collateral ligaments are lax. (This causes stiffness of the joints in extension.)

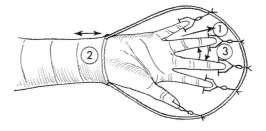

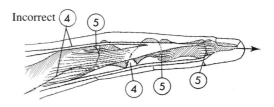

Incorrect

LIGAMENTOUS INJURIES AND FRACTURE-DISLOCATIONS OF THE THUMB

Carpometacarpal Joint

REMARKS

The thumb is the most mobile component of the hand; in fact, through the carpometacarpal joint, it is capable of almost universal motion. This great range of mobility is necessary in order that the hand can function effectively as a prehensile organ.

The bony architecture of the carpometacarpal joint provides little stability; the stability of this joint is chiefly provided by the capsule and the collateral ligaments.

The very nature of the position of the thumb and its function renders it vulnerable to abnormal stresses capable of producing sprains of varying degrees, ranging from simple sprains to complete disruption of part of the ligamentous apparatus of all the joints of the thumb.

The type of injury is determined by the direction of the force. Forceful hyperextension produces lesions of the anterior portion of the capsule, whereas forceful hyperflexion involves the dorsal portion of the capsule; laterally or medially directed forces produce lesions of the collateral ligaments opposite to the side of application of the violence. The most frequent mechanism is that of hyperextension producing subluxation or dislocation of the carpometacarpal joint. When the joint is dislocated the metacarpal bone may pierce the anterior capsule allowing the thumb to be on the dorsum of the wrist. Generally spontaneous relocation occurs, or someone pulls on the thumb and effects a relocation.

Inadequate treatment of a subluxated or dislocated thumb results in painful hypermobility of the joint and even a chronic subluxated joint.

MANAGEMENT OF A SIMPLE SPRAIN OF THE THUMB

In this lesion the capsule and ligaments are stretched and some of the fibers may be torn but the continuity of the structures is intact.

Apply a strapping of ½ inch strips of adhesive.

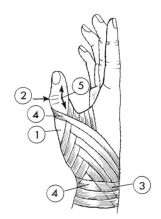

1. The strapping encircles the meta-carpophalangeal joint.
2. The interphalangeal joint is free.
3. The basket-weave strapping extends above the wrist.
4. Anchor the strips of adhesive encircling the thumb by strips encircling the wrist.
5. The thumb is strapped in the grasp position.

Reapply the strapping every week if it becomes loose.

Remove the strapping after three weeks but protect the joint against excessive strains.

MANAGEMENT OF SEVERE SPRAINS OF THE THUMB

The capsular structures are more severely implicated than in simple sprains and demand a greater period of immobilization.

Immobilize the thumb in a nonpadded plaster cast.

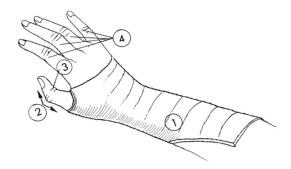

1. It extends above the wrist.
2. The interphalangeal joint is free.
3. The thumb is in the grasp position.
4. The unaffected fingers are free.

Maintain the thumb in plaster for three weeks.

Allow free use of the unaffected fingers.

Remove the cast after three weeks but protect the thumb for three more weeks with adhesive strapping.

Page 1039

SUBLUXATION OF THE CARPOMETACARPAL JOINT OF THE THUMB

In this lesion the capsular structures are attenuated and enough of the fibers are torn to permit some displacement of the articular surfaces of the joint.

Examination reveals hypermobility and instability of the joint. The type of treatment depends upon whether or not the subluxation tends to recur after it is reduced, and the thumb is placed in the grasp position with some pressure over the base of the metacarpal bone. If this can be achieved, immobilize the thumb in a nonpadded cast.

Apply a nonpadded cast:
1. Cast extends above the wrist.
2. The interphalangeal joint is free.
3. The thumb is in the grasp position.
4. The unaffected fingers are free.

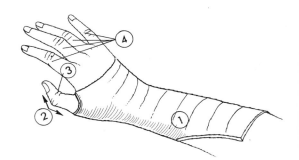

Note: Mold the cast firmly against the base of the metacarpal bone.

Maintain the thumb in plaster for six weeks.
Allow free use of the unaffected fingers.
After six weeks remove the cast.
Protect the joint with a basket-weave adhesive strapping for several more weeks.

FOR UNSTABLE SUBLUXATION OF THE CARPOMETACARPAL JOINT OF THE THUMB

REMARKS

If the capsular tissues are severely disrupted the joint is very unstable and may subluxate even in plaster.

It is most essential that the tissues heal with the articular surfaces of the joint in the normal anatomic position.

Incongruity of the joint surfaces predisposes to chronic subluxation with marked impairment of function; secondary osteoarthritic changes may develop subsequently, necessitating an arthrodesis of the joint.

Treat unstable lesions by traction.

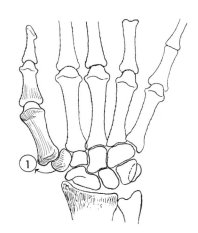

Prereduction X-Ray

1. The metacarpal is subluxated upward and dorsally.

Reduction by Skeletal Traction

1. Pass a threaded wire through the proximal phalanx.

2. While traction is made on the abducted and opposed thumb,

3. Apply a nonpadded plaster cast extending from below the elbow to just distal to the metacarpophalangeal joints—include the proximal phalanx of the thumb.

4. Mold the plaster carefully and firmly against the base of the metacarpal.

5. Incorporate a wire loop in the plaster cast, using a coat hanger wire.

6. Make continuous traction with rubber bands.

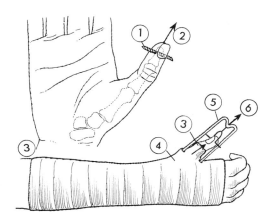

Postreduction Management

Keep the rubber bands taut at all times.

Take x-rays on the fifth and tenth days; check the position of the articular surfaces of the joint.

Encourage active exercises for the unaffected fingers.

At the end of three weeks remove the wire and apply a similar plaster cast.

Remove the second cast at the end of three more weeks.

Protect the joint with a basket-weave strapping for several more weeks.

DISLOCATION OF THE CARPOMETACARPAL JOINT OF THE THUMB

REMARKS

This is not a common lesion—when it does occur, spontaneous reduction follows, or someone pulls the joint into normal position.

Manipulative reduction is readily achieved but maintenance of the reduction is difficult; the joint tends to subluxate or even dislocate.

Prereduction X-Ray

1. The metacarpal is displaced upward and backward.
2. The metacarpal rests on the posterior aspect of the trapezium.

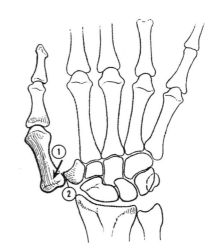

Manipulative Reduction

1. A bandage is first looped around the patient's thumb and then around the operator's hand.
2. While traction is made in the long axis of the thumb, the thumb is gradually abducted and, at the same time,
3. Direct pressure is exerted against the head of the metacarpal bone.
4. As the thumb is pulled downward and outward,
5. The head of the metacarpal is pushed forward and inward.

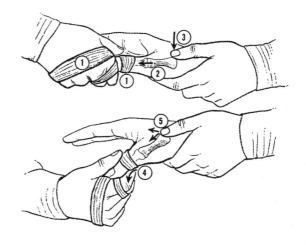

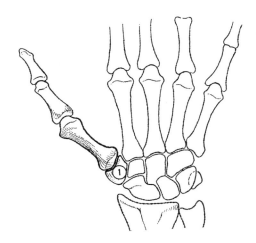

Postreduction X-Ray

1. The head of the metacarpal is in normal relationship to the trapezium.

Immobilization

1. Apply a circular plaster cast from the lower forearm to just distal to the interphalangeal joint.

2. The thumb is slightly flexed at the metacarpophalangeal joint and is in an abducted and opposed position. (Mold the plaster carefully at the base of the thumb.)

3. The wrist is slightly dorsiflexed and in the neutral position.

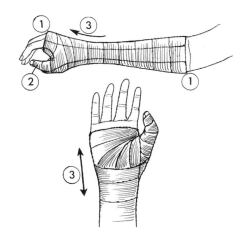

Postreduction Management

Take x-ray on the fifth and tenth days. Check the position of the articular surfaces of the joint.

Encourage active exercises of the unaffected fingers.

Remove the cast at the end of six weeks.

Institute physical therapy and active exercises to restore normal function.

Note: If displacement of the ends of the bones occurs in plaster, internal fixation of the bones must be done.

REDUCTION AND INTERNAL FIXATION

REMARKS

If the carpometacarpal joint is unstable or displacement of the bones occurs while in plaster, internal fixation becomes necessary.

Failure to achieve complete anatomic restoration of the articular surfaces results in a chronic subluxated joint which is painful and causes marked impairment of function.

Procedure of Reduction and Internal Fixation

1. An assistant makes traction on the abducted thumb and, at the same time,

2. Makes inward pressure on the metacarpal with his thumb.

3. While this position is maintained pass a threaded wire through the base of the metacarpal and into the adjacent metacarpals. Cut the wire below the level of the skin.

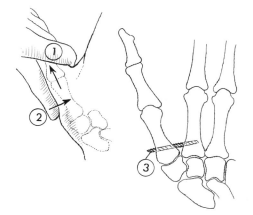

External Immobilization

Apply a circular nonpadded plaster cast from the lower forearm to just proximal to the metacarpophalangeal joints.

1. The cast includes the proximal phalanx of the thumb but the interphalangeal joint is free.

2. The thumb is abducted and opposed.

3. The metacarpophalangeal joint of the thumb is slightly flexed.

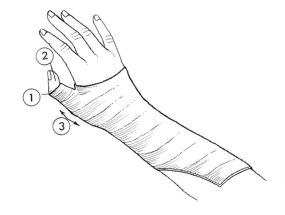

Postoperative Management

During the period of immobilization encourage free exercises of the remaining fingers.

Remove the wire after three weeks.

Reapply a similar cast, firmly molded against the base of the metacarpal.

Remove the second cast after three weeks (the total period of immobilization is six weeks).

Institute a program of physical therapy and active exercises to restore normal motion of the thumb.

FRACTURE-DISLOCATION OF THE CARPOMETACARPAL JOINT OF THE THUMB (BENNETT'S FRACTURE)

REMARKS

Essentially this is an oblique fracture through the base of the first metacarpal with dislocation of the radial portion of its articular surface while the medial portion (which is triangular in shape and smaller than the radial fragment) remains in normal relationship with the trapezium.

It is usually produced by direct violence applied to the end of the metacarpal, which drives the shaft proximally and dorsally.

The dislocated portion of the metacarpal disrupts the dorsal capsular structures.

It is most essential to restore the fragments to their normal anatomic position and to maintain this position until bony healing is complete.

Inadequate reduction and immobilization result in malunion; such a joint may develop secondary osteoarthritic changes causing pain and impairment of function.

Conservative measures, especially plaster immobilization alone, fail to maintain anatomic reduction of the fragments.

I prefer to treat this lesion by open reduction, internal fixation and repair of the dorsal capsule.

If open reduction is contraindicated or refused, traction is the next best method of treatment.

Prereduction X-Ray

1. The proximal fragment is displaced upward and backward.

2. The distal medial fragment maintains its normal position in relation to the trapezium.

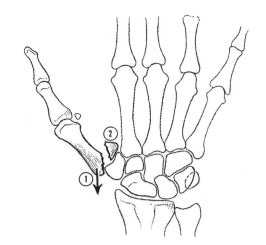

Operative Procedure

1. Make a 2 inch incision centered over the dorsum of the first metacarpal bone. It extends from the conjuncture of the distal and middle thirds of the metacarpal to the distal limits of the anatomic snuffbox.

2. Divide the periosteum longitudinally between the abductor pollicis brevis and the extensor pollicis longus and expose the bone by subperiosteal dissection.

3. At the proximal end of the wound, divide the capsule of the carpometacarpal joint and expose the interior of the joint.

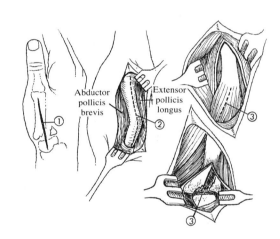

1. Make traction on the abducted thumb.

2. Approximate the proximal and distal fragments and hold them in normal position with a towel clip.

3. Transfix both fragments with one or two fine threaded wires. Cut the wire below the level of the skin.

Note: Repair the dorsal capsule.

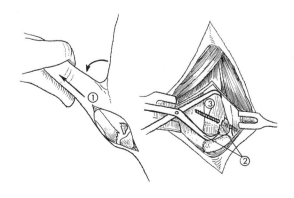

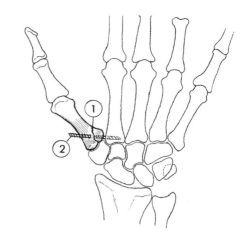

Postoperative X-Rays

1. The fracture is adequately reduced.

2. A wire stabilizes the fragments in normal anatomic position.

Immobilization

Apply a circular plaster cast from the lower forearm to just proximal to the interphalangeal joint.

1. The interphalangeal joint is free.

2. The thumb is abducted and opposed.

3. The metacarpophalangeal joint is slightly flexed.

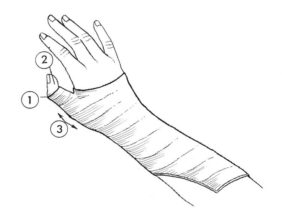

Postoperative Management

During the period of immobilization encourage active exercises of the remaining fingers.

Remove the wire after three weeks.

Reapply the plaster cast.

Remove the second cast after three more weeks (the total period of immobilization is six weeks).

Institute a program of physical therapy and active exercises.

Alternate Method

1. Pass a threaded wire through the proximal phalanx.

2. While traction is made on the abducted and opposed thumb,

3. Apply a nonpadded plaster cast extending from the lower forearm to the metacarpophalangeal joints.

4. Mold the plaster firmly against the base of the metacarpal.

5. Incorporate a wire loop in plaster.

6. Make continuous traction with rubber bands.

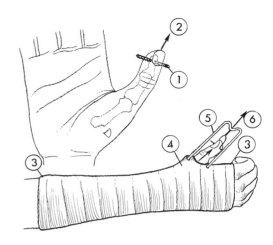

Postreduction Management

Keep the rubber bands taut at all times.

Take x-ray on the fifth and tenth days; check the position of the fragments.

Remove the traction apparatus after three weeks and apply a similar cast extending to just proximal to the interphalangeal joint.

Remove the second cast after three weeks (the total period of immobilization is six weeks).

During the period of immobilization allow and encourage free use of the unaffected fingers.

After immobilization institute a program of physical therapy and active exercises to restore normal function of the thumb.

Metacarpophalangeal Joint of the Thumb

REMARKS

Ligamentous injuries to the metacarpophalangeal joint occur more frequently than to the carpometacarpal joint of the thumb.

Although this articulation functions primarily as the interphalangeal joints it does also possess some lateral motion made possible by the broad lateral convex surfaces of the proximal end of the metacarpal bone.

Chronic instability of this joint is a common occurrence after injury and is due to inadequate management.

The types of injuries are determined by the direction of the force applied to the thumb; hyperextension injuries are by far the most frequent and cause varying degrees of implication of the anterior capsule and also of one of the collateral ligaments. Lateral violence causes disruption of the collateral ligaments opposite the side of the application of the force. The dorsoradial structures are involved more often than those on the ulnar side.

Injuries to the ligaments and capsule vary from simple sprains to complete disruption of the structures.

It is most essential to determine the severity of the injury; instability of the joint indicates tearing of the stabilizing ligaments and capsule.

Subluxations and dislocations may reduce spontaneously; or immediately after the injury, someone may pull on the deformed finger effecting reduction of the joint. In this event it is difficult to determine the extent of injury; however, the presence of abnormal motion in any direction indicates severe disruption of the soft tissues.

In severe hyperextension injuries the head of the metacarpal is thrust through the base of the anterior palmar ligament, detaching it from the metacarpal bone. The metacarpal head projects between the tendons of the two heads of the flexor pollicis brevis. The proximal phalanx is driven backward and comes to rest vertically on the dorsum of the metacarpal. In this position the detached palmar ligament lies anterior to the head of the metacarpal.

Traction on the metacarpal in line with the forearm may cause the palmar ligament to be displaced between the two bones, producing an irreducible or complex dislocation (McLaughlin).

Always suspect a complex dislocation when the long axis of the phalanx is parallel to that of the metacarpal instead of a right angle.

1. Normal arrangement of the collateral ligaments and the palmar ligament of the metacarpophalangeal joint.

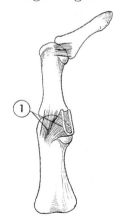

Simple Dislocation

1. The phalanx sets on the back of the metacarpal in a vertical position.

2. The palmar ligament hangs in front of the head of the metacarpal.

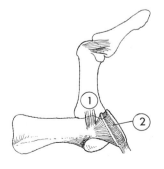

Page 1049

Complex Dislocation
(McLaughlin)

As the result of traction on the thumb, the phalanx pivots on the intact collateral ligaments.

1. The proximal phalanx is in the same plane as the metacarpal.

2. The palmar ligament is interposed between the bones.

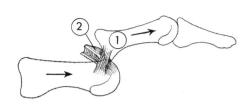

The pivot mechanism is reinforced by the action of the intrinsic muscles of the thumb.

1. Proximal phalanx.

2. Protruding head of the metacarpal.

3. Intrinsic muscles of the thumb.

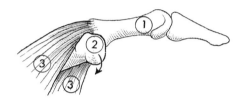

MANAGEMENT OF SIMPLE SPRAINS OF THE METACARPOPHALANGEAL JOINT OF THE THUMB

Apply a strapping of ½ inch strips of adhesive.

1. The strapping encircles the metacarpophalangeal joint.

2. The interphalangeal joint is free.

3. The basket-weave strapping extends above the wrist.

4. Anchor the strips of adhesive encircling the thumb by strips encircling the wrist.

5. The thumb is strapped in the grasp position.

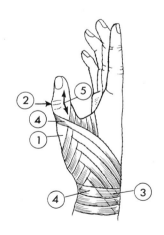

Reapply the strapping every week.

Remove the strapping after three weeks but protect the joint against excessive strains.

MANAGEMENT OF SEVERE SPRAINS OF THE METACARPOPHALANGEAL JOINT OF THE THUMB

Immobilize the thumb in a nonpadded cast.

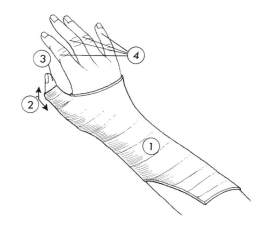

1. The cast extends above the wrist.
2. The interphalangeal joint is included in the cast.
3. The thumb is in the grasp position.
4. The unaffected fingers are free.

Maintain the thumb in plaster for three weeks.

Allow free use of the unaffected fingers.

Remove the cast after three weeks and apply a basket-weave adhesive strapping.

MANAGEMENT OF DISLOCATION OF THE METACARPOPHALANGEAL JOINT OF THE THUMB

REMARKS

If the dislocation has reduced spontaneously immobilize the thumb in a plaster cast as described above.

If the thumb is dislocated effect a reduction by the manipulative maneuvers described on page 1052 and then immobilize the thumb in a plaster cast.

If reduction is not possible after one or, at the most, two attempts by the manipulative procedure, then open reduction is indicated.

Do not inflict more damage to the capsule and ligaments by repeated and futile attempts at closed reduction.

Prereduction X-Ray

1. The phalanx is hyperextended and displaced upward and backward.

2. The base of the phalanx rests on the head of the metacarpal at a right angle.

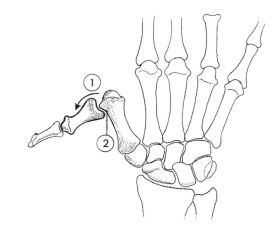

Manipulative Reduction (Under General Anesthesia)

1. A bandage is looped around the patient's thumb and then around the operator's hand.

2. Grasp the patient's thumb with your thumb and index finger and make traction in the long axis of the thumb (not in the axis of the forearm). While traction is maintained,

3. Push the base of the thumb distalward to a position opposite the head of the metacarpal.

4. Flex the thumb.

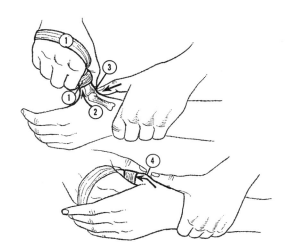

Postreduction X-Ray

1. The base of the phalanx is in normal relationship to the head of the metacarpal.

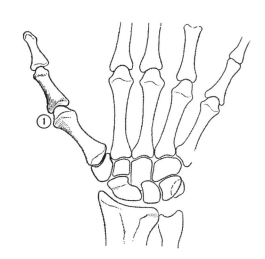

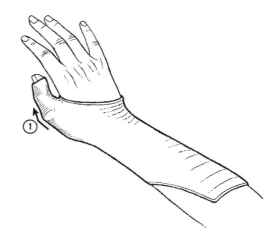

Immobilization

Apply a plaster cast from the lower portion of the forearm to the base of the thumbnail.

1. The thumb is slightly flexed at the metacarpophalangeal joint. The hand is in the grasp position.

Postreduction Management

Remove the cast after three weeks.

Apply a basket-weave strapping around the metacarpophalangeal joint with the interphalangeal joint free for three more weeks.

Protect the thumb from excessive stresses for several more weeks.

During the period of immobilization allow free use of the unaffected fingers.

OPEN REDUCTION OF DISLOCATION OF THE METACARPOPHALANGEAL JOINT OF THE THUMB

INDICATIONS

The metacarpal head may pierce the capsule, which in turn constricts around the metacarpal neck, preventing reduction.

The short flexor tendons of the thumb may preclude reduction.

Open Reduction

1. Make a 2 inch incision over the radial and volar aspects of the thumb centered over the metacarpophalangeal joint.

2. Divide the articular capsule, exposing the articular surfaces of the phalanx and the metacarpal bone.

3. Enlarge the hole in the articular capsule or disengage the tendons of the flexor pollicis brevis and retract them forward.

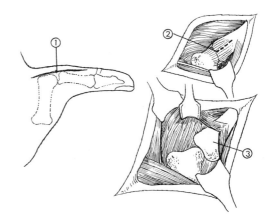

Page 1053

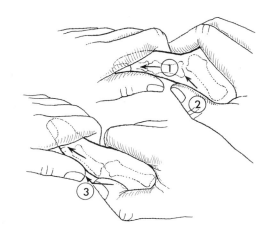

Open Reduction (Continued)

1. Apply traction to the hyperextended thumb.

2. Push the phalanx off the metacarpal bone.

3. Flex the thumb, completing the reduction.

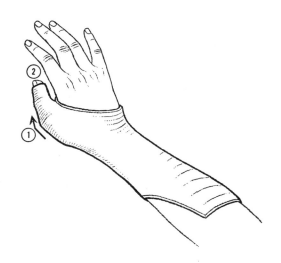

Immobilization

Apply a circular plaster cast from the lower forearm to the tip of the thumb.

1. The thumb is slightly flexed at the metacarpophalangeal joint.

2. The thumb is abducted and opposed.

Postreduction Management

Remove the plaster cast at the end of three weeks.

Apply a basket-weave adhesive strapping around the metacarpophalangeal joint, with the interphalangeal joint free.

Maintain the thumb strapped for three more weeks.

Protect the thumb from forceful hyperextension for several more weeks.

During the period of immobilization allow free and full use of the unaffected fingers.

FRACTURE-DISLOCATION OF THE METACARPOPHALANGEAL JOINT OF THE THUMB

REMARKS

One of the sesamoid bones situated in the anterior portion of the capsular ligament may be fractured from direct violence. This lesion can be treated by a simple basket-weave strapping; however, the joint will remain painful and stiff for many months.

Lateral injury of the ligament may be associated with avulsion fracture of the proximal phalanx; this involves the articular surfaces of the phalanx and indicates severe involvement of the affected ligament.

If there is no displacement, ignore the fracture and treat the lesion as a severe sprain (see page 1051).

If there is displacement of the fragment, the treatment depends on its size; remove a small fragment and repair the ligament; replace a large fragment and fix it with a fine Kirschner wire.

The dislocation may reduce spontaneously or may be reduced by someone pulling on the finger before medical aid is sought.

If the dislocation is still present, it is reduced by the techniques described for simple or complex dislocations of this joint (see page 1052).

The associated fracture should be treated as noted above.

Preoperative X-Ray

1. Small fragment avulsed from the dorsoradial margin of the proximal phalanx.

2. Ulnar deviation of the proximal phalanx.

Note: Remove this fragment and repair the ligament; then treat as a severe sprain.

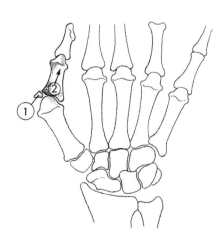

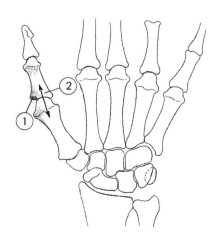

Postoperative X-Ray

1. Defect after removal of the fragment.

2. Phalanx is in normal alignment with head of the metacarpal.

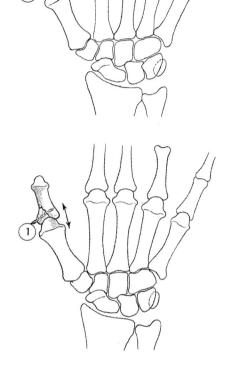

Preoperative X-Ray

1. Large triangular fragment avulsed from the proximal phalanx.

2. Ulnar deviation of the proximal fragment.

Note: Replace this fragment and fix it with a fine Kirschner wire.

Postoperative X-Ray

1. Fragment has been reduced and fixed with a fine Kirschner wire. Normal alignment between the phalanx and the metacarpal is restored.

Dislocation and Fracture-dislocation of the Interphalangeal Joint of the Thumb

REMARKS

These are not common lesions; they are produced by lateral violence causing rupture of the collateral ligament on the side opposite that to which the force was applied. They may also be produced by hyperextension mechanisms.

Many of these lesions are underdiagnosed or missed completely, resulting in a deformed painful thumb.

This is a hinge joint functioning in one plane; if lateral motion is present it indicates rupture of the collateral ligament opposite the direction of the abnormal motion.

A marginal piece of bone may be avulsed from the proximal phalanx; especially in lateral mechanisms indicating a detachment of the collateral ligament.

Small undisplaced fragments are ignored; treat the lesion by adequate immobilization.

Displaced small fragments are removed—the ligament is reattached; large displaced fragments should be replaced and fixed with a fine Kirschner wire.

If the dislocation is present at the time of the initial examination, it should be reduced promptly; if the dislocation is complicated by marginal fractures of the proximal phalanx, the fractures are treated as noted above.

Management of:

Severe sprain of the interphalangeal joint of the thumb.
Rupture of one of the collateral ligaments.
Marginal fracture without displacement.

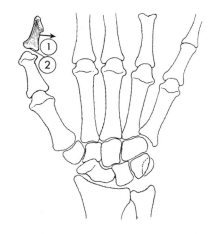

X-RAY: RUPTURE OF ONE OF THE COLLATERAL LIGAMENTS

1. Lateral deviation of the distal phalanx.
2. Widening of the interphalangeal joint.

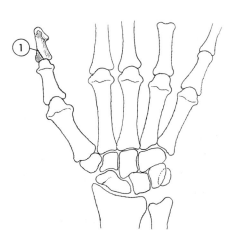

X-RAY: FRACTURE WITHOUT DISPLACEMENT

1. Marginal fracture without displacement.

Page 1057

Immobilization

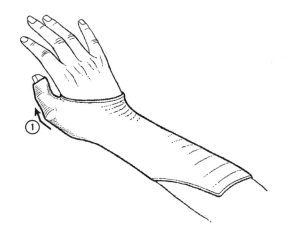

Apply a nonpadded plaster cast from the wrist to the tip of the thumb.

1. The thumb is flexed slightly at the metacarpophalangeal joint and interphalangeal joint.

Mold the cast well around the interphalangeal joint.

Remove the cast after three weeks.

Apply basket-weave strapping around the thumb to the proximal joint; protect the thumb with this type of strapping for two to three more weeks.

During the period of immobilization allow free use of all the unaffected fingers.

Note: These joints remain painful for many weeks.

MANAGEMENT OF DISLOCATION OF THE INTERPHALANGEAL JOINT OF THE THUMB

Prereduction X-Ray

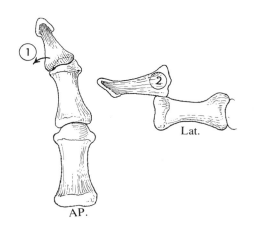

ANTEROPOSTERIOR VIEW

1. The distal phalanx is displaced laterally.

LATERAL VIEW

2. The distal phalanx sits on the dorsum of the proximal phalanx.

Note: In this type of lesion the capsule and the collateral ligaments must be disrupted.

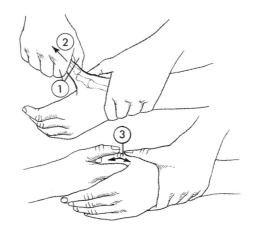

Reduction

1. Grasp the patient's thumb with your thumb and index finger.

2. Make steady traction in the line of deformity of the distal phalanx.

3. While traction is maintained flex the interphalangeal joint.

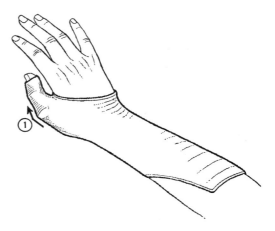

Immobilization

Apply a nonpadded plaster cast from above the wrist to the tip of the thumb.

1. The thumb is flexed slightly at the metacarpophalangeal and interphalangeal joints.

Mold the plaster well around the interphalangeal joint.

Remove the cast after three weeks.

Apply a basket-weave strapping around the interphalangeal joint; leave the metacarpal joint free; protect the thumb with this type of strapping for two to three more weeks.

During the period of immobilization allow free use of the unaffected fingers.

FRACTURE-DISLOCATIONS OF THE INTERPHALANGEAL JOINT OF THE THUMB WITH DISPLACEMENT OF THE FRAGMENTS

Preoperative X-Ray

1. Small displaced fragment lying within the joint.

2. Deviation of the distal phalanx.

Note: Remove the fragment and repair the ligament.

Postoperative immobilization and management is the same as that for dislocation of the thumb without fracture of the distal phalanx.

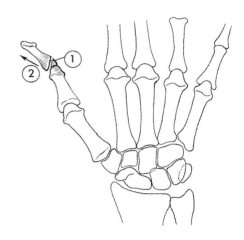

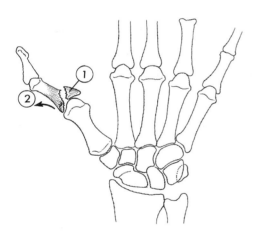

Preoperative X-Ray

1. Large triangular fragment avulsed from the proximal phalanx.

2. Deviation of the finger.

Note: Replace this fragment and fix it with a fine Kirschner wire.

Postoperative X-Ray

1. Fragment is in its normal position and

2. Fixed with a fine Kirschner wire.

Note: Postoperative immobilization and management are the same as for a simple dislocation.

Remove the wire at the end of the third week.

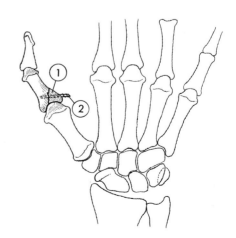

DISLOCATIONS AND FRACTURE-DISLOCATIONS OF THE FINGER METACARPALS

Carpometacarpal Joints

REMARKS

Dislocation of the carpometacarpal joints occurs infrequently because the carpus and the bases of the metacarpal bones are firmly bound together by the dorsal and palmar ligaments.

Severe hyperextension or hyperflexion of the wrist may cause a rupture of the ligaments and permit either a dorsal or a volar dislocation; the former is more common than the latter.

Generally all the metacarpals are dislocated; however, single bones may be involved; when this occurs it is usually the second or the fifth metacarpal because they are more mobile than the middle two metacarpals.

In early lesions reduction is readily achieved and maintained by conservative methods.

The dislocations may be associated with avulsion fractures of the bases of the metacarpals; for these lesions the treatment is the same as that for uncomplicated dislocations. The fracture-dislocation may be unstable and difficult to hold by simple plaster fixation; in this event internal fixation should be employed.

Prereduction X-Ray (Dorsal Dislocation)

1. The four metacarpals are displaced en masse dorsally.
2. The bases of the metacarpals lie on the dorsum of the distal row of carpal bones.

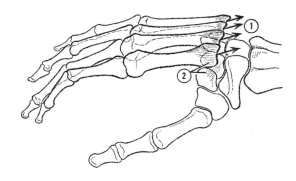

Prereduction X-Ray (Volar Dislocation)

1. The four metacarpals are displaced volarly.

2. The bases of the metacarpals are in the palm.

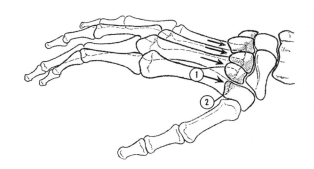

Reduction by Traction and Manipulation (For Dorsal Dislocation)

1. One hand of the operator encircles the wrist while the other encircles the hand.

2. The wrist is slightly dorsiflexed.

3. The fingers are flexed.

4. While counter traction is made on the wrist, make strong traction on the hand.

5. While the thumb of the proximal hand makes first downward pressure over the bases of the metacarpal bones, the fingers of the distal hand make upward pressure on the shafts of the metacarpals, and at the same time,

6. Dorsiflex the wrist further.

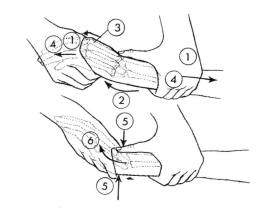

Prereduction X-Ray

1. The bases of the metacarpals are now in normal relationship with the distal row of carpal bones.

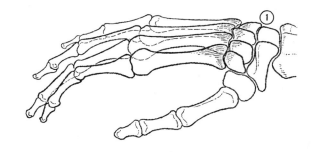

Immobilization

While traction is maintained,

1. Place a felt pad over the bases of the metacarpals.

2. Apply anterior and posterior plaster splints directly to the skin, extending from the upper portion of the forearm to just proximal to the metacarpophalangeal joint.

3. Mold the plaster carefully over the dorsum of the wrist and in the palm.

4. Make firm even pressure over the bases of the metacarpals.

5. The wrist is dorsiflexed.

6. The metacarpophalangeal joints are free; also the thumb and the interphalangeal joints are free.

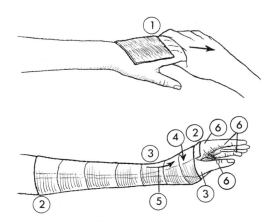

Postreduction Management

Institute active exercises for all fingers immediately.

Remove the cast at the end of the fourth week.

Encourage free use of the hand.

Note: For volar dislocations, the manipulative maneuvers recorded above are reversed and the wrist is immobilized in the neutral position.

Fracture-dislocations of the Carpometacarpal Joints

REMARKS

Carpometacarpal dislocations may be accompanied by marginal avulsion fractures of the bases of the metacarpals.

The treatment for these lesions is the same as that for uncomplicated dislocations, except for the unstable fracture-dislocations.

If one or two fractured metacarpals are dislocated and unstable, reduction can be maintained by transfixion of the metacarpals to the adjacent undisplaced metacarpals by threaded Kirschner wires.

Prereduction X-Ray

1. Fracture of the base of the fourth metacarpal.

2. Dorsal displacement of the shaft of the metacarpal.

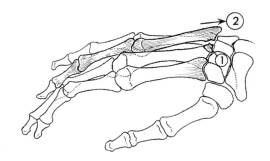

Postreduction X-Ray

1. The base of the fourth metacarpal is fixed to the adjacent metacarpals by Kirschner wires.

2. The fracture-dislocation is reduced.

Note: This procedure does not require exposing the fracture site.

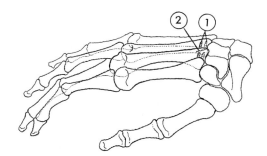

ALTERNATE METHOD

This method is employed when open reduction is necessary to reduce the fracture-dislocation.

Operative Procedure

1. Make a 2 inch longitudinal incision centered over the dorsum of the base of the fractured metacarpal.

2. Displace the extensor tendon to one side and expose the fracture site by subperiosteal dissection. Open the articular capsule to expose the carpometacarpal joint.

3. Make traction on the metacarpal and with a small curette pry the bone fragments into anatomic position.

4. Hold the fragments with a towel clip and transfix them with two threaded wires crossing each other; cut the wires below the level of the skin.

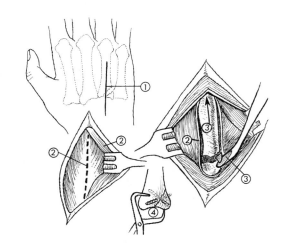

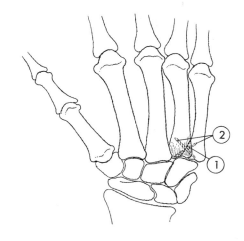

Postreduction X-Ray

1. The fragments are in anatomic position.
2. The fragments are fixed by two threaded Kirschner wires.

Immobilization

Apply a nonpadded plaster cast from the upper portion of the forearm to just proximal to the metacarpophalangeal joints.
1. The wrist is slightly dorsiflexed.
2. The thumb is free.
3. The fingers are free.

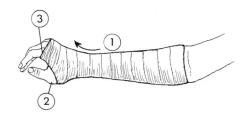

Postreduction Management

Remove the cast and wires at the end of three weeks.
During the period of immobilization allow free use of all the fingers.

Metacarpophalangeal Joints

REMARKS

Dislocations of the metacarpophalangeal joints of the fingers rarely occur—the index finger is more frequently involved.

The usual mechanism is one of hyperextension resulting in a simple or complex dislocation as described for dislocation of the metacarpophalangeal joint of the thumb (see page 1048).

Generally, reduction is readily effected by traction in the long axis of the finger followed by flexion.

If this maneuver fails it indicates that the detached anterior ligament is interposed between the bones, and open reduction is indicated.

Repeated attempts at reduction inflict further damage on the capsule and collateral ligaments—do not make more than two attempts.

There may be an avulsion fracture of the base of the phalanx.

If the fragment is small and displaced, it should be removed and the ligament repaired; if it is large and displaced, it should be replaced and fixed by a fine Kirschner wire.

If open reduction is necessary to reduce the dislocation, the technique is the same as that depicted for irreducible dislocation of the thumb (see page 1053).

Prereduction X-Ray (Simple Dislocation)

1. The base of the phalanx sits on the dorsum of the head of the metacarpal at a right angle.

Note: When the phalanx is in this position it can be assumed that the anterior capsule is not interposed between the bones.

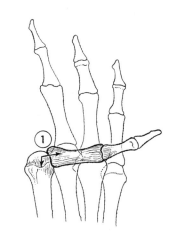

Manipulative Reduction

1. A bandage is first looped around the patient's finger and then around the operator's hand.

2. Grasp the finger with your thumb and index finger and make traction along the axis of the hyperextended phalanx (not along the axis of the metacarpal).

3. While traction is maintained push the base of the dislocated phalanx distalward to a position opposite the head of the metacarpal.

4. Flex the metacarpophalangeal joints.

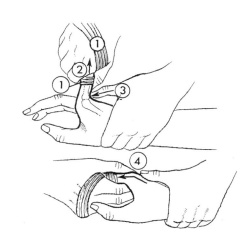

Prereduction X-Ray (Complex Dislocation)

1. The base of the phalanx lies on the dorsal surface of the head of the metacarpal.

2. The axis of the phalanx is almost parallel to that of the metacarpal.

Note: When the phalanx lies in this position it can be assumed that the anterior palmar ligament is interposed between the bones.

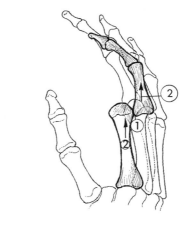

Manipulative Reduction

1. A bandage is first looped around the patient's finger and then around the operator's hand.

2. Grasp the finger with your thumb and index finger and with gentle traction hyperextend the phalanx.

3. Make traction on the hyperextended finger and at the same time push the base of the phalanx opposite the head of the metacarpal.

4. Flex the metacarpophalangeal joint.

Note: If two attempts of this maneuver fail to achieve a reduction, open reduction is indicated.

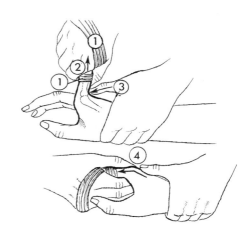

Immobilization

1. Apply a posterior plaster slab over the dorsum of the wrist, hand and finger as far as the proximal interphalangeal joint.

2. The wrist is slightly dorsiflexed.

3. The metacarpophalangeal joint is slightly flexed.

4. The interphalangeal joints are free.

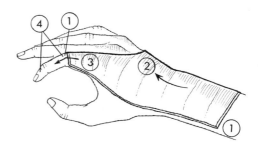

Postreduction Management

During the period of immobilization actively exercise the unaffected fingers.

The plaster slab is removed at the end of three weeks.

Protect the joint with a basket-weave adhesive strapping for two or three more weeks.

Institute physical therapy to restore normal function to the wrist and affected finger.

FRACTURE-DISLOCATIONS OF THE METACARPOPHALANGEAL JOINT

X-Ray Appearance: Small Displaced Fragment

1. Small avulsed fragment from the base of the phalanx.

2. Fragment is displaced.

Note: Remove this fragment and repair the torn ligament.

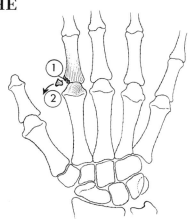

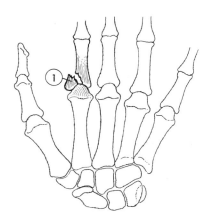

X-Ray Appearance: Large Displaced Fragment

1. Large triangular fragment from volar aspect of the base of the phalanx.

Note: Replace this fragment and fix it with a fine Kirschner wire.

Postreduction X-Ray

1. Fragment is fixed in its normal position with fine Kirschner wire.

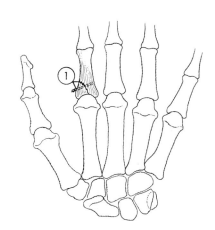

DISLOCATIONS AND FRACTURE-DISLOCATIONS OF THE PHALANGES OF THE FINGERS

REMARKS

Dislocation of the interphalangeal joints is relatively common and may be produced by lateral or hyperextension mechanisms.

Like the metacarpophalangeal joints, the interphalangeal joints are stabilized by a strong palmar ligament and collateral ligaments.

Hyperextension injuries always implicate the anterior capsule and palmar ligament; one or both collateral ligaments may also be involved. In lateral injuries the collateral ligament opposite the side to which the force was applied is involved.

The structure of the collateral ligaments is such that in flexion they are taut and in extension they are relaxed.

Inadequate treatment of a tear of a collateral ligament results in lateral deviation of the distal phalanx toward the opposite side and marked impairment of function due to pain and restricted motion.

In severe hyperextension injuries, the head of the proximal phalanx may penetrate the anterior capsule and become trapped in this position by the capsule or by the flexor tendon so that reduction is impossible.

In most instances the dislocation reduces spontaneously or is readily reduced by manipulative maneuver; those that cannot be reduced by closed methods require open reduction in order to disengage the head of the proximal phalanx.

It is possible to have a hyperextension type of dislocation without rupture of the anterior or collateral ligaments. When this occurs the joint exhibits no instability after reduction.

After reduction the joint should be carefully examined for the presence or absence of instability. If instability is present an estimate of its severity should be made.

In most instances immobilization of the affected joint in the correct position suffices to permit healing of the ligaments so that no deformity or instability of the joint occurs and function is only minimally impaired. However, if gross lateral instability is demonstrable, surgical repair of the collateral ligaments is indicated.

Dislocations of the interphalangeal joints may be accompanied by fracture of the base of the distal phalanx; the management of these fractures depends upon the size of the fragment and the amount of displacement.

Management of Lateral Dislocations of the Interphalangeal Joints

REMARKS

In lateral subluxation or dislocation of the interphalangeal joint the collateral ligament on the same side the force was applied is ruptured.

Spontaneous reduction usually occurs or the dislocation is reduced before medical aid is sought.

The joint should be carefully examined for evidence of instability.

If unreduced, reduction is readily achieved by closed methods.

Prereduction X-Ray

1. Lateral dislocation of the distal phalanx of the proximal interphalangeal joint.

2. There is no anterior or posterior displacement of the phalanx.

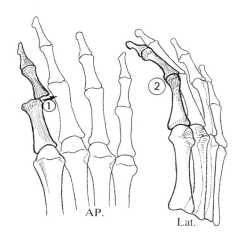

Manipulative Reduction

1. Loop a gauze bandage around the end of the injured finger and around the operator's hand.

2. Grasp the end of the finger with your thumb and index finger.

3. Make steady traction in the axis of the finger.

4. While traction is being maintained bring the distal phalanx in line with the proximal phalanx.

5. Squeeze the sides of the joint to correct any residual lateral displacement.

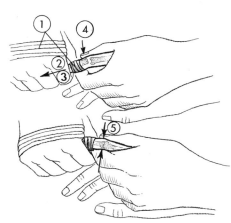

Immobilization

1. Apply anterior and posterior plaster slabs directly to the skin.

2. The plaster extends from just distal to the metacarpophalangeal joint to the base of the nail.

3. The interphalangeal joints are extended.

Note: This lesion must be treated in extension because the collateral ligaments are taut in flexion; if allowed to heal in flexion, the ligament would be redundant, therefore causing instability of the joint.

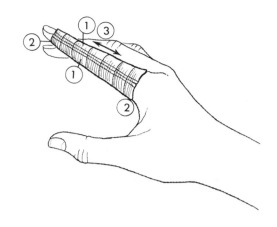

Postreduction Management

Remove the plaster splints at the end of two weeks.

During the period of immobilization actively exercise the unaffected fingers.

After removal of the splints do not permit full flexion for three or four more weeks—never perform passive stretchings or allow forced motions of the affected joint.

Some restriction of motion usually ensues; the joint may be painful and stiff for many weeks.

Management of Hyperextension Dislocations of the Interphalangeal Joints

REMARKS

If the patient presents with the finger dislocated it indicates that the head of the proximal phalanx is trapped in this position, either by the torn anterior capsule or the flexor tendon.

Prereduction X-Ray

1. The base of the distal phalanx of the interphalangeal joint lies on the dorsal aspect of the proximal phalanx.

2. The distal phalanx is deviated laterally.

Note: this deformity indicates a tear of the anterior capsule and of the collateral ligament opposite the side toward which the phalanx deviates.

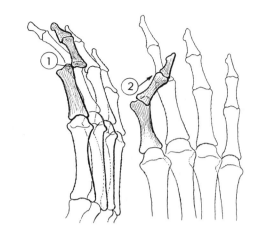

Manipulative Reduction (Local Anesthesia)

1. A bandage is first looped around the end of the injured finger and then around the operator's hand.

2. Grasp the dislocated finger with your thumb and index finger and make gentle traction along the axis of the dislocated phalanx; at the same time,

3. Bring the phalanx into the hyperextended position.

4. While traction is being maintained,

5. Slide the base of the phalanx distalward to a position opposite the head of the proximal phalanx; then,

6. Flex the interphalangeal joint.

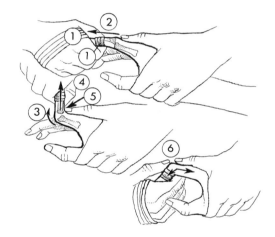

Immobilization

1. Apply anterior and posterior plaster slabs directly to the skin.

2. The metacarpophalangeal joint is free.

3. The interphalangeal joints are slightly flexed.

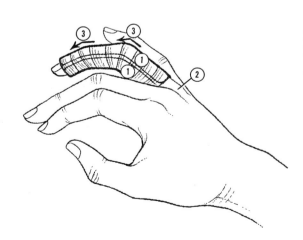

Postreduction Management

Take x-rays after the manipulative reduction to ascertain evidence of uncorrected lateral displacement.

Take x-rays on the fifth and tenth days to note any evidence of displacement (this may occur in plaster).

Remove the plaster splints after three weeks.

Exercise actively all unaffected fingers during the period of immobilization.

After removal of the external immobilization, allow free use of the finger and encourage active exercise. Never perform passive stretchings or allow forced motion of the affected joint.

Fracture-dislocations of the Interphalangeal Joints

REMARKS

Dislocation of the interphalangeal joints may be complicated by marginal avulsion fractures of the dislocated phalanx. These lesions are similar to fracture-dislocations of the metacarpophalangeal joints and are treated in a similar manner.

Undisplaced fractures are ignored and the treatment is directed to the dislocation.

Small displaced fragments should be removed and the ligament repaired.

Large displaced fragments should be replaced and fixed with a fine Kirschner wire.

X-Ray of Undisplaced Fracture

1. Small undisplaced fracture of the palmar aspect of the base of the middle phalanx.

Note: This fracture can be ignored.

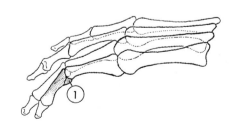

X-Ray of Small Displaced Fracture

1. Small marginal fracture of the ulnar aspect of the base of the middle phalanx.

Note: This fragment should be removed and the ligament repaired.

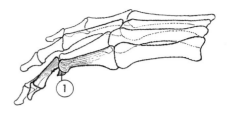

X-Ray of Large Displaced Fragment

1. Large triangular fragment from the palmar aspect of the base of the middle phalanx with marked displacement.

Note: This is a very unstable fracture; the fragment should be replaced and fixed with a fine Kirschner wire.

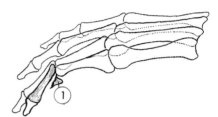

Postoperative X-Ray

1. Fragment is reduced and fixed with a Kirschner wire.

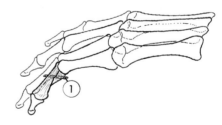

FRACTURES OF THE METACARPALS

Fractures of the Base of the Metacarpal of the Thumb

REMARKS

Fractures of the base of the shaft of the metacarpal of the thumb may be transverse, oblique or comminuted.

Generally they occur in adult males, but they may occur in children, in whom the lesion is essentially an epiphyseal separation with a triangular fragment of the diaphysis displaced with the epiphysis.

Usually the deformity is posterior with outward bowing.

Most lesions are readily reduced by traction and manipulative maneuvers and are stable; these can be treated by immobilizing the thumb in abduction.

Unstable fractures should be treated by open reduction and internal fixation by one or two Kirschner wires.

In the event that open reduction is contraindicated, continuous traction may be employed as in the treatment of Bennett's fracture.

MANAGEMENT OF STABLE FRACTURES OF THE BASE OF THE SHAFT OF THE METACARPAL OF THE THUMB

A. *Prereduction X-Ray (Adult Male)*

1. Fracture through the base of the metacarpal.

2. The distal fragment is displaced upward and backward.

3. The usual deformity is posterior with outward bowing.

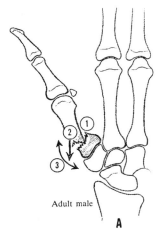

Adult male

A

B. Prereduction X-Ray (Child 13 Years Old)

1. Epiphyseal fracture with detachment of the triangular portion of the diaphysis.

2. The deformity is posterior with outward bowing.

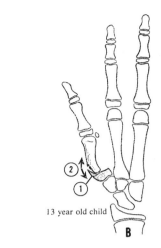

13 year old child

B

Manipulative Reduction

1. Apply strong traction to the abducted thumb.

2. The surgeon places the thumb of his other hand at the base of the metacarpal.

3. While traction is maintained,

4. Firm pressure is made over the proximal end of the distal fragment.

5. The thumb is hyperabducted.

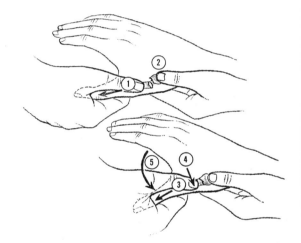

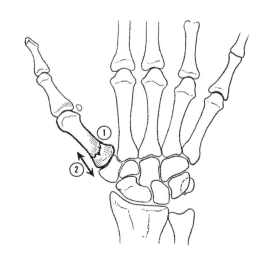

Postreduction X-Ray

1. The fragments are engaged and in normal alignment.

2. The posterior and outward bowing is corrected.

Immobilization

Apply a plaster slab from the lower forearm to the tip of the thumb.

1. The thumb is abducted and opposed.

2. The metacarpophalangeal joint is slightly flexed.

3. Mold the cast well at the base of the thumb.

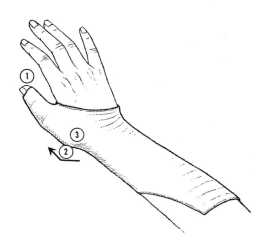

Postreduction Management

Check the position by x-ray on the fifth and fourteenth days.

Encourage the patient to use the remaining fingers of the hand during the period of immobilization.

Reapply a new cast at the end of ten to 14 days if the original cast becomes loose.

Active exercises that flex and extend completely all joints of the fingers should be executed daily on a regulated program.

Remove the cast at the end of six weeks.

Now institute physical therapy and active exercises to restore normal function in all joints of the thumb.

Note: In the case of comminuted or unstable fractures, employ skeletal traction as described under the treatment of Bennett's fracture.

MANAGEMENT OF UNSTABLE FRACTURES OF THE BASE OF THE SHAFT OF THE METACARPAL OF THE THUMB

Prereduction X-Ray

1. The fracture does not implicate the carpometacarpal joint.

2. The base of the metacarpal is severely comminuted.

3. The distal fragment is displaced upward and backward.

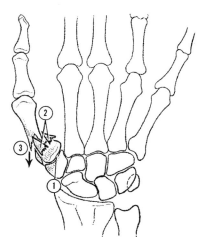

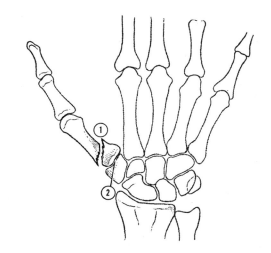

Prereduction X-Ray

1. Oblique fracture through the base of the metacarpal.

2. The carpometacarpal joint is not involved.

Note: Plaster fixation failed to hold this fracture.

Operative Reduction

1. Make a 2 inch incision centered over the dorsum of the first metacarpal. It extends from just proximal to the metacarpophalangeal joint to the distal limit of the anatomic snuffbox.

2. Divide the periosteum longitudinally between the abductor pollicis brevis and the extensor pollicis longus and expose the bone by subperiosteal dissection.

3. If it is necessary to visualize the carpometacarpal joint divide the capsule of the joint at the proximal end of the wound.

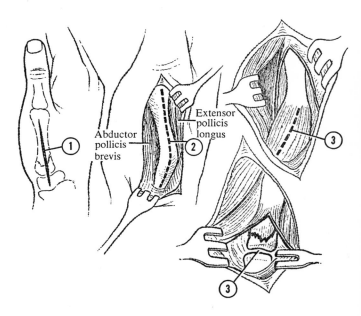

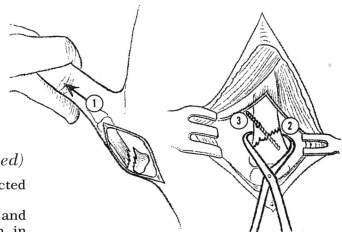

Operative Reduction (Continued)

1. Make traction on the abducted thumb.

2. Approximate the proximal and distal fragments and hold them in normal position with a towel clip.

3. Transfix the fragments with one or two five-threaded Kirschner wires— cut the wires below the level of the skin.

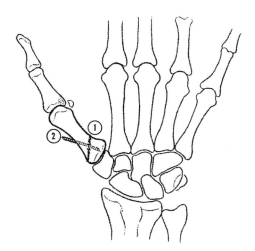

Postoperative X-Ray

1. The fracture is reduced.

2. The wire stabilizes the fragments.

Immobilization

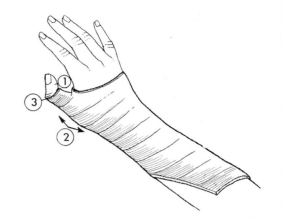

Apply a plaster cast from the lower forearm to just proximal to the interphalangeal joint.

1. The thumb is abducted and opposed.

2. The metacarpophalangeal joint is slightly flexed.

3. The interphalangeal joint is free.

Postoperative Management

During the period of immobilization encourage active exercises of the remaining fingers.

Remove the wire after three weeks.

Reapply a nonpadded cast.

Remove the cast after three weeks (the total period of immobilization is six weeks).

Institute a program of physical therapy and active exercises.

Alternate Method of Management (Continuous Skeletal Traction)

This method is employed only when open reduction and internal fixation are contraindicated; it should never be the first choice of treatment.

The method is the same as that employed for Bennett's fracture (see page 1048).

Fractures of the Shaft of the Metacarpal of the Thumb

REMARKS

In general what has been noted for fractures of the base of the first metacarpal is applicable to fractures of the shaft.

They can be grouped into stable and unstable fractures.

Stable fractures are treated by plaster immobilization with the thumb in abduction.

Unstable fractures should be treated by open reduction and internal fixation. If this method is contraindicated continuous skeletal traction should be employed.

MANAGEMENT OF STABLE FRACTURES OF THE SHAFT OF THE METACARPAL OF THE THUMB

Prereduction X-Ray

1. Fracture of the shaft of the thumb metacarpal with no displacement.

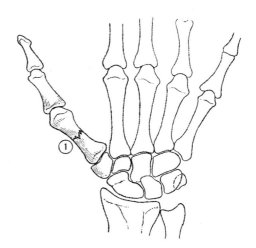

Prereduction X-Ray

1. Fracture of the shaft of the thumb metacarpal with backward displacement.
2. The proximal fragment is tilted forward.
3. The distal fragment is displaced upward and backward.

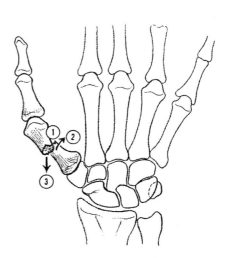

Manipulative Reduction (For Displaced Fractures)

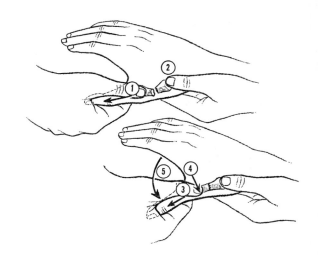

1. Apply strong traction on the abducted thumb.
2. Place the thumb of your other hand over the end of the proximal fragment.
3. While traction is maintained,
4. Make firm pressure on the proximal end of the distal fragment and
5. Hyperabduct the thumb.

Postreduction X-Ray

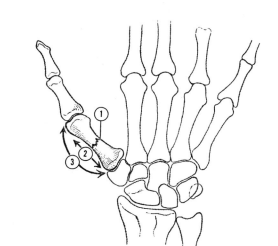

1. The fragments are engaged and in normal alignment.
2. The posterior angulation is corrected.
3. The length of the shaft is restored.

Immobilization

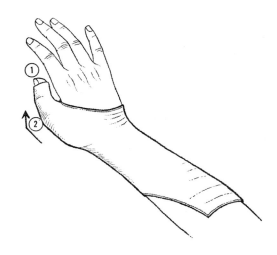

Apply a plaster cast from the lower forearm to the tip of the thumb.
1. The thumb is abducted and opposed.
2. The metacarpophalangeal joint is slightly flexed.

Postreduction Management

Check the position by x-rays on the fifth and fourteenth days.

Encourage the patient to use the remaining fingers of the hand during the period of immobilization.

Reapply a new cast at the end of ten or 14 days if the original cast becomes loose.

Active exercises which flex and extend completely all joints of the fingers should be executed daily on a regulated program.

Remove the cast at the end of six weeks.

Now institute physical therapy and active exercises to restore normal function in all joints of the thumb.

MANAGEMENT OF UNSTABLE FRACTURES OF THE SHAFT OF THE METACARPAL OF THE THUMB

REMARKS

Open reduction and internal fixation with one or two fine threaded Kirschner wires is the procedure of choice.

If open reduction is contraindicated use continuous skeletal traction.

Prereduction X-Ray

1. Oblique fracture of the shaft of the metacarpal.

2. The metacarpal is shortened.

3. The distal fragment is displaced upward and backward.

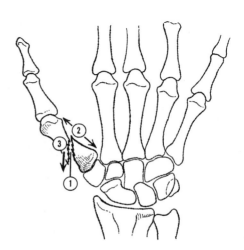

Page 1083

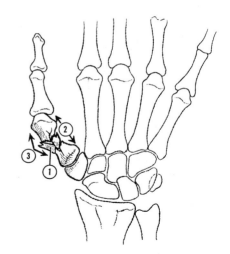

Prereduction X-Ray

1. Comminuted fracture of the shaft of the metacarpal.
2. The metacarpal is shortened
3. Posterior bowing is marked.

Operative Reduction

The technique is the same as that employed for unstable fractures of the base of the first metacarpal (see page 1046).

Skeletal Traction

Employ the same technique used for unstable fractures of the base of the first metacarpal (see page 1048).

Fractures of the Metacarpals of the Fingers

REMARKS

These are common lesions of the hand; in frequency they are second only to fractures of the phalanges.

Fractures of the metacarpals are serious lesions which require meticulous attention to all the details of treatment, otherwise severe deformity and marked impairment of the hand results.

Following fractures of the metacarpals the delicate muscle balance of the hand is disturbed. If malunion occurs, normal muscle balance is not restored, thus resulting in clawing of the finger affected (dorsiflexing the proximal joint and flexing the two distal joints).

Malunion with rotation of the distal fragment results in overlapping of the fingers.

Malunion with acute volar displacement of the distal fragment forces the metacarpal head into the palm interfering with the grasping function of the hand.

Contracture and shortening of the collateral ligaments of the metacarpophalangeal joint resulting from immobilization of the joint in extension produces marked stiffness.

Stiffness of the proximal finger joint may also be the result of fixation of the interossei muscles and tendons by inflammatory exudates associated with fractures of the metacarpals.

MECHANISMS OF FRACTURE

Fractures are produced by one of two mechanisms:

1. By a direct blow to the end of this knuckle such as when the clenched fist strikes a firm object, or

2. By direct crushing violence to the dorsum of the hand; this may produce comminuted fractures of more than one metacarpal. The resulting fracture may involve the base, the shaft or the neck of the metacarpal; at all levels the fracture may be transverse oblique, spiral or comminuted. The factures may or may not be displaced. When displacement occurs, at all levels, the intrinsic muscle action produces a constant deformity—the distal fragment is displaced volarward producing a backward angulation.

1. Lumbrical and

2. Interossei muscles inserting into the dorsal expansion.

3. Extensor digitorum communis.

4. Flexor digitorum profundus.

5. Flexor digitorum sublimis.

Note: All these muscles function in perfect balance.

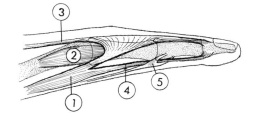

1. Fracture of the shaft or fracture of the neck of the metacarpal.

2. Muscle pull of the intrinsic muscles.

3. Volar displacement of the distal fragment.

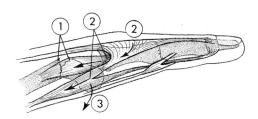

Page 1085

FRACTURES OF THE BASE OF THE FINGER METACARPALS

REMARKS

The bases of the metacarpals are firmly bound together by the palmar and dorsal ligaments so that displacement of the fragments rarely occurs — except when the fracture is associated with a carpometacarpal dislocation.

Many of these fractures are impacted so that x-ray visualization may be very difficult; the fractures are frequently missed.

MANAGEMENT OF UNDISPLACED FRACTURES OF THE BASE OF THE FINGER METACARPALS

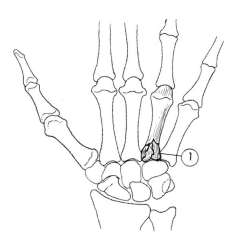

X-Ray Appearance

1. Comminuted fracture of the fourth metacarpal.

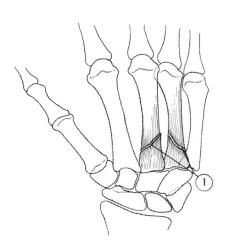

X-Ray Appearance

1. Undisplaced fractures of the third and fourth metacarpal.

Management

Apply a nonpadded plaster cast from the lower part of the forearm to just proximal to the metacarpophalangeal joints.

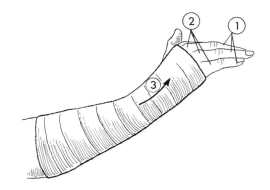

1. The fingers are free.
2. The metacarpophalangeal joints of the fingers are free.
3. The wrist is slightly dorsiflexed.

Remove the cast after three weeks.

During the period of immobilization encourage free use of all the unaffected fingers.

MANAGEMENT OF DISPLACED FRACTURES OF THE BASE OF THE FINGER METACARPALS

These essentially are fracture-dislocations of the carpometacarpal joints. Their management is described on page 1063.

FRACTURES OF THE SHAFT OF THE FINGER METACARPALS

REMARKS

Fractures of the shaft of the inner metacarpals (the third and the fourth) rarely are displaced or angulated, whereas the second and fifth are very likely to exhibit displacement and angulation of the fragments.

Displacement and angulation are usually corrected by traction and pressure over the apex of the deformity. If the fracture following reduction remains stable plaster immobilization suffices; if the fracture is unstable internal fixation with Kirschner wires transfixing the fractured metacarpal to adjacent metacarpals or transfixing the fragments only should be performed.

Traction should never be used if it can possibly be avoided; it predisposes to nonunion and to stiffness of the joints of the fingers.

Traction is employed in the treatment of unstable fractures only when internal fixation is contraindicated.

Page 1087

MANAGEMENT OF FRACTURES OF THE SHAFT OF THE FINGER METACARPALS WITHOUT DISPLACEMENT OR WITH ONLY MINIMAL DISPLACEMENT

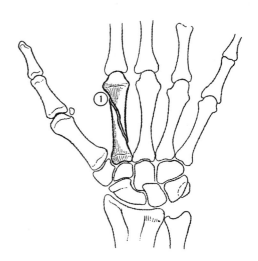

X-Ray (No Displacement)

1. Spiral fracture of the second metacarpal with no displacement.

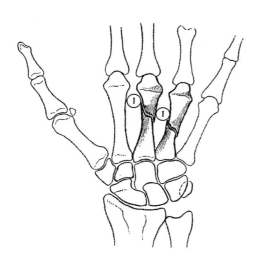

X-Ray (Minimal Displacement)

1. Spiral fracture of the third and fourth metacarpal with minimal displacement and shortening.

Note: This amount of shortening is acceptable.

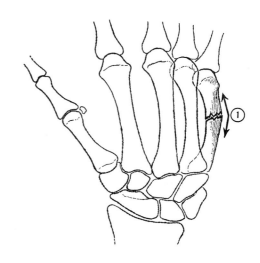

X-Ray (Minimal Displacement)

1. Fracture of the fifth metacarpal with slight posterior angulation.

Note: This degree of angulation is acceptable.

Immobilization

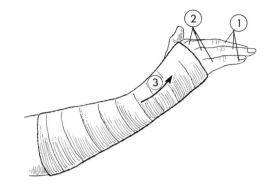

Apply a nonpadded plaster cast extending from the upper forearm to just proximal to the metacarpophalangeal joints.

1. The fingers are free.
2. The metacarpophalangeal joints are free.
3. The wrist is slightly dorsiflexed.

Management

During the period of immobilization all fingers are actively exercised.

The initial plaster cast is replaced at the end of three weeks by a similar cast extending to the metacarpophalangeal joints.

The second cast is removed at the end of two or three weeks.

Institute physical therapy and active exercises to restore normal function in the hand and the wrist.

MANAGEMENT OF STABLE FRACTURES OF THE SHAFT OF THE FINGER METACARPALS

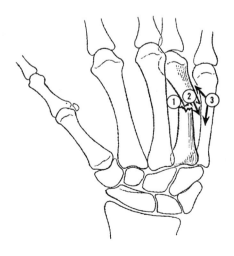

Prereduction X-Ray

1. Transverse fracture of the fourth metacarpal.
2. The head of the metacarpal is displaced volarly.
3. Posterior angular deformity is marked.

Reduction

1. One hand of the operator encircles the wrist while the other grasps the finger of the fractured metacarpal.

2. The wrist is dorsiflexed and the finger is flexed.

3. Make strong traction on the finger; while traction is maintained,

4. The thumb of the proximal hand makes firm downward pressure over the apex of the deformity and,

5. The index finger of the distal hand pushes the head of the metacarpal upward.

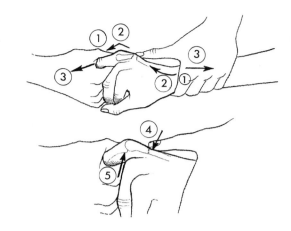

Immobilization

While traction is maintained place a felt pad over the fracture site and apply anterior and posterior plaster splints directly to the skin.

1. The wrist is dorsiflexed.

2. The thumb and fingers are free.

3. Mold the plaster carefully in the palm and over the dorsum of the hand.

Note: Maintain the traction and pressure over the fracture site manually until the plaster has set.

4. Add a padded wire extension to the cast to support the finger.

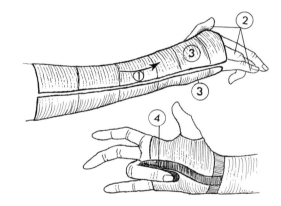

1. The finger is flexed 45 degrees at the metacarpophalangeal joint.

2. The proximal interphalangeal joint is flexed 90 degrees.

3. The center of the nail of the injured finger points to the tubercle of the scaphoid bone.

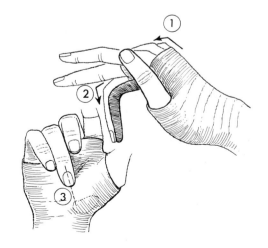

Postreduction Management

During the period of immobilization permit active exercises of all the unaffected fingers.

Take x-rays on the fifth and tenth day; look for displacements of the fragments.

Remove the plaster cast at the end of four weeks.

Allow free use of the affected finger and institute a program of physical therapy to restore normal function in all joints of the hand and wrist.

Note: If following reduction as described above, the position of the fragments cannot be maintained without traction, either traction should be added or the position of the fragments should be maintained by some form of internal fixation. The latter method, if not contraindicated, is by far more effective.

TRACTION FOR UNSTABLE FRACTURES OF THE FINGER METACARPALS

After the fracture is reduced by traction and a cast has been applied with a padded aluminum splint bent to support the finger:

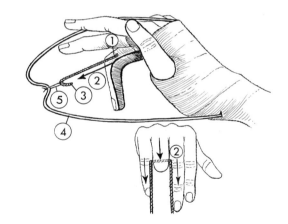

1. Drill a fine Kirschner wire through the head of the proximal phalanx. (Don't penetrate the joint or the dorsal expansion.)

2. Bend each end of the wire so that it is parallel with the finger; cut the ends of the wire ½ to ¾ inch from the tip of the finger.

3. The ends of the wire end in a hook.

4. Add a wire extension loop to the cast.

5. Apply elastic traction between the wire loop and the hooks at the end of the Kirschner wire.

Postreduction Management

Remove the traction apparatus after four weeks.

During the period of immobilization encourage active exercise of the unaffected fingers.

After the cast is removed institute physical therapy to restore motion to all joints. Prolonged stiffness of the finger usually follows this form of treatment.

MANAGEMENT OF UNSTABLE FRACTURES OF THE SHAFT OF THE FINGER METACARPALS – PREFERRED METHOD (TRANSFIXION OF FRACTURED METACARPAL TO THE ADJACENT METACARPALS)

REMARKS

This method is especially applicable to displaced fractures for the third and fourth metacarpals when it is obvious that plaster immobilization without traction will not maintain the reduction.

The fracture site is not opened except when reduction cannot be achieved by closed methods.

Prereduction X-Ray

1. Transverse fracture of the fourth metacarpal.
2. The distal fragment is displaced volarly and proximally, forming
3. A posterior angular deformity.

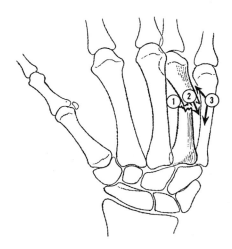

Prereduction X-Ray

1. Oblique fracture of the third metacarpals with posterior bowing.
2. The shaft of the metacarpal is shortened.

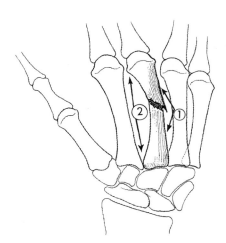

Reduction and Fixation of the Fracture

1. An assistant grasps the wrist in one hand and the affected finger in the other.

2. The wrist is held in dorsiflexion and the finger in flexion.

3. While the proximal hand makes counter traction on the wrist, the distal hand makes longitudinal traction on the finger.

4. While traction is maintained the proximal thumb makes firm downward pressure over the apex of the deformity and the distal thumb and fingers push upward on the metacarpal head.

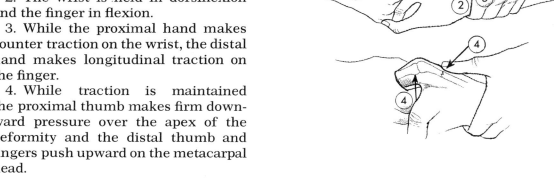

1. While this position is maintained,

2. Transfix the fractured metacarpal to the adjacent metacarpals with Kirschner wires.

Note: One wire passes through the bones above the level of the fracture and one wire passes below.

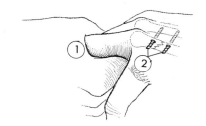

Postreduction X-Ray

1. The fracture of the fourth metacarpal is reduced.

2. The wires pass through the metacarpals above and below the fracture site.

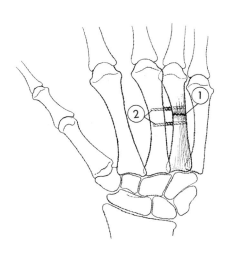

Postreduction X-Ray

1. Fracture of the third metacarpal is reduced.

2. Length of the third metacarpal is restored.

3. Wires pass through the bones above and below the fracture site.

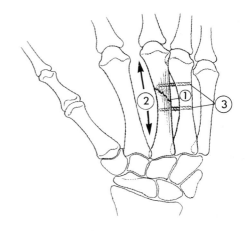

PREFERRED METHOD FOR DISPLACED FRACTURES OF THE SECOND AND FIFTH METACARPALS

REMARKS

Fractures of the fifth and second metacarpals may be fixed by numerous methods—my preference is intermedullary fixation by a Kirschner wire drilled through the head of the metacarpal or by open reduction and fixation of the fragments with two Kirschner wires crossing each other.

Prereduction X-Ray

1. Oblique fracture of the fifth metacarpal.

2. Volar displacement of the head.

3. Posterior angulation of the fragments.

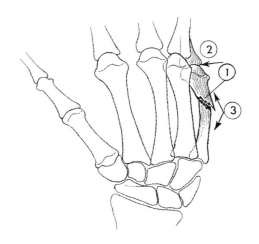

Reduction and Transfixion

1. An assistant flexes the metacarpophalangeal joint to a right angle and,

2. With the finger flexed makes direct pressure upward on the metacarpal head in the long axis of the proximal phalanx.

3. At the same time strong downward pressure is made over the apex of the deformity.

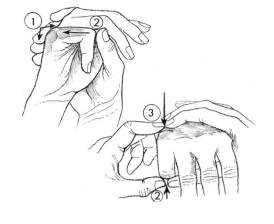

While this position is maintained,

1. Pass a fine threaded wire through the metacarpal head and into the distal fragment—cut the wire ¼ inch from the skin.

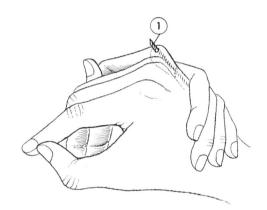

Postreduction X-Ray

1. The backward angulation is corrected.

2. Wire maintains normal alignment.

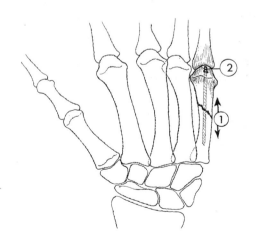

Immobilization

Apply a posterior plaster splint directly to the skin.

1. The cast extends from the lower forearm to the tip of the finger.

2. The metacarpophalangeal joint and interphalangeal joint are semiflexed.

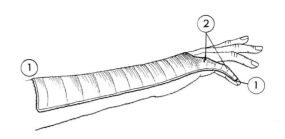

Postreduction Management

Remove the cast and wire at the end of three weeks.

During the period of immobilization encourage free use and exercises of the unaffected fingers.

Alternate Method

1. Make a 1½ inch longitudinal incision centered over the dorsum of the fractured metacarpal.

2. Displace the extensor tendon to one side and expose the fracture site by subperiosteal dissection.

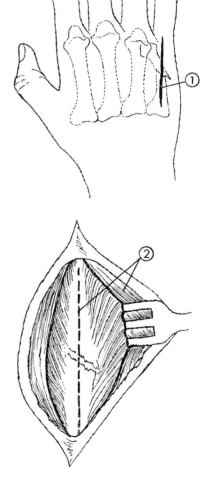

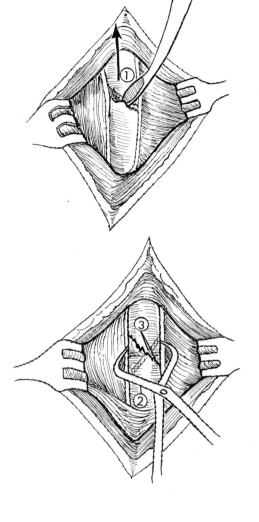

Alternate Method (Continued)

1. Make traction on the finger and with a small curette pry the fragments into alignment.

2. Hold the fragments with a towel clip.

3. Transfix the fragments with two fine threaded Kirschner wires which cross each other—cut the wires below the level of the skin.

Postreduction X-Ray

Two wires stabilize the fragments.

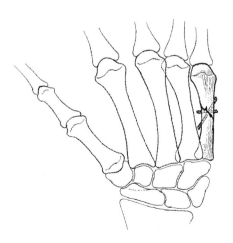

Immobilization

Apply nonpadded anterior and posterior plaster splints.

1. The fingers are free.
2. The metacarpophalangeal joints and interphalangeal joints are free.
3. The wrist is dorsiflexed.

Note: Usually there is no need to immobilize the fifth metacarpophalangeal joint. However, if the fracture is not firmly stabilized with the transfixion wires, the cast can be extended on the fifth finger to the middle of the proximal phalanx.

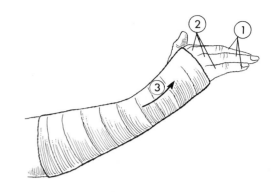

Postreduction Management

Remove the cast and the wires after four weeks.

During this period encourage exercise of all the affected fingers.

After removal of the wires and cast institute an active program of physical therapy and exercises to restore normal motion.

FRACTURES OF THE NECK OF THE FINGER METACARPALS

REMARKS

These are very common lesions, the fifth metacarpal is more frequently involved than the other four metacarpals.

If the deformity is not corrected and union occurs with volar displacement of the head of the metacarpal, pronounced disability may ensue, particularly when the third and fourth metacarpals are implicated. These two bones are not very mobile; however, because of the greater mobility of the second and fifth metacarpals, malunion following fractures of the neck of these metacarpals does not produce severe functional impairment of the hand.

The fracture may or may not be impacted; an impacted fracture is readily reduced by making upward pressure on the head of the metacarpal through the long axis of the proximal phalanx flexed 90 degrees. Impacted fractures may require considerable force to achieve a reduction.

Some of these fractures are stable after reduction while others are not.

The conventional plaster cast employed to treat unstable fractures fails to prevent redisplacement of the fragments and it is poorly tolerated by the patient—these fractures are best treated by internal fixation.

Stable fracture can readily be treated by plaster immobilization with the finger in the functional position.

MANAGEMENT OF STABLE FRACTURES OF THE NECK OF THE FINGER METACARPALS

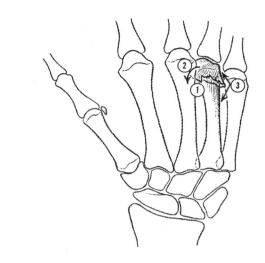

Prereduction X-Ray

1. Fracture of the fourth metacarpal.
2. The head of the bone is tilted volarly.
3. The fracture is angulated backward.

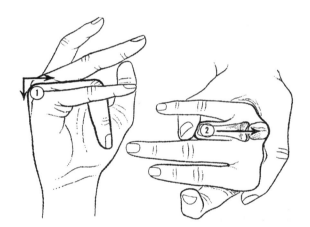

Reduction (General Anesthesia)

1. Flex the metacarpophalangeal joint to the right angle.
2. With finger flexed make direct strong pressure backward on the metacarpal head in the axis of the proximal phalanx.

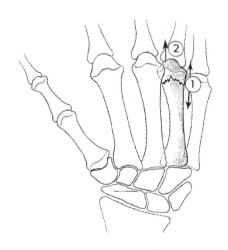

Postreduction X-Ray

1. The backward angulation is corrected.
2. The head of the metacarpal is directed forward.

Page 1099

Immobilization

Apply a nonpadded posterior plaster splint.

1. The splint extends from the lower forearm to the tip of the affected finger.

2. The metacarpophalangeal joint and interphalangeal joints are semiflexed.

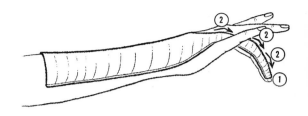

Postreduction Management

Take x-rays on the fifth and tenth days to note any displacements of the fragments.

Remove the cast at the end of three weeks.

During the period of immobilization encourage active use of the unaffected finger.

After removal of the cast institute physical therapy and exercises to restore normal motion of the affected finger.

MANAGEMENT OF UNSTABLE FRACTURES OF THE NECK OF THE FINGER METACARPALS

Prereduction X-Ray

1. Fracture of the neck of the fourth metacarpal.

2. The head of the metacarpal is tilted forward toward the palm.

3. The fracture is angulated backward.

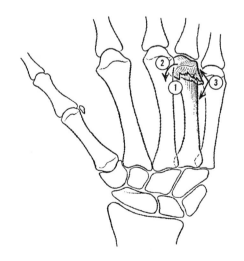

Reduction and Transfixion

1. Flex the metacarpophalangeal joint to the right angle.

2. With the finger flexed make direct pressure backward on the metacarpal head in the axis of the proximal phalanx.

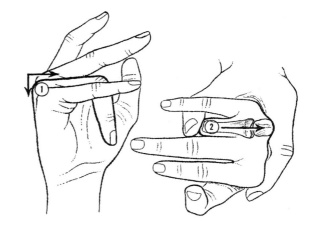

1. While an assistant maintains pressure on the metacarpal head,

2. Pass a fine threaded wire through the metacarpal head and into the distal fragment.

Cut the wire ¼ inch from the skin.

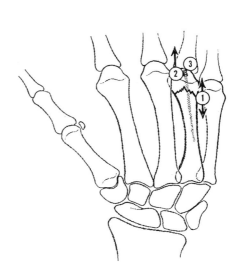

Postreduction X-Ray

1. The backward angulation is corrected.

2. The head of the metacarpal is directed forward.

3. A wire maintains alignment.

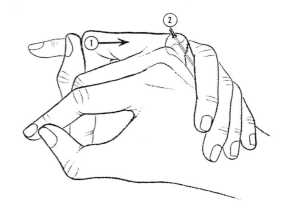

Immobilization

Apply a posterior plaster slab directly to the skin.

1. The cast extends from the lower forearm to the tip of the finger.

2. The metacarpophalangeal joint and interphalangeal joints are slightly flexed.

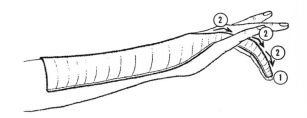

Postreduction Management

Remove the wire and cast at the end of three weeks.

Institute physical therapy and active exercises to restore normal function in the joint of the affected finger.

During the period of immobilization actively exercise the unaffected fingers.

FRACTURES OF THE SHAFTS OF THE PHALANGES

REMARKS

Fractures of the phalanges are the most common lesions of the hand.

The characteristics of fractures of the proximal, middle and distal phalanges differ because the phalanges possess different anatomic arrangements of the tendons which motorize them.

Because of these differences the methods of management of the different phalanges also differ.

Fractures of the phalanges are the result of either direct trauma or of hyperextension injuries—direct trauma usually produces comminuted fractures with little or no displacement whereas hyperextension injuries produce varying degrees of angulation and displacement of the fragments.

In the management of fractures of the phalanges great care must be taken to correct any rotatory displacements of the fragments; failure to observe this rule results in overlapping of the fingers when the fingers are completely flexed as in making a fist.

ANATOMIC CONSIDERATIONS

Fractures of the shaft of the proximal phalanx are characterized by volar angulation of the fragments. Such angulation is due to the action of the extensor and intrinsic muscles which buckle the fragments.

1. Fracture of the middle of the shaft of the proximal phalanx.

2. Pull of the extensor and intrinsic muscles buckle the fragments; the apex of the angular displacement points volarly.

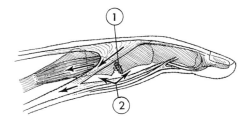

The type of deformity produced by fractures of the middle phalanx depends upon the relationship of the site of the fracture to the insertion of the tendon of the flexor digitorum sublimis.

If the fracture site is proximal to the insertion of the tendon, the action of the extensor slip on the proximal fragment and the action of the flexor digitorum sublimis on the distal fragment produce a dorsal angulation of the fragments.

1. Fracture of the middle phalanx.
2. The cental slip of the extensor tendon extends the proximal fragment.
3. The flexor digitorum sublimis flexes the distal fragment, producing
4. Dorsal angulation of the fragments.

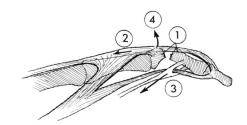

If the fracture site is distal to the insertion of the flexor sublimis tendon, the extensor tendon extends the distal fragment and the flexor digitorum sublimis flexes the proximal fragment, producing a volar angulation of the fragments.

1. Fracture of the middle phalanx distal to the insertion of the flexor digitorum sublimis tendon.
2. The proximal fragment is flexed.
3. The distal fragment is extended, producing
4. Volar angulation of the fragments.

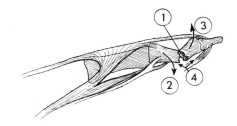

MANAGEMENT OF UNDISPLACED FRACTURES OF THE PROXIMAL PHALANX

REMARKS

These fractures need nothing more than immobilization of the affected finger with the joints of the fingers flexed.

Be sure to correct any rotation of the fragments.

These fractures are usually the result of direct violence.

X-Ray Appearance

1. Comminuted fracture of the proximal phalanx.

2. There is no displacement of the fragments.

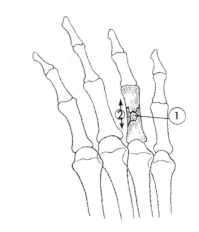

Immobilization

Apply a nonpadded plaster splint from the lower forearm to the base of the nail.

1. The wrist is slightly dorsiflexed.

2. The metacarpophalangeal joint is flexed 45 degrees.

3. The proximal interphalangeal joint is flexed 90 degrees, and the distal interphalangeal joint is flexed 45 degrees.

Note: Never immobilize this fracture with a tongue blade or a straight splint.

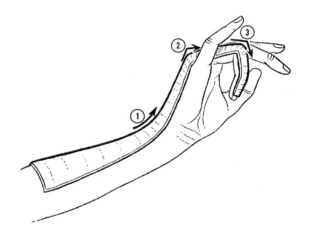

Postimmobilization Management

Remove the splint after three weeks.

Institute physical therapy and exercises to restore motion of the joints of the affected finger; don't stretch the joints passively!

During the period of immobilization allow free use of the unaffected fingers.

MANAGEMENT OF DISPLACED FRACTURES OF THE PROXIMAL PHALANX

REMARKS

These fractures are usually the result of severe hyperextension of the finger; they may be transverse, oblique or spiral fractures.

The apex of the angular deformity points volarly.

Most of these fractures are stable after reduction and can be immobilized with the joints of the finger in flexion.

If the fractures are unstable traction must be employed.

MANAGEMENT OF STABLE FRACTURES OF THE PROXIMAL PHALANX

Prereduction X-Ray

1. Fracture of the proximal phalanx of the fourth finger.

2. Typical anterior angulation at the fracture site.

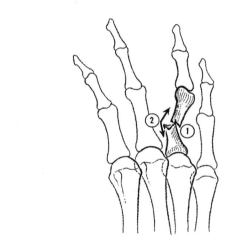

Manipulative Reduction

1. Loop a gauze bandage around the end of the finger and around the operator's hand.

2. Grasp the finger between your thumb and index finger.

3. Make steady traction in the line of the finger.

4. While traction is maintained,

5. Flex the finger over

6. The index finger of the opposite hand which pushes upward at the apex of the angular deformity.

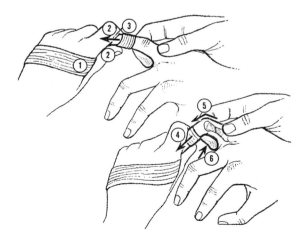

Postreduction X-Ray

1. The fragments of the proximal phalanx are engaged and in normal alignment.

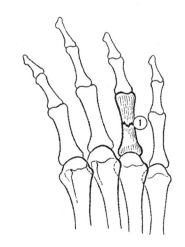

Immobilization

Apply a posterior plaster slab from the lower portion of the forearm to the tip of the finger.

1. The wrist is slightly dorsiflexed.
2. The metacarpophalangeal joint is flexed 45 degrees.
3. The proximal interphalangeal joint is flexed 90 degrees.

Note: Never immobilize this fracture with a tongue blade or a straight splint.

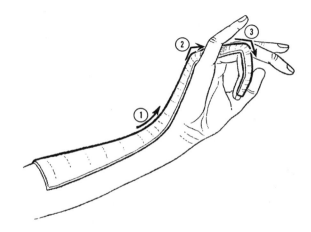

Postreduction Management

Repeat x-rays on the fifth and tenth days; check for position.

During the period of immobilization encourage active exercises of all uninvolved fingers.

Remove the plaster cast at the end of three weeks.

Institute physical therapy and active exercises to restore normal function.

Never employ forced motions or stretching to hasten recovery. These will delay recovery.

MANAGEMENT OF UNSTABLE FRACTURES OF THE PROXIMAL PHALANX

REMARKS

In addition to manual reduction traction is necessary to maintain the anatomic position of the fragments.

Traction should be maintained until healing has progressed sufficiently to stabilize the fragments—usually three weeks. In addition to the volar buckling of the fragments, the fragments may be angulated and rotated; all these aspects of the deformity must be corrected.

Be sure that the center of the nail of the affected finger points to the tubercle of the scaphoid while traction is maintained.

Reduction and Application of Traction

1. First apply a circular plaster cast extending from the lower portion of the forearm to the distal palmar crease anteriorly and to just proximal to the metacarpophalangeal joints dorsally; the thumb is free; the wrist is dorsiflexed.

2. Next, pass a fine threaded wire through the base of the distal phalanx. Now reduce the fracture by the same manipulation technique employed for stable fractures (see page 1106).

3. Pull the finger over a padded aluminum splint previously molded to fit the configuration of the flexed finger; incorporate the splint in the cast.

4. Make traction with rubber bands stretching from the threaded wire traversing the distal phalanx to a wire loop incorporated in the cast.

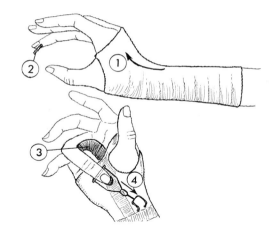

1. The metacarpophalangeal joint is flexed 45 degrees.

2. The proximal interphalangeal joint is flexed 90 degrees.

3. The distal interphalangeal joint is flexed 45 degrees.

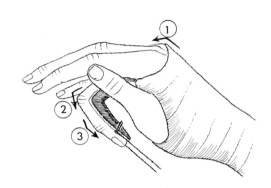

Postreduction Management

Take check x-rays on the fifth and tenth days.

Remove the wire and the cast at the end of three weeks.

During the period of immobilization encourage active use of the uninvolved fingers.

After removal of the cast permit free use of the finger.

Refrain from passive stretchings and forced motions.

The convalescent period is usually protracted.

FRACTURES OF THE DISTAL END OF THE PROXIMAL PHALANX

REMARKS

Two types of fracture occur at this site: (1) the head of the phalanx may be snapped off and displaced volarly; (2) in addition to a fracture through the base, the condyles of the head may be split vertically, producing a T-type fracture. The latter carries a poor prognosis because the congruity of the articular surface is disturbed; therefore it is most essential that anatomic replacement of the condyle is achieved.

MANAGEMENT OF FRACTURE AT THE DISTAL END OF THE PROXIMAL PHALANX

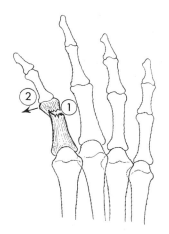

Prereduction X-Ray

1. Fracture through the neck of the distal end of the proximal fragment.

2. The head is displaced volarly.

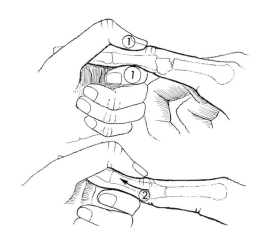

Reduction

1. Grasp the finger distal to the proximal interphalangeal joint.

2. Hyperextend the middle phalanx.

Note: Once reduced this fracture is usually stable.

Postreduction X-Ray

1. The head of the proximal phalanx is in normal alignment with the shaft.

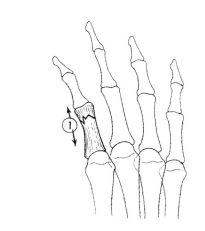

Immobilization

A. Apply a padded aluminum splint extending to the metacarpophalangeal joint.

1. The finger is in extension.

Note: The finger is in extension at both interphalangeal joints.

Don't maintain this position for more than two weeks.

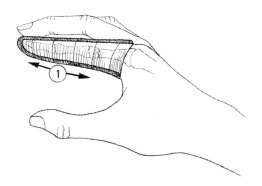

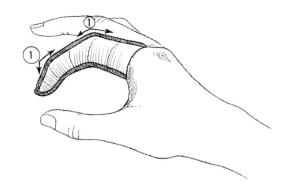

Immobilization *(Continued)*

B. At the end of two weeks apply a padded aluminum splint extending to the metacarpophalangeal joint.

1. The interphalangeal joints are semiflexed.

Postreduction Management

At the end of seven to ten days remove the second splint.

Institute a program of gentle exercises to restore normal motion to the affected finger.

Don't employ passive stretching maneuvers—these will delay recovery.

MANAGEMENT OF "T" FRACTURE OF THE DISTAL END OF THE PROXIMAL PHALANX

REMARKS

The complete congruity of the articular surface must be restored; this is achieved by open reduction.

Failure to restore the fragments to their normal position results in a painful stiff joint with lateral deviation of the middle phalanx.

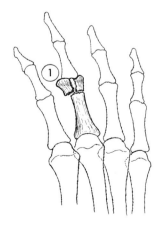

Prereduction X-Ray

1. "T" fracture of the end of the proximal phalanx of the third finger.

Operative Reduction

1. Make a 1½ inch incision over the fracture site.

2. By sharp subperiosteal dissection expose the fracture site.

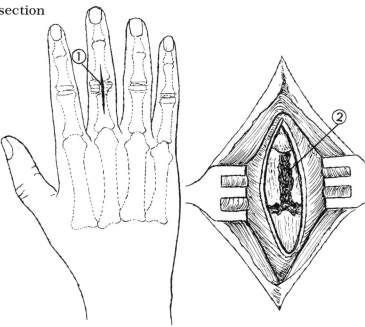

1. With a small curette lever the fragments into normal position.

2. Fix the fragments in the desired position with a towel clip.

3. Transfix the fragments with a fine threaded Kirschner wire.

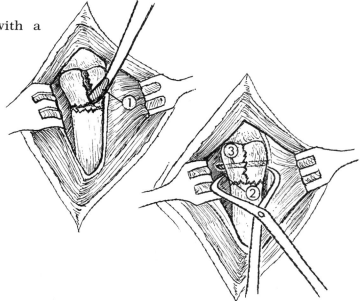

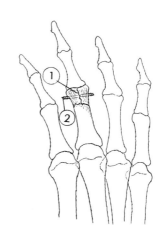

Postreduction X-Ray

1. The fragments are in normal alignment.
2. The fragments are stabilized by a threaded wire.

Immobilization

1. Apply a posterior nonpadded plaster splint over the dorsum of the wrist, hand and finger.
2. All the finger joints are semiflexed.

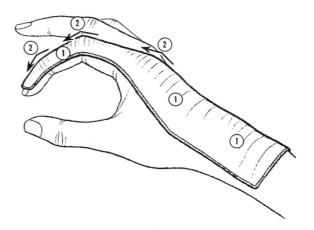

Postreduction Management

Remove the wire at the end of three weeks.

During the period of immobilization actively exercise the unaffected fingers.

After removal of the wire and splint institute a program of gentle exercises to restore normal motion to the affected finger.

FRACTURES OF THE SHAFT OF THE MIDDLE PHALANX

REMARKS

Fractures of the middle phalanx without displacement present no problems in management; however, displaced fractures demand careful study and their management is governed by the types of deformity they present.

As noted previously, the configuration of the deformity of displaced fractures of the middle phalanx is determined by the location of the fracture in relation to the insertion of the flexor digitorum sublimis tendon (see page 1104).

In the management of unstable fractures particular attention must be given to the correction of any rotation of the distal fragment.

Union with residual rotation of the distal fragment produces overlapping of the fingers when a fist is made.

Unstable fractures are usually of the comminuted or spiral variety; in order to achieve and maintain an anatomic reduction, traction must be employed.

MANAGEMENT OF UNDISPLACED FRACTURES AND DISPLACED FRACTURES DISTAL TO THE INSERTION OF THE FLEXOR DIGITORUM SUBLIMIS WHICH ARE STABLE FOLLOWING REDUCTION BY SIMPLE MANUAL TRACTION AND FLEXION OF THE DISTAL FRAGMENT

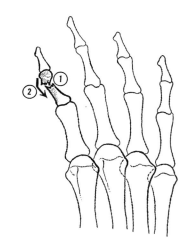

Prereduction X-Ray

1. Fracture of the distal end of the middle phalanx.
2. Typical volar angulation.

Reduction and Immobilization

1. Apply directly to the skin a posterior plaster slab extending from the lower forearm to the tip of the finger.
2. The wrist is slightly dorsiflexed.
3. The metacarpophalangeal joint is slightly flexed.
4. The interphalangeal joints are completely flexed.

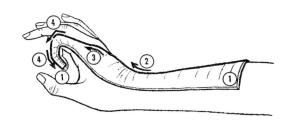

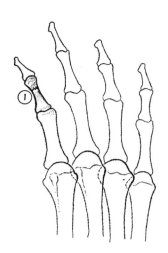

Postreduction X-Ray

1. The fragments of the middle phalanx are in normal alignment.

MANAGEMENT OF FRACTURES PROXIMAL TO THE INSERTION OF THE FLEXOR SUBLIMIS DIGITORUM

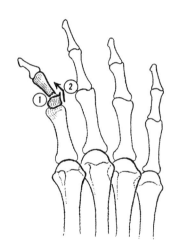

Prereduction X-Ray

1. Fracture of the proximal end of the middle phalanx.
2. Typical dorsal angulation.

Reduction and Immobilization

Apply directly to the skin a posterior plaster slab which extends from the lower portion of the forearm to the tip of the finger.

1. The metacarpophalangeal joint is slightly flexed.
2. The interphalangeal joints are extended.

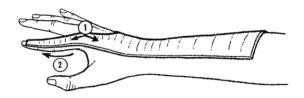

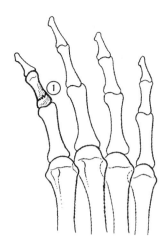

Postreduction X-Ray

1. The fragments of the middle phalanx are in normal alignment.

Postreduction Management

During the period of immobilization actively exercise the uninvolved fingers.

Remove the cast at the end of three weeks.

Allow free use of the finger and encourage active exercises.

Never execute forced motions or passive stretchings of the finger.

MANAGEMENT OF UNSTABLE FRACTURES OF THE MIDDLE PHALANX

REMARKS

These fractures are best managed by traction; the type of traction employed is the same as that described and depicted for unstable fractures of the proximal phalanx (see page 1108).

Fractures of the Distal Phalanx

REMARKS

Comminution of the phalanx with minimal displacement or no displacement of the fragments is the rule.

In children and adolescents the epiphyses of the distal phalanges may be separated. These lesions require reduction.

Occasionally there is wide separation of the fragments. These lesions also require reduction.

Most of these fractures can be reduced and immobilized as depicted here.

Occasionally the fractures are unstable and require internal fixation to maintain the reduction. This is best achieved by transfixing the fragments with a Kirschner wire.

The pulp of the end of the finger is frequently severely traumatized and in some instances lost; if the bone end is exposed, a primary full thickness graft should be applied after adequate débridement and cleansing of the wound.

Appearance on X-Ray

1. Severe comminution of the distal phalanx with minimal displacement of fragments.

Note: This fracture requires no reduction.

2. Fracture of the terminal phalanx with upward, backward and lateral displacement of the distal fragment.

Note: This fracture should be reduced.

3. Epiphyseal separation of the terminal phalanx of the index finger.

Note: This epiphyseal fracture should be reduced.

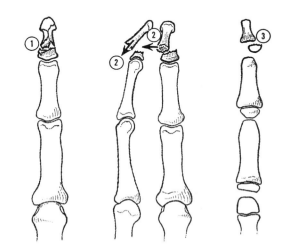

Manipulative Reduction

1. Make traction and mold the fragments by squeezing the end of the finger between your thumb and index finger.

2. Correct the lateral displacement by compressing the lateral borders of the terminal phalanx between your index finger and thumb.

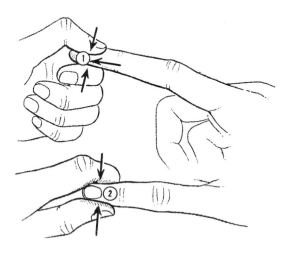

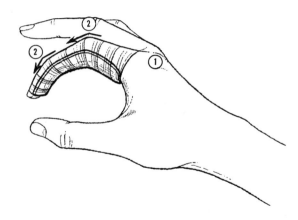

Immobilization

Apply an anterior plaster slab directly to the skin.

1. The metacarpophalangeal joint is free.

2. The interphalangeal joints are slightly flexed.

Postreduction Management

Allow free, active use of the uninvolved fingers. Remove the plaster cast at the end of two weeks. Institute active exercises to restore joint function.

MANAGEMENT OF UNSTABLE FRACTURES OF THE SHAFT OF THE DISTAL PHALANX

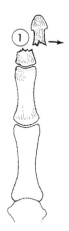

Prereduction X-Ray (I)

1. Fracture of the shaft with lateral displacement of the distal fragment.

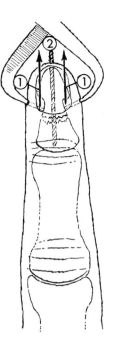

Reduction

1. Grasp the distal fragment with a towel clip and make straight traction — this realigns the fragments.

2. Pass a threaded wire through the distal end of the finger into the proximal fragment.

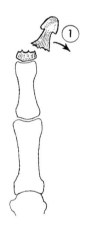

Prereduction X-Ray (II)

1. Fracture through the base of the phalanx with lateral deviation of the distal fragment.

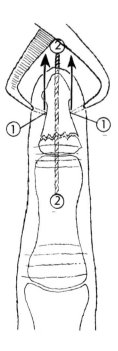

Reduction

1. Grasp the distal fragment with a towel clip and make straight traction.

2. Pass a threaded wire through both fragments, across the distal joint and into the middle phalanx.

Postreduction Management

Apply plaster splints directly to the skin.

1. The metacarpophalangeal joint is free.

2. The interphalangeal joints are slightly flexed.

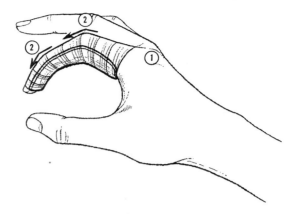

Remove the wire at the end of two weeks and apply plaster splints for one more week.

The total period of immobilization is three weeks.

Institute a program of gentle exercises to restore normal motion to the joints of the affected finger.

AVULSION FRACTURE OF THE DORSAL SURFACE OF THE BASE OF THE DISTAL PHALANX

REMARKS

These are relatively common lesions, especially in athletes; the extensor mechanism pulls off a fragment of bone from the base of the terminal phalanx.

The conventional methods of closed treatment by splinting rarely produce a satisfactory result.

The lesions are best managed by open reduction and internal fixation.

If the avulsed fragment of bone is large it can readily be reduced and fixed to the distal phalanx by a fine Kirschner wire.

If the fragment is small, together with the extensor tendon it should be anchored to the base of the phalanx with a pull-out wire suture passing through the distal phalanx and the end of the finger.

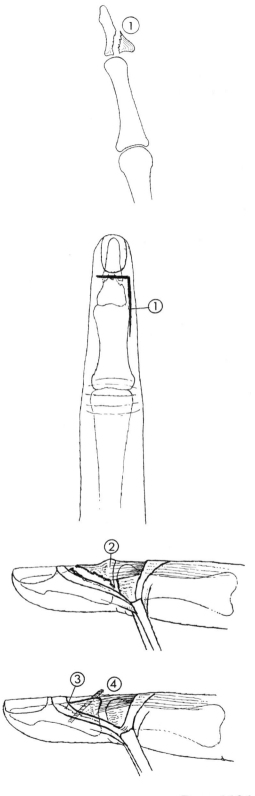

Prereduction X-Ray

1. Large fragment of bone avulsed from the dorsum of the base of the distal phalanx.

Operative Reduction

1. Make an L-shaped incision crossing the dorsum of the finger just distal to the distal interphalangeal joint.

2. Expose the fracture site and identify the loose fragment.

3. Approximate the fragment to the fracture surface of the phalanx.

4. Fix the fragment to the phalanx with a fine threaded Kirschner wire.

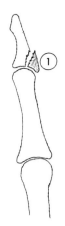

Prereduction X-Ray

1. Small fragment of bone is avulsed from the dorsum of the distal phalanx.

Operative Reduction

Expose the fracture in the same manner as just depicted.

1. Identify the avulsed fragment of bone and the attached extensor tendon.

2. Identify the area on the phalanx from which the bone was avulsed.

3. Through the distal phalanx make two drill channels which enter its tip and emerge at the site from which the bone was avulsed.

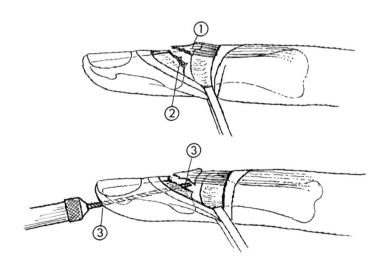

Operative Reduction (Continued)

1. Pass a wire suture through the fragment and the attached tendon; the wire pierces the fragment from the fracture surface, then passes through the tendon transversely and finally again pierces the fragment to emerge on the fracture surface.

2. Pass the wires through the channels in the distal phalanx to emerge at the end of the finger. Pull the fragment snugly against the phalanx and

3. Tie the ends of the wire over a button.

4. Engage the wire passing through the tendon with a second wire whose ends are tied over a button on the dorsum of the finger.

Note: The second wire is looped around the first before the latter is tied. Don't tie the wires over the buttons too tightly less necrosis of the underlying skin ensues.

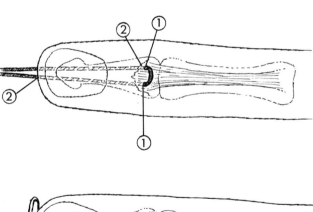

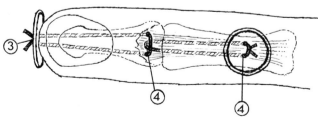

Immobilization

Apply an anterior nonpadded plaster splint.

1. The proximal interphalangeal joint is flexed 90 degrees.

2. The distal interphalangeal joint is hyperextended.

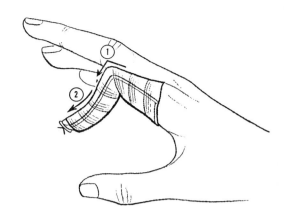

Postoperative Management

During the period of immobilization exercise actively all uninvolved fingers.

In the case of a large fragment which was transfixed with a wire, remove the wire at the end of four weeks.

In the case of a small fragment anchored with a pull-out wire, also remove the wire at the end of four weeks.

Institute a program of active exercises to restore joint function to the involved finger.

DISLOCATIONS OF THE HIP AND FRACTURES OF THE ACETABULUM

ANATOMIC FEATURES AND CLASSIFICATION OF INJURIES

Knowledge of the anatomy of the hip is essential in order to comprehend the tissues involved as the result of the different mechanisms capable of producing fractures and dislocations of the hip.

ANATOMY OF THE HIP JOINT

Anterior Superficial Structures

1. Iliacus.
2. Psoas major.
3. Pectineus.
4. Femoral nerve, artery, vein.
5. Adductor longus.

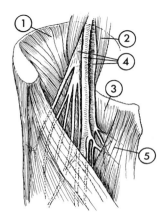

Anterior Deep Structures

1. Iliofemoral (Y) ligament.
2. Rectus femoris.
3. Iliopsoas tendon.
4. Thin or defective portion of the anterior capsule.
5. Obturator externus.
6. Obturator nerve (anterior and posterior divisions).

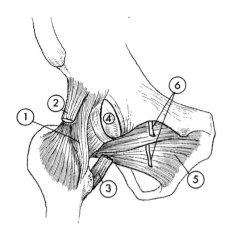

Posterior Superficial Structures

1. Superior gluteal artery.
2. Inferior gluteal artery.
3. Piriformis.
4. Sciatic nerve.
5. Obturator internus and gemelli.
6. Quadratus femoris.

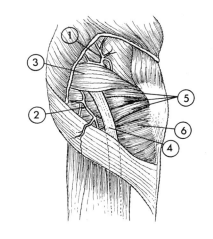

Posterior Deep Structures

1. Piriformis.
2. Gemelli.
3. Obturator internus.
4. Obturator externus.
5. Sciatic nerve.
6. Spiral fibers of posterior capsule.

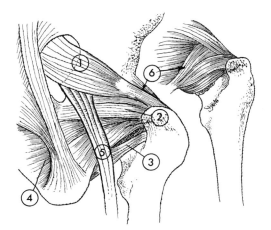

Blood Supply of the Femoral Capital Epiphysis and Neck of the Femur in Childhood

1. Femoral capital epiphysis.
2. Epiphyseal plate—this plate precludes anastomosis of the epiphyseal and metaphyseal vessels.
3. Lateral epiphyseal vessels.
4. Nutrient vessels.
5. Superior metaphyseal vessels.

Note: The blood supply coming through the ligamentum teres at this age is very inadequate and confined to a small segment of the epiphysis.

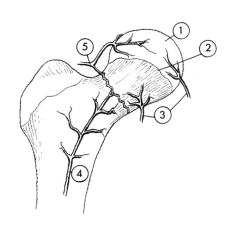

ANATOMY OF THE ACETABULUM

From a functional and surgical point of view the acetabulum consists of three distinct areas which correspond to the three original centers of ossification, the pubis, the ilium and the ischium.

The acetabulum forms the dome of a bony arch made up of an anterior and posterior column of bone. The anterior column consists of a portion of the ilium and of the pubis (iliopubic column) and is directed downward, forward and anteriorly, making an angle of 60 degrees with the posterior column (ilioischial column), which is composed of a portion of the ilium and the vertical segment of the ischium.

The roof of the acetabulum is the dome of the bony arch and is composed of thick, compact iliac bone. The anterior articular surface and the anterior rim of the acetabulum are situated on the posterolateral surface of the anterior column. The posterior articular surface and the posterior rim of the acetabulum are located on the anterolateral surface of the posterior column.

The roof or dome of the acetabulum is strong, compact and voluminous and is the weight-bearing portion of the acetabulum.

The posterior portion of the acetabulum is also thick and strong and is primarily concerned with providing stability to the hip joint.

The anterior portion, comprising the inner wall and the anterior rim of the acetabulum, is relatively thin and may be disrupted by minimal forces as compared to the forces required to fracture the superior or posterior portions of the acetabulum.

The close proximity of the sciatic nerve to the posterior portion of the acetabulum has much clinical significance; it is frequently traumatized by displaced fragments of this portion of the acetabulum.

Bony Composition of the Acetabulum (In Youth)

1. Ilium.
2. Pubis.
3. Ischium.
4. Triradiate synchondrosis.

Note: The three bones meet at the triradiate cartilage in the acetabulum. These three parts roughly correspond to the superior, posterior and anterior segments of the acetabulum which are involved in fractures of the acetabulum.

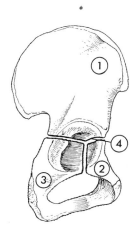

Bony Columns Forming the Acetabulum

1. Ilioischial column (posterior arm of the arch).
2. Iliopubic column (anterior arm of the arch).
3. Roof of the acetabulum (dome of the arch).

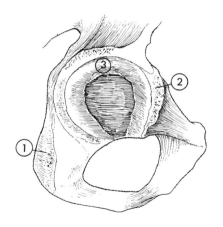

CLASSIFICATION OF TRAUMATIC DISLOCATIONS OF THE HIP AND ACETABULAR FRACTURES

Anterior dislocation.
Posterior dislocation.
Acetabular fractures.
    a. Linear undisplaced acetabular fractures.
    b. Posterior acetabular fracture.
    c. Inner wall fracture.
    d. Superior and bursting fractures.

Note: The above classification of acetabular fractures, evolved by Rowe and Lowell, is by far the simplest and the most practical classification.

REMARKS

Because of the ever increasing number of traffic accidents, the incidence of dislocations and fracture-dislocations of the hip is increasing steadily and rapidly.

The great majority of these lesions are the result of high velocity injuries.

The lesions occur in all age groups, although they are rarely encountered in children under four years.

Frequently the injuries are associated with other severe injuries which in some instances take priority of treatment.

In the presence of other severe injuries the lesions of the hip may be overlooked; this is particularly true when the associated lesion is a fracture of the ipsilateral femur. This complication occurs in 2 to 4 per cent of hip dislocations.

Always take an x-ray of the pelvis of a patient with a fractured femur in order to rule out the presence of dislocation of the hip.

All dislocations must be reduced promptly; these are true emergencies. The longer the head remains out of the acetabulum the higher the incidence of aseptic necrosis of the femoral head. Very few femoral heads survive if they remain dislocated over 24 hours.

Always perform the reduction under general anesthesia; complete muscle relaxation is essential to achieve an atraumatic reduction.

All manipulative maneuvers must be performed with gentleness; don't use great force and leverage to effect a reduction; don't subject the patient to repeated attempts at reduction. These methods inflict greater damage to the soft tissues of the joint, to the vascular supply of the femoral head and to the cartilage of the femoral head.

Failure to achieve reduction of the dislocation by gentle closed methods is an indication for open reduction.

Before reduction always check the motor and sensory functions of the sciatic nerve; the sciatic nerve is injured in 10 to 12 per cent of all dislocations; the deficit in the nerve may be complete or incomplete.

A complete deficit in the nerve from which the patient does not show evidence of recovery after reduction should be explored early.

An incomplete nerve deficit from which the patient does not show evidence of improvement within 10 to 12 weeks should also be explored.

There is no correlation between the time weight bearing is started and the development of aseptic necrosis of the femoral head; however, weight bearing is a factor in the severity of the aseptic necrosis and also the degree of subsequent hip disability. Protection from weight bearing for 12 weeks tends to reduce the severity of the lesion and the disability at the hip.

There is definite correlation between the severity of the original trauma and the incidence of aseptic necrosis of the femoral head.

ANTERIOR DISLOCATIONS OF THE HIP

Anterior dislocation of the hip is not common, occurring in 10 to 12 per cent of all traumatic dislocations of the hip.

The femoral head is forced through the anteroinferior portion of the capsule and it moves either toward the obturator foramen or toward the pubis.

Generally reduction is readily achieved by closed methods, but occasionally open reduction is necessary. In these instances the head may be firmly gripped by the capsule, preventing its reduction, or the head may pierce the iliopsoas muscle which now encircles the head and prevents its reduction.

As a rule, if anterior dislocations are reduced promptly the results are uniformly excellent; however, occasionally aseptic necrosis of the femoral head occurs (8 to 9 per cent). If the femoral head remains outside of the acetabulum for more than 24 hours, aseptic necrosis of the head will develop in most instances.

MECHANISMS OF ANTERIOR DISLOCATION

REMARKS

In anterior dislocation the femoral head may assume one of two positions; it may move toward the obturator foramen or it may move toward the pubis.

Obturator dislocation may be produced by three different forces:

1. With the limb abducted, externally rotated and flexed the force passes from the knee through the femur and drives the head out of the acetabulum.

2. With the limb in the flexed position the force is applied to the inner side of the thigh, forcing the limb into severe abduction and external rotation. In this mechanism the limb is also forced into extension, causing the posterior surface of the neck of the femur to impinge against the acetabulum. The head of the femur is actually levered out of the joint through a rent in the anteroinferior portion of the capsule.

3. With the limb abducted, externally rotated and flexed a force is applied to the posterior aspect of the thigh, driving the head of the femur out of the joint.

1. The limb is abducted, externally rotated and flexed.

2. Force is applied to the back of the thigh.

3. The head of the femur is forced out of the joint.

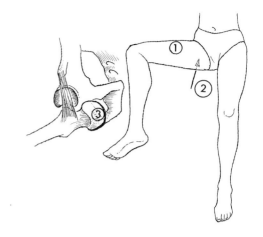

1. The limb is abducted, externally rotated and flexed.

2. Force applied to the inner side of the thigh increases the abduction and extends the limb.

3. The head of the femur is levered out of the joint.

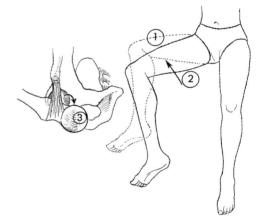

1. The limb is abducted, externally rotated and flexed.

2. Force applied to the knee passes through the femur.

3. The head of the femur is forced out of the joint through a rent in the capsule.

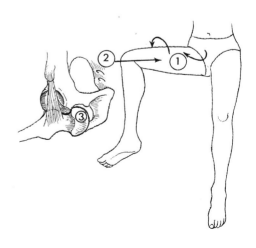

MECHANISM OF PUBIC DISLOCATION

Note: This type of anterior dislocation occurs less frequently than the obturator dislocation and, in some instances, is very difficult to reduce. The dislocating mechanism is severe hyperextension and external rotation, forcing the head of the femur directly forward; the limb is in the neutral position or only slightly abducted.

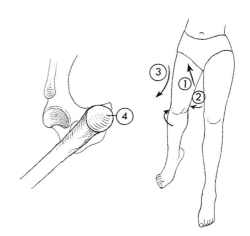

1. The limb is only slightly abducted and externally rotated.
2. Force applied to the front of the thigh forces the limb into
3. Severe hyperextension.
4. The head of the femur is forced out of the joint through a tear in the anterior aspect of the joint capsule.

REDUCTION OF ANTERIOR DISLOCATION

Both obturator and pubic dislocations are reduced by the same manipulative maneuvers.

Some pubic dislocations cannot be reduced by these methods and will offer considerable resistance to flexion of the limb. In these instances employ hyperextension, traction and internal rotation; these maneuvers usually are successful.

Most anterior dislocations can be reduced by closed methods, but occasionally closed methods fail. This is an indication for open reduction (see page 1139).

Typical Deformity (Obturator Dislocation)

1. The hip is slightly flexed.
2. The limb is externally rotated.
3. The thigh is abducted.

Note: In pubic dislocation, there is little or no abduction, the hip is extended and the limb is externally rotated.

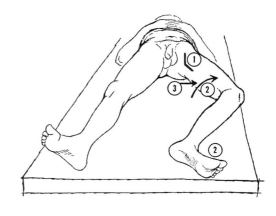

Prereduction X-Ray (Obturator Dislocation)

1. The femoral head rests on the obturator foramen.
2. The femur is widely abducted and
3. Flexed and
4. Externally rotated.

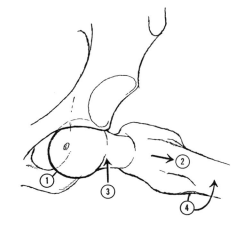

Typical Deformity (Pubic Dislocation)

1. The extremity is in severe external rotation (90 degrees).
2. The extremity is abducted only slightly (15 to 20 degrees) and it is extended.
3. The femoral head can readily be palpated in the inguinal region.

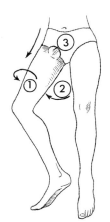

Prereduction X-Ray (Pubic Dislocation)

1. The femoral head lies on the pubic bone, distal, lateral and inferior to the acetabulum.
2. The femur is extended.
3. The femur is externally rotated and
4. Abducted slightly (15 to 20 degrees).

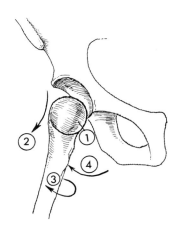

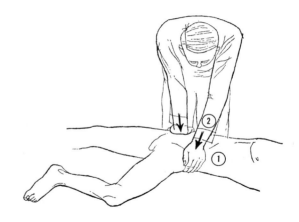

Manipulative Reduction (Always Under General Anesthesia)

1. The patient is placed on the floor in the supine position.

2. An assistant makes downward pressure on the anterosuperior iliac spines.

3. Grasp the affected limb and flex the hip and knee to a right angle.

4. Rotate the limb to a neutral position. (This position converts an anterior to a posterior dislocation.)

5. Make steady traction on the leg directly upward, lifting the head of the femur into the acetabulum.

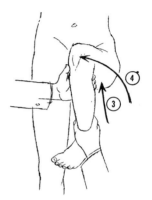

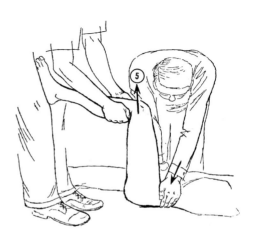

Page 1135

Manipulative Reduction (Always Under General Anesthesia) (Continued)

1. While upward traction is maintained,

2. Lower the thigh to the floor to the extended position.

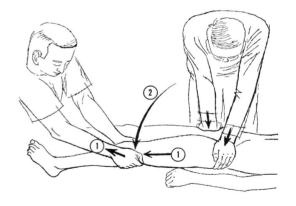

If reduction is not achieved by the depicted maneuvers:

1. Apply traction to the limb in the position of deformity, which is that of flexion and abduction.

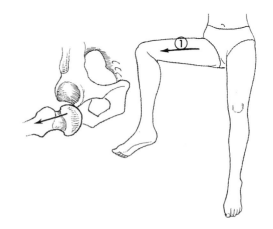

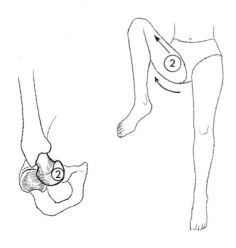

2. While traction is maintained gently bring the limb to a vertical position. This lifts the femoral head onto the anterior rim of the acetabulum.

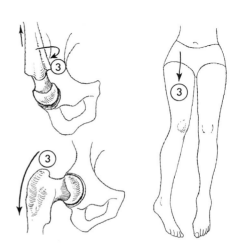

3. While traction is maintained, internally rotate the limb and lower the thigh to the extended position.

Postreduction X-Ray

1. The head of the femur is seated in the acetabulum.
2. The shaft of the femur is in the neutral position.
3. Shenton's line is intact.
4. The lesser trochanter is well visualized.

Note: Check carefully for the presence or absence of any bony fragments within the joint.

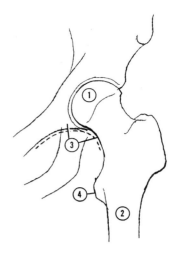

Immobilization

Apply skin traction to the lower leg. The hip is extended and the leg is slightly abducted.

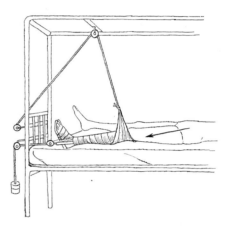

Postreduction Management

Maintain skin traction for three weeks.

During this period institute, within a few days, passive and active motion at the hip joint and muscle-setting exercises.

At the end of three weeks ambulate the patient on crutches without weight bearing on the affected limb.

During this period institute a regulated program of active exercises to restore joint function and develop muscle tone and power.

Permit unprotected weight bearing at the end of 12 weeks.

Light work can be resumed in 14 to 16 weeks and full activity six to ten months after injury.

Follow the patient for at least two years. X-rays should be taken every four to six months; examine the hip carefully at these periodic evaluations and note and record the motions of the hip joint.

Caution: Although rare, aseptic necrosis of the femoral head does occur in 8 to 9 per cent of anterior dislocations.

Page 1137

REDUCTION OF PUBIC DISLOCATION

REMARKS

Occasionally a pubic dislocation cannot be reduced by the maneuvers described to reduce anterior dislocations of the hip.

In these instances the head is forced out of the anterior aspect of the capsule by severe hyperextension and external rotation of the hip joint, and any attempt to flex the hip is met by the firm resistance offered by the posterior capsule which binds the head firmly on the pubis.

This dislocation is readily reduced by first hyperextending the hip, then internally rotating the limb.

Reduction

1. Place the patient on a fracture table.
2. Fasten the unaffected limb to the foot plate.
3. Make longitudinal traction in the line of the deformity.

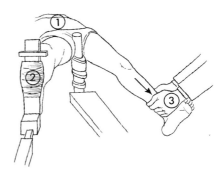

While traction is maintained:
1. Hyperextend the hip and
2. Gently rotate the femur internally and externally to disengage the femoral head; at the same time,
3. An assistant makes direct downward pressure on the femoral head.

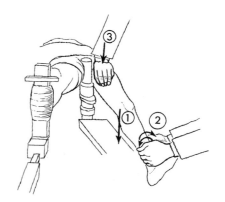

Postreduction Management

This is the same as for uncomplicated anterior dislocation (see page 1137).

Unreducible Anterior Dislocations of the Hip (Fresh Dislocations)

REMARKS

In rare instances, the usual manipulative maneuvers employed to reduce anterior dislocations fail.

The uncomplicated anterior dislocation offers little or no resistance to reduction.

If resistance is met, force must not be used. This is an indication for open reduction.

Failure of reduction may be caused by (1) penetration of the iliopsoas muscle by the femoral head and (2) extrusion of the femoral head through a buttonhole in the anterior capsule.

Operative Reduction

1. Beginning 4 inches from the anterosuperior spine make an incision over the iliac crest, then continue it straight downward on the thigh for 6 inches.

2. Divide the deep fascia over the iliac crest and develop the interval between the tensor fasciae latae and the sartorius muscles.

3. Deepen the incision on the crest to the bone.

4. Reflect by subperiosteal dissection the tensor fasciae latae, gluteus medius and gluteus minimus muscles from the outer surface of the ilium.

5. Identify and ligate the lateral circumflex artery in the interval between the sartorius and the rectus femoris muscles.

6. Identify and divide the two heads of the origin of the rectus femoris muscle and displace the muscle downward.

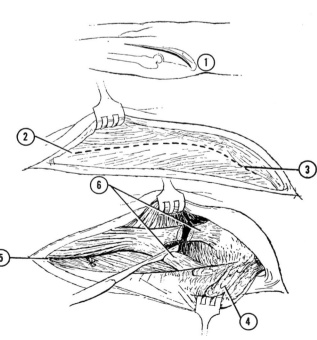

Operative Reduction
(Continued)

When the femoral head has pierced the iliopsoas muscle:

1. Divide one limb of the iliopsoas muscle surrounding the neck of the femur; if necessary enlarge the hole in the capsule surrounding the femoral neck.

2. Make straight longitudinal traction on the limb.

3. While traction is maintained, internally rotate the limb and

4. Make direct pressure on the head to effect a reduction.

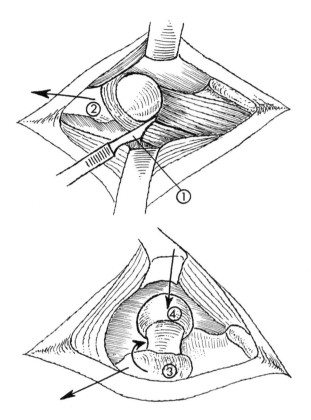

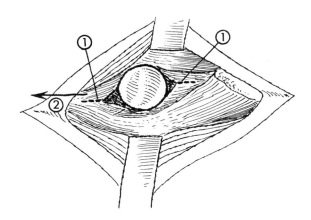

Operative Reduction
(Continued)

When the head has buttonholed the anterior portion of the capsule:

1. Extend the opening in the capsule proximally and distally.

2. Make straight longitudinal traction on the limb.

3. While traction is maintained, internally rotate the limb and

4. Make direct pressure on the head to effect a reduction.

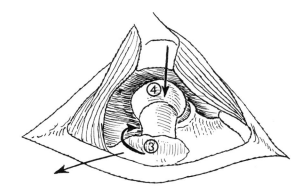

Postoperative Management

This is the same as for uncomplicated anterior dislocation reduced by the closed method (see page 1137).

POSTERIOR DISLOCATIONS OF THE HIP

Posterior Dislocation of the Hip (Uncomplicated)

REMARKS

These lesions are associated with severe soft tissue damage; the patient may be in severe shock.

Always take lateral and oblique views of the hip to determine the presence or absence of a fracture of the posterior rim of the acetabulum; anteroposterior views will show a dislocation but may fail to show a fracture of the posterior rim.

Always check for deficit of the sciatic nerve before and after reduction; the sciatic nerve is involved in 10 to 12 per cent of all dislocations.

Effect reduction as soon as possible; the greater the delay, the more difficult the reduction.

Delay in reduction, even in terms of minutes, may produce severe vascular impairment of the femoral head and also increases the incidence of aseptic necrosis of the head.

Posterior dislocation of the hip may complicate a fracture of the shaft of the femur; always x-ray the hip when there is a fracture of the femur; this complication occurs in 2 to 4 per cent of hip dislocations.

Always check for possible fractures of the lower leg, especially the patella, tibial plateaus and upper end of the shaft of the tibia.

Perform all manipulative maneuvers gently; failure to achieve a reduction by closed methods is an indication for open reduction. Approximately 20 per cent of posterior dislocations require open reduction.

The prognosis should be guarded in all cases because of the possibility of late complications, such as disturbance of the circulation of the femoral head producing aseptic necrosis, traumatic arthritis and myositis ossificans.

MECHANISM OF INJURY

Posterior dislocation of the hip is usually the result of a force driving the femur backward while the thigh is flexed and adducted, such as when the knee strikes the dashboard of an automobile.

The femoral head is thrust through the capsule onto the dorsum of the ilium.

The external rotators of the hip (the piriformis, gemelli and obturator internus) are usually disrupted.

The femoral head may assume a high (iliac) or low (ischiatic) position depending on the degree of flexion of the thigh at the time of the dislocation.

1. Knee strikes the dashboard.
2. The thigh is flexed and adducted.
3. The femoral head is driven backward out of the acetabulum.

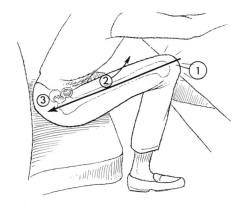

Typical Deformity (Iliac Dislocation)

1. Hip is flexed.
2. Hip is adducted.
3. Hip is internally rotated.
4. Affected extremity appears shortened.
5. Greater trochanter and buttock on affected side are unusually prominent.
6. Knee of the affected extremity rests on the opposite thigh.

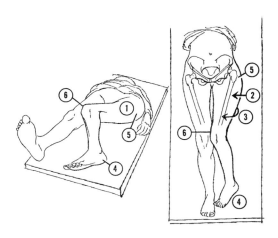

Prereduction X-Ray (Iliac Type)

1. Femoral head is displaced upward and back.
2. Head lies on dorsum of the ilium.
3. Head lies above and posterior to the acetabulum.
4. Femur is adducted and internally rotated.

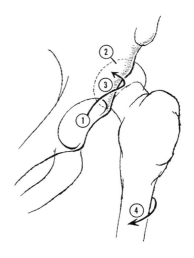

Typical Deformity (Ischiatic Dislocation)

1. The hip is flexed.
2. The hip is markedly adducted so that the knee of the affected limb lies on the opposite thigh.
3. The limb is in extreme internal rotation.
4. The greater trochanter and buttock on the affected side are unusually prominent.

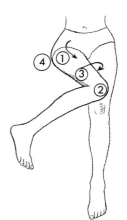

Prereduction X-Ray (Ischiatic Type)

1. The femoral head lies inferior to, lateral to and behind the acetabulum.
2. The lesser tuberosity is not seen.
3. The femoral shaft is in extreme adduction; the findings resemble those of coxa vara.

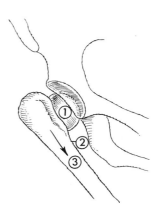

Page 1144

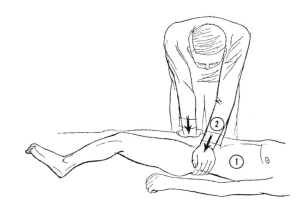

Manipulative Reduction (Under General Anesthesia)

1. The patient lies on the floor in the supine position.

2. An assistant makes downward pressure on the anterosuperior iliac spines.

3. Grasp the affected limb and flex the hip and knee to a right angle.

4. Rotate the limb to the neutral position.

5. Make steady traction on the leg directly upward, lifting the femoral head into the acetabulum.

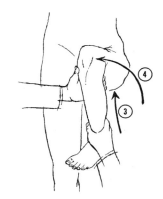

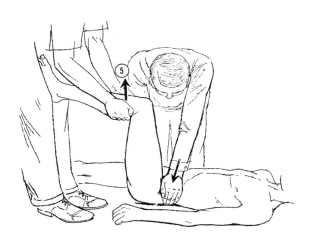

Manipulative Reduction (Under General Anesthesia)
(Continued)

1. While upward traction is maintained
2. Lower the thigh to the floor to the extended position.

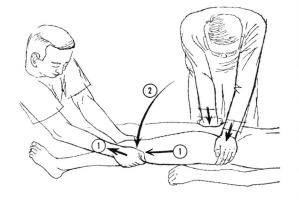

If reduction is not achieved by the preceding maneuvers:

1. An assistant makes downward pressure on the anterosuperior iliac spines.
2. With the knee flexed make traction on the limb in the line of the deformity and

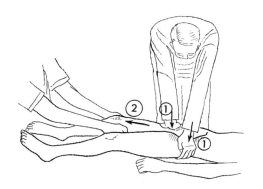

1. Slowly bring the thigh to 90 degrees of flexion.
2. Gently rotate internally and externally and rock the thigh gently backward and forward to disengage the head from the external rotator muscles and posterior capsule.
3. Relocate the femoral head by (a) further internal rotation and extension of the thigh or (b) by external rotation and extension of the thigh.

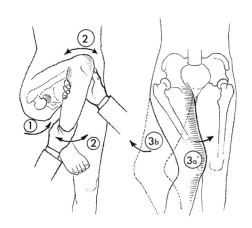

Page 1146

ALTERNATE METHOD (Stimson)

REMARKS

This method utilizes the weight of the limb and gravity to reduce the dislocation.

It is nontraumatic and should be employed more often.

Reduction

1. The patient is placed on a table face downward.

2. The affected thigh hangs directly downward; the knee is flexed at a right angle.

3. An assistant hold the unaffected thigh horizontally.

4. The operator may make steady downward pressure at the flexed knee.

This position is maintained until the muscles relax and the head of the femur drops into the acetabulum. Occasionally slight rocking of the thigh will enhance the reduction.

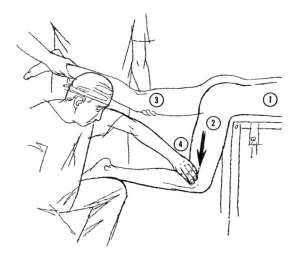

Postreduction X-Ray

1. The head of the femur is in the acetabulum.

2. The shaft of the femur is in a neutral position.

3. Shenton's line is intact.

4. The lesser trochanter is well visualized.

Note: If Shenton's line is broken or the lesser trochanter is not visualized, it means that the head lies behind the acetabulum.

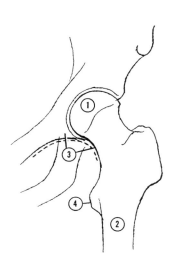

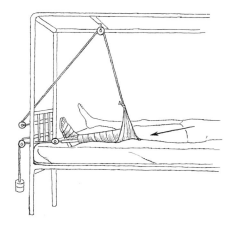

Immobilization

Apply skin traction to the lower leg. The hip is extended and the extremity is slightly abducted.

Postreduction Management

Maintain the traction for three weeks; during this period institute, within a few days after reduction, passive and active motion at the hip joint and muscle-setting exercises.

At the end of three weeks ambulate the patients on crutches without weight bearing on the affected limb.

Institute a regulated regimen of active exercises to restore joint motion and muscle power.

Permit unprotected weight bearing at the end of 12 weeks.

Light work can be resumed in 14 to 16 weeks and full activity 6 to 10 months after injury.

Follow the patient for two years (every three months); at each examination check and record the range of motion in the hip; take x-rays to note any changes in the femoral head and acetabulum.

Unreducible Posterior Dislocations of the Hip (Fresh Dislocations)

REMARKS

Occasionally posterior dislocations without fracture of the posterior rim of the acetabulum or of the femoral head cannot be reduced by closed methods.

In posterior dislocations the femoral head extrudes through the posteroinferior portion of the capsule and may even penetrate the external rotator muscles.

The soft tissues surrounding the femoral neck may prevent relocation of the femoral head; this is particularly true of the edges of the capsule, which may be tightly looped around the neck.

In rare instances the labrum of the acetabulum may be torn from its attachment with or without a fragment of bone by the dislocating femoral head; upon reduction the labrum may be pulled into the joint in front of the head preventing concentric seating of the head in the acetabulum. The torn labrum may simulate a bucket handle tear in a meniscus of the knee joint.

Always suspect soft tissue interposition or loose bodies in the joint following reduction of a posterior dislocation when the femoral head is not concentrically seated in the acetabulum.

These cases are best managed by early open reduction through a posterior approach to the hip joint.

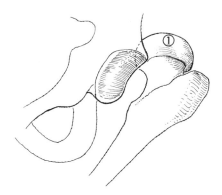

Prereduction X-Ray

1. The femoral head is superior, posterior and lateral to the acetabulum.

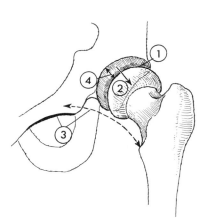

Postreduction X-Ray

1. The femoral head is not concentrically seated.

2. The femoral head is slightly low and laterally in the acetabulum.

3. Shenton's line is broken.

4. The interval between the head and the acetabulum is greater than normal.

Note: These features are indicative of soft tissue lying between the head and the acetabulum.

OPERATIVE REDUCTION

Posterior Exposure of the Hip Joint

The patient is placed in the lateral position.

1. Begin the skin incision 1¾ inches distal and lateral to the posterosuperior iliac spine and extend it laterally and distally parallel with the fibers of the gluteus maximus muscle to the posterosuperior aspect of the greater trochanter. Continue the incision distally in line with the posterior border of the trochanter for 5 inches.

2. Deepen the incision through the gluteus maximus by separating its fibers parallel to the skin incision.

3. Divide the insertion of the gluteus maximus into the fasciae latae for 2 inches in line with the vertical limb of the skin incision.

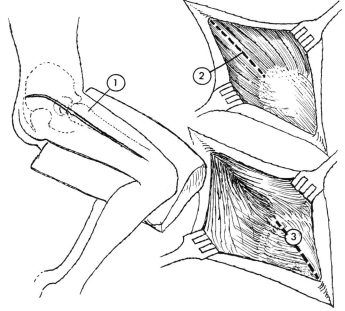

Note: For cases in which the capsule or the external rotators preclude closed reduction:

At this stage of the operation, if the rotator muscles are intact a prominence made by the femoral head can be seen and felt under the muscles; or if the muscles have been penetrated by the femoral head, the head is clearly visible.

Posterior Exposure of the Hip Joint *(Continued)*

1. Visualize the sciatic nerve.

2. Sever the tendons of the piriformis, gemelli and obturator internus at their line of insertion into the greater trochanter.

3. Retract the rotator muscles together with the sciatic nerve posteriorly.

4. Identify the capsule surrounding the femoral neck and, if necessary, enlarge the tear proximally and distally in order to free the neck and head of the femur.

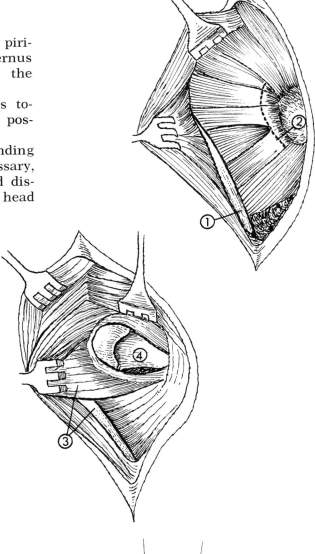

Reduction of the Dislocation

1. Make traction on the thigh along its longitudinal axis with

2. The hip flexed 90 degrees and adducted.

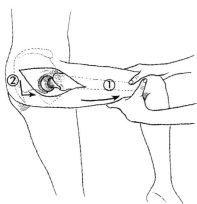

Reduction of the Dislocation
(Continued)

Note: For cases in which concentric reduction is precluded by the labrum being pulled in the acetabulum in front of the head during closed reduction:

1. Flex the hip 90 degrees.
2. Adduct the hip.
3. Dislocate the head posteriorly by internal rotation of the thigh.

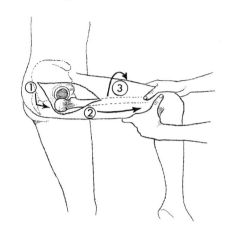

1. Make strong longitudinal traction on the femur.
2. Visualize the cartilaginous labrum inside the acetabulum.
3. Pull the labrum out of the acetabulum with a blunt hook.
4. Excise the detached portion of the labrum.
5. Reduce the femoral head by making longitudinal traction on the flexed and adducted femur.

Note: Before reducing the head inspect the acetabulum carefully for any loose bony fragments; if present remove them.

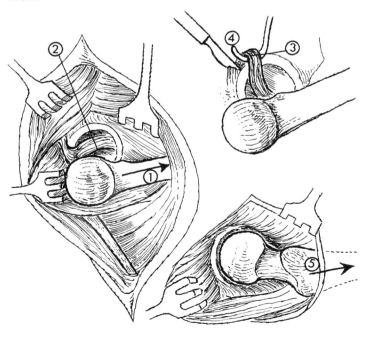

Immobilization

Apply skin traction to the lower leg. The hip is extended and the extremity is slightly abducted.

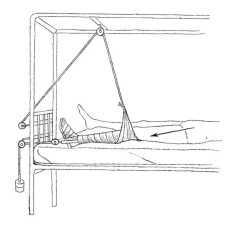

Postreduction Management

Maintain the traction for three weeks; during this period institute, within a few days after reduction, passive and active motion at the hip joint and muscle-setting exercises.

At the end of three weeks permit crutch walking without weight on the affected extremity.

Institute a regulated program of active exercises to restore joint motion and muscle power.

Permit unprotected weight bearing at the end of 12 to 14 weeks.

Return the patient to full activity six to ten months after surgery.

Follow the patient for two years (every three months); at each examination record the arcs of motion of the hip and take x-rays to note the presence or absence of aseptic necrosis of the femoral head.

FRACTURES OF THE
ACETABULUM

REMARKS

The type of fracture of the acetabulum depends upon the direction and intensity of the force passing through the femoral head to the acetabulum.

In general, two types of forces produce these lesions: (1) a force produced by a direct blow to the lateral aspect of the greater trochanter and (2) a force produced by a blow on the anterior aspect of the knee, which travels along the shaft, neck and head of the femur and is expended on the acetabulum.

The portion of the acetabulum affected by the second force depends upon the degree of flexion of the hip and the relative position of adduction or abduction of the femur.

The acetabulum, for clinical purposes, may be divided into three parts: (1) the superior portion or the dome, which is the weight-bearing area of the acetabulum, (2) the posterior portion, which provides stability to the hip and (3) the anterior portion or inner wall.

1. Dome or superior portion of the acetabulum.
2. Posterior portion.
3. Inner wall.

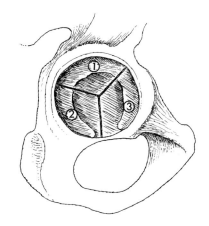

Linear Fractures of the Acetabulum
(Undisplaced Fractures)

REMARKS

This lesion is usually the result of a blow of minimal intensity on the lateral aspect of the greater trochanter.

In general the prognosis is good; rarely encountered are any complications such as aseptic necrosis, traumatic arthritis or myositis ossificans.

Mechanism of Injury

1. Blow on the lateral aspect of the trochanter.
2. Linear undisplaced fractures of the acetabulum.

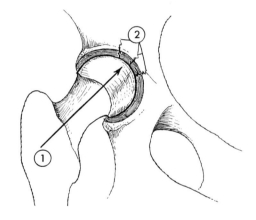

X-Ray

1. The fracture is readily demonstrable by anteroposterior x-rays.

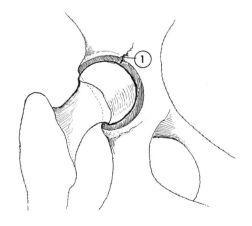

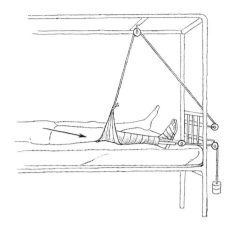

Immobilization

Apply skin traction.
The hip is extended.
Apply 5 to 10 pounds of weight.

Management

Maintain the traction for two to three weeks.

During this period permit active motion of the hip joint and institute a program of muscle-setting exercises.

Permit protected weight bearing with crutches after the third week. (If partial weight bearing produces pain, no weight bearing should be permitted for several more weeks.)

If patient is free of pain, discard the crutches after eight weeks.

Return to full activity after 12 weeks.

Check the patient every four to six months for two years. At these examinations record any limitation of motion in the hip joint and take x-rays to determine any changes in the hip joint.

Rim Fractures of the Acetabulum

REMARKS

Rim fractures usually occur through the posterior portion of the acetabulum.

The size of the fragment depends on the degree of adduction or abduction of the flexed femur when it drives the femoral head backward against the acetabulum. The less the adduction the greater the size of the fragment; if the femur is abducted, the fragment is usually large enough to produce instability of the joint.

Displaced large fragments following closed reduction are an indication for immediate open reduction.

Posterior rim fractures are frequently associated with implication of the sciatic nerve. Complete functional loss of the sciatic nerve is another indication for early exploration. Incomplete functional loss associated with displaced fragments also demands early exploration. The peroneal portion of the sciatic nerve is usually involved.

Displaced small fragments can be disregarded following closed reduction, provided the hip is stable and no evidence of sciatic nerve irritation is demonstrable.

All posterior dislocations must be reduced immediately; after 12 hours without reduction the incidence of aseptic necrosis of the femoral head rises sharply; after 24 hours rarely does a femoral head fail to develop aseptic necrosis.

Anteroposterior roentgenograms may fail to reveal posterior rim fractures; oblique views of the affected hip are mandatory in order to visualize adequately the position of the fragment. These views should be taken before and after reduction.

Always check for fractures of the patella or tibial plateau of the same limb.

The incidence of poor results in these lesions is relatively high (35 to 40 per cent). The poor results are due to instability of the hip, late reductions, and initial injury to the cartilaginous and bony elements of the femoral head.

The single most important factor in the prevention of poor results is early concentric relocation of the femoral head; if bony fragments remain displaced such fragments can be replaced by operation, if necessary later.

Mechanism of Injury

1. The femur is flexed.
2. A force applied to the knee is transmitted to the femoral head via the femur (as in a dashboard injury).
3. Posterior portion of the acetabulum is sheared off.

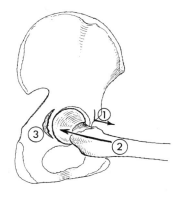

X-Ray (Oblique View)

1. The femoral head is out of the acetabulum and lies posterior.
2. The lesser trochanter is not visible, indicating internal rotation of the femur.
3. Small fragment of the posterior rim is displaced upward and backward.

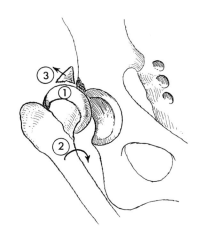

Reduction

Reduce the hip by the same manipulative maneuvers employed for uncomplicated posterior dislocation (see page 1145).

Postreduction X-Ray (Oblique View)

1. The femoral head is concentrically seated in the acetabulum.
2. The posterior fragment is reduced satisfactorily.

Note: The hip is stable after reduction.

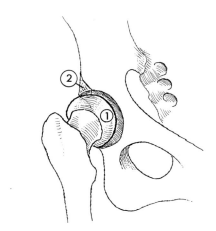

Immobilization

Apply skin traction to the leg in balanced suspension (Russell traction).

1. The extremity is in balanced suspension but with minimal flexion.
2. Apply 10 to 15 pounds of weight for traction.

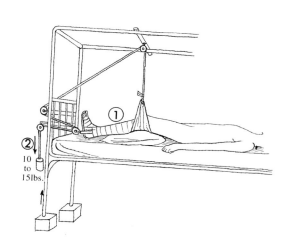

Postreduction Management (For Stable Hip with a Small Posterior Rim Fracture)

Maintain traction for six weeks.

During this period permit active motion at the hip and knee, permitting only minimal flexion at the hip. (This favors adequate nourishment to the cartilage of the femoral head and acetabulum.)

Institute a program of muscle-setting exercises for the quadriceps muscle.

At the end of six weeks permit crutch walking without weight bearing on the affected hip, but encourage motion in the hip and active exercises of all muscle groups.

Permit unprotected weight bearing at the end of 12 weeks.

Return patient to full activity six to ten months after injury.

Follow the patient for two years (every three months); at each examination check and record the range of motion in the hip and take x-rays to determine the presence or absence of aseptic necrosis of the femoral head or degenerative arthritis of the hip.

OPERATIVE REDUCTION OR EXPLORATION

REMARKS

Operative intervention is indicated for the following reasons:

Instability of the hip following closed reduction.

Displaced large fragments demonstrated on oblique x-ray views.

Clinical evidence of a complete deficit of the sciatic nerve.

A partial sciatic nerve deficit which is increasing or from which the patient does not show evidence of recovery.

The presence of loose fragments within the joint after closed reduction.

Prereduction X-Ray

1. Posterior dislocation of the femoral head.

2. Large acetabular fragment tilted outward.

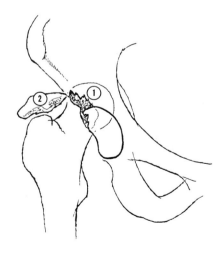

Postreduction X-Ray

1. Dislocation of the femoral head is reduced.

2. The acetabular fragment is still displaced; it is tilted outward and upward.

Note: This fragment can be replaced only by operative intervention.

Operative Technique

Posterior exposure of the hip joint:

1. Make a vertical incision on the lateral aspect of the thigh beginning 5 inches below the tip of the greater trochanter, then extend the incision posteriorly for 5 inches more along the anterior margin of the gluteus maximus muscle.

2. Deepen the incision through the deep fascia.

1. Divide the gluteus maximus along its line of insertion into the fascia lata and displace the muscle mass posteriorly.

2. Visualize the sciatic nerve and examine it for any injury.

3. Divide the tendons of the piriformis, superior gemellus, internal obturator and inferior gemellus muscles.

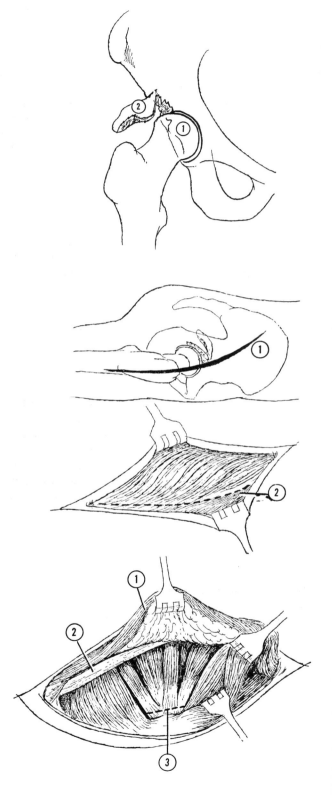

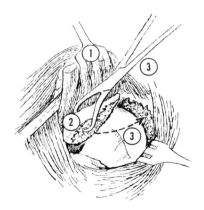

Operative Technique
(Continued)

1. Retract the detached external rotators of the hip joint and the sciatic nerve posteriorly.

2. Locate the detached acetabular fragment.

3. Grasp the acetabular fragment with a towel clip and pull it down into its anatomic position.

4. Fix the fragment in place with one or two screws.

Note: Small bony fragments are discarded.

Inspect the femoral head for any evidence of cartilaginous or osseous damage.

Make sure that the head is concentrically reduced; if not, inspect the inside of the joint for loose bony fragments.

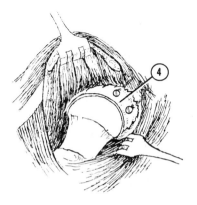

Postreduction X-Rays

1. The dislocation is reduced.
2. The fragment is fixed by two screws.

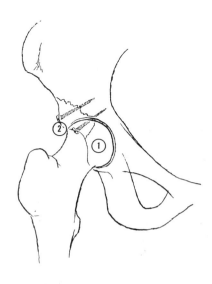

Immobilization

Apply skin traction to the leg in balanced suspension.

1. The extremity is in balanced suspension, but with minimal flexion.

2. Apply 10 to 15 pounds of weight for traction.

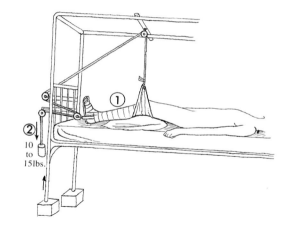

Maintain traction for six weeks.

During this period permit active motion at the hip and knee, permitting only minimal flexion at the hip.

Institute a program of muscle-setting exercises for the quadriceps muscle.

Start crutch walking at the end of six weeks but without weight bearing on the affected limb; encourage motion in the hip and active exercises of all muscle groups.

Permit unprotected weight bearing at the end of 12 to 14 weeks.

Return the patient to light activity six to eight months after injury and to full activity in 10 to 12 months.

Follow the patient for two years (every three months); at each examination check and record the range of motion in the hip and take x-rays to determine the presence or absence of aseptic necrosis of the femoral head or degenerative arthritis of the hip.

Superior and Bursting Fractures of the Acetabulum

REMARKS

These lesions are produced by severe violence; there may be total disruption of the acetabulum.

In uncomplicated fractures of the superior portion of the acetabulum the disrupting force is directed upward; in bursting fractures, which are explosive in nature, the disrupting force is directed upward and inward.

These lesions are responsible for the highest incidence of poor results in all acetabular fractures (45 to 50 per cent of these injuries result in poorly functioning hips).

In general, the end result in simple fractures of the superior portion of the acetabulum is good, provided healing occurs with the fragment in its anatomic position and the relationship of the dome of the acetabulum to the femoral head is a normal one.

Failure to reduce anatomically a large fragment or to reassemble multiple fragments so that the articular surfaces of the femoral head and the dome are congruous invariably is followed by a poor result.

Routine x-rays often fail to reveal the nature and the extent of displacement of the fragments in these lesions; oblique views of the affected hip must be taken in order to visualize the true relationship of the displaced fragments and the acetabulum.

In bursting fractures the two most important factors determining the fate of the hip joint are: (1) the relationship of the dome with the weight-bearing surface of the femoral head (if this relationship is anatomically correct and the articular surfaces are congruous, a good result can be anticipated; if not, a poor result is inevitable); (2) an intact superior acetabular dome (the relationship of the fragments comprising the rest of the acetabulum has no bearing on the end result).

Injury to the sciatic nerve in these lesions is a relatively common finding; it occurs in 20 to 25 per cent of the cases.

If open reduction is done, always inspect the sciatic nerve; it may be contused by bony fragments; it may be compressed by fragments; it may be lacerated or even severed.

The clinical results do not always parallel the anatomic results; not infrequently patients with poor anatomic or roentgenographic results have good functional results.

Always follow these patients for at least two years; in general, the fate of the hip is determined in one year; few hips develop changes in the femoral head and acetabulum which are not already evident at the end of the first year.

In view of the fact that many disrupted hips are capable of good function regardless of the anatomic and roentgenographic evaluation, primary arthrodesis or arthroplasty is rarely indicated. These measures should be reserved for failures following conservative treatment.

Injuries to the femoral head associated with these lesions signify a poor prognosis.

Mechanism of Injury

For fractures of the dome of the acetabulum (as an isolated lesion):

1. The femur is almost completely extended.

2. Force is transmitted directly upward onto the dome of the acetabulum.

3. A large fragment of the dome is sheared off and displaced upward and slightly backward.

4. The femoral head is dislocated upward.

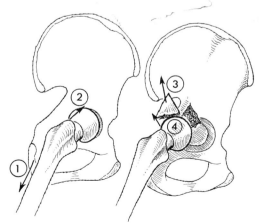

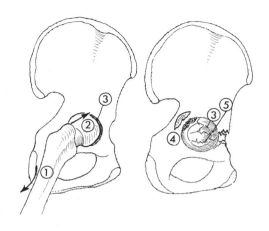

For superior and bursting fractures of the acetabulum (the dome is preserved):

1. Femur is almost completely extended and slightly abducted.

2. Force is transmitted upward and inward onto the acetabulum.

3. The superior dome is intact.

4. Fracture of the posterior portion of the acetabulum.

5. Fracture of the inner wall.

or

1. The dome is comminuted.

2. The inner wall is disrupted.

3. The femoral head is displaced inward.

or

1. The dome is comminuted.

2. The inner wall is markedly disrupted.

3. The femoral head is displaced inward.

4. Fracture of the superior and inferior pubic rami.

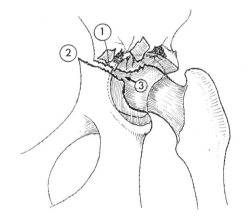

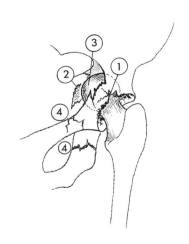

MANAGEMENT OF SUPERIOR DOME AND BURSTING FRACTURES OF THE ACETABULUM (WHEN THE SUPERIOR DOME AND THE FEMORAL HEAD ARE IN NORMAL RELATIONSHIP)

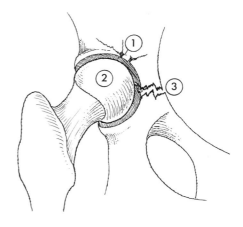

X-Ray — First Example

1. Fracture of the superior dome without displacement.

2. Femoral head is in normal relationship with articular surface of the dome.

3. Fracture of the inner wall.

or

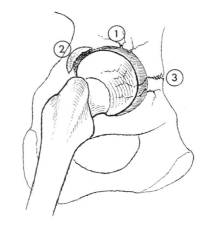

X-Ray — Second Example

1. Fracture of the superior dome without displacement.

2. Fracture of posterior rim in acceptable position.

3. Fracture of inner wall.

Reduction

These fractures need no reduction.

Immobilization

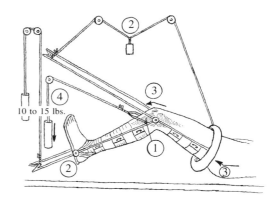

Apply skeletal traction:

1. Insert a threaded wire immediately below the tibial tubercle.

2. Place the limb in a Thomas splint with a Pearson attachment balanced from an overhead frame.

3. Hip and knee are slightly flexed.

4. Apply 10 to 15 pounds of weight.

10 to 15 lbs.

Page 1165

Immobilization (Continued)

Maintain the traction for six weeks.

During this period permit active gentle exercises of the hip and knee and muscle-setting exercises for the quadriceps muscle.

After six weeks permit crutch walking without weight bearing on the affected limb.

After 12 to 16 weeks, depending on the severity of the bone injury, permit unprotected weight bearing on the affected extremity.

Return the patient to light activity in six to eight months and full activity 10 to 12 months after injury.

Follow the patient for two years (every three months); at each examination record the range of motion in the hip and take x-rays to determine the presence or absence of aseptic necrosis in the femoral head or other degenerative changes in the hip.

MANAGEMENT OF SUPERIOR DOME AND BURSTING FRACTURES OF THE ACETABULUM (WHEN THE SUPERIOR DOME IS DISPLACED OR COMMINUTED)

REMARKS

Closed manipulative maneuvers rarely restore a displaced acetabular dome to its anatomic position. It is most essential that the normal relationship between the femoral head and the dome be restored.

The degree of comminution and the extent of displacement of the fragments of the dome cannot be determined by x-ray examination. Replacement of the fragments and restoration of congruity between the articular surface of the acetabulum and the femoral head must be achieved in order to attain a good functioning hip joint.

These lesions should be treated by open reduction.

If the femoral head is dislocated superoposteriorly it is most essential to relocate the head immediately. This is accomplished by the closed methods described for simple posterior dislocations of the hip (see page 1145). Open reduction of the dome can be performed later (five to ten days later if necessary).

Inward displacement of the femoral head must also be reduced immediately, although reduction of this lesion is not as urgent as when the head is outside the acetabulum.

Page 1166

Prereduction X-Ray (Oblique View)

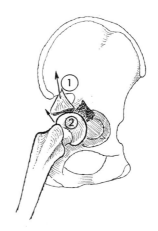

1. Large fragment of the dome is displaced upward and backward.

2. The femoral head is dislocated upward and slightly backward.

Note: Following closed reduction the head is relocated but the fragment remains displaced.

Postreduction X-Ray

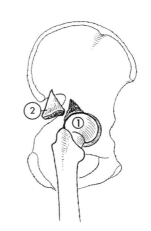

1. The femoral head is reduced.

2. The superior acetabular fragment remains displaced.

Prereduction X-Ray (Oblique View)

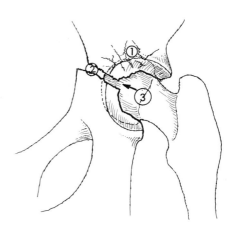

1. The dome is comminuted.
2. The inner wall is disrupted.
3. The femoral head is displaced inward.

OPERATIVE MANAGEMENT

The patient is in the lateral position.

Posterior Exposure of the Hip Joint

1. Begin the skin incision 1¾ inches distal and lateral to the posterosuperior iliac spine and extend it laterally and distally, parallel to the fibers of the gluteus maximus muscle, to the posterosuperior aspect of the greater trochanter. Continue the incision distally for 5 inches in line with the posterior border of the trochanter.

2. Deepen the incision through the gluteus maximus muscle by separating its fibers parallel to the skin incision.

3. Divide the insertion of the gluteus maximus into the fascia lata for 2 inches in line with the vertical limb of the skin incision.

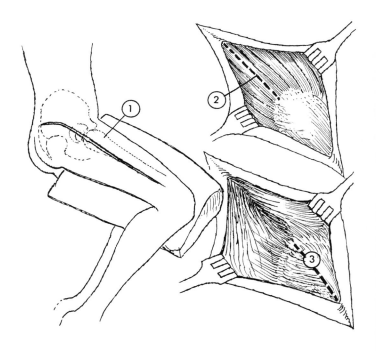

Posterior Exposure of the Hip Joint (*Continued*)

1. Visualize the sciatic nerve.

2. Sever the tendons of the piriformis, gemelli and obturator internus at their site of insertion into the greater trochanter.

3. Retract the rotator muscles together with the sciatic nerve posteriorly. This brings into view:

4. The femoral head.

5. Disrupted capsule.

6. Detached fragment of the dome.

7. Raw surface of the superior portion of the acetabulum.

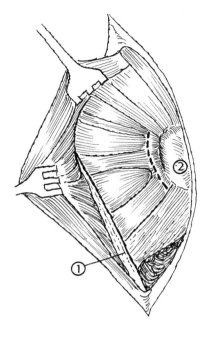

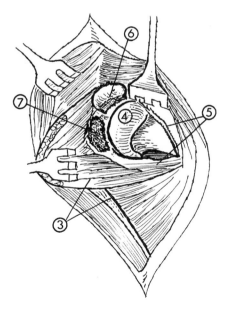

Posterior Exposure of the Hip Joint (*Continued*)

1. Insert a flat blade retractor into the pelvis opposite the acetabulum between the greater sciatic notch and the ischial spine.

2. By subperiosteal dissection reflect the gluteus minimus muscle superiorly. This brings into view:

3. Superior and posterior portions of the acetabulum.

Note: Beyond this stage of the operation the technique depends upon the pathologic condition found.

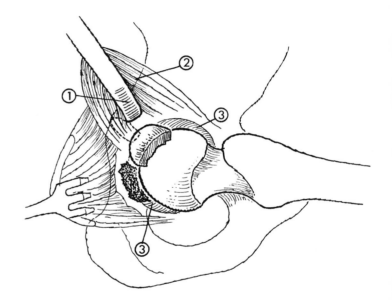

Posterior Exposure of the Hip Joint (Continued)

When the lesion comprises a large single bony fragment:

Clean the raw surfaces of the detached fragment and the acetabulum of any debris.

1. Replace the fragment in its anatomic position.

2. Fix it to the ilium with one or two screws.

3. Direct the screws obliquely upward to engage the thick portion of the ilium.

Note: Flush out the wound thoroughly before closing the capsule.

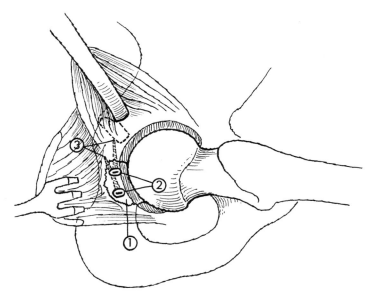

Posterior Exposure of the Hip Joint (Continued)

When the displaced dome comprises several fragments:

1. If there is some inward displacement of the head, make traction on the femur downward and laterally. (The head must be concentrically reduced.)

2. Reassemble the large fragments. (Small loose fragments can be discarded; large fragments must be replaced.)

3. Fix them in the anatomic position to the ilium with screws. (Inspect the femoral head. Remove all small fragments of bone and cartilage which lie in the joint and might interfere with accurate reduction.)

Note: Flush out the wound before repairing and closing the capsule.

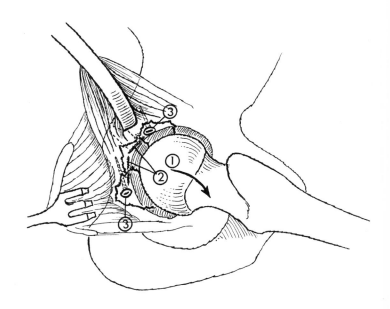

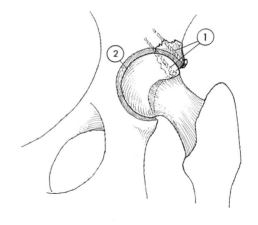

Postreduction X-Rays

1. The large acetabular fragment is reduced and fixed with two screws.

2. The head and roof of the acetabulum are congruous.

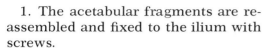

1. The acetabular fragments are re-assembled and fixed to the ilium with screws.

2. The femoral head and roof of the acetabulum are in normal relationship.

3. The fracture of the inner wall is not completely reduced; this is of no significance.

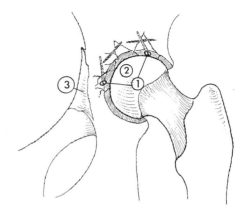

Immobilization

Apply skeletal traction:

1. Insert a threaded wire immediately below the tibial tubercle.

2. Place the limb in a Thomas splint with a Pearson's attachment balanced from an overhead frame.

3. The hip and knee are slightly flexed.

4. Apply 20 to 25 pounds of weight.

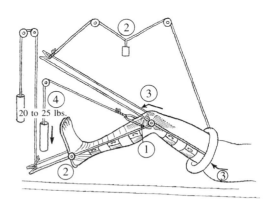

Page 1173

Begin quadriceps setting exercises immediately but do not allow motion at the hip for three weeks.

At the end of three weeks begin knee and hip motion.

Maintain skeletal traction for 10 to 12 weeks.

After 10 to 12 weeks permit crutch walking with partial weight bearing on the affected extremity.

After 16 to 20 weeks (depending on the severity of the bone injury) permit unprotected weight bearing on the affected limb.

Return the patient to light activity in six to eight months.

Return the patient to full activity in 10 to 12 months after injury.

Follow the patient for two years (every three months); at each examination record the range of motion in the hip and take x-rays to ascertain the presence or absence of aseptic necrosis of the femoral head or other degenerative abnormalities in the hip.

MANAGEMENT OF FRACTURES WITH MARKED DISRUPTION OF THE ENTIRE ACETABULUM AND INTRAPELVIC DISPLACEMENT OF THE HEAD

These are very unstable fractures; closed reduction rarely restores the fragments of the dome to their normal position.

However, a closed reduction should be attempted; if this fails, open reduction is indicated to reassemble the dome.

These fractures, because of their instability, require skeletal traction both in the longitudinal and lateral directions, either to maintain the reduction (after closed or open reduction) or to achieve reduction if the initial closed attempt was unsuccessful.

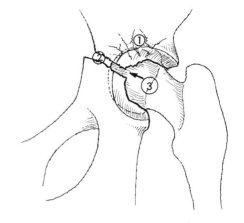

Prereduction X-Ray

1. Fracture of the dome with some comminution.

2. Disruption of the inner wall.

3. Intrapelvic displacement of the femoral head.

Closed Reduction

1. Place the patient on a fracture table.

2. Fasten the unaffected foot to a foot plate.

3. Make longitudinal traction on the limb.

4. Make lateral traction on the upper end of the thigh.

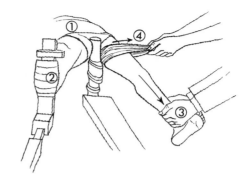

Postreduction X-Ray

1. Femoral head is not in normal relation to the dome.

2. The dome is fragmented; some of the fragments are displaced.

3. The fragments of the inner wall are not completely reduced. (This is of no significance.)

Note: This patient requires open reduction to reassemble the acetabular dome.

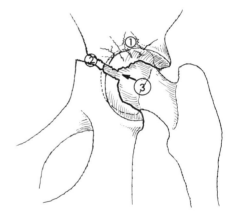

Technique of open reduction is described on page 1168.

Following open reduction apply skeletal traction to the limb in the longitudinal and lateral directions to maintain the reduction.

Application of Skeletal Traction

1. Insert a threaded wire immediately below the tibial tubercle.

2. Insert a second threaded wire through the greater trochanter in an anteroposterior plane.

3. Apply a Thomas splint without a perineal ring but with a Pearson attachment.

4. Apply 25 to 40 pounds of traction in a longitudinal direction (depending on the size of the patient and the severity of bony disruption of the acetabulum) to the wire in the tibia, and

5. Apply 10 to 15 pounds of lateral traction in the line of the femoral neck to the wire through the trochanter.

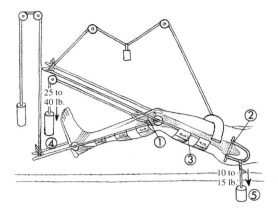

Note: Check by x-ray every 24 hours the position of the fragments and the relation of the femoral head to the dome.

If reduction is maintained:

After 10 to 12 days reduce the longitudinal traction to 10 to 15 pounds but don't disturb the lateral traction.

After three weeks discontinue the lateral traction but maintain the longitudinal traction.

During this period institute quadriceps setting exercises but no hip motion.

After three weeks institute gentle active motion at the hip and knee and continue the quadriceps exercises.

Maintain skeletal traction for 10 to 12 weeks or until there is definite roentgenographic evidence of solid bony union of the acetabular fractures.

After 10 to 12 weeks permit crutch walking with partial weight bearing on the affected hip.

After 16 to 20 weeks (depending on the severity of the bony injury) permit unprotected weight bearing on the affected limb.

Return the patient to light activity in six to eight months and to full activity 10 to 12 months after injury.

Follow the patient for two years (every three months); at each examination record the range of motion in the hip and take x-rays to ascertain the presence or absence of aseptic necrosis of the femoral head or other degenerative abnormalities in the hip.

MANAGEMENT OF STABLE INNER WALL FRACTURES WITHOUT DISPLACEMENT OF THE FEMORAL HEAD

REMARKS

These lesions comprise the largest group of all fractures of the acetabulum.

Because the inner acetabular wall is thin, minimal violence to the lateral aspect of the trochanter is capable of producing displaced fractures.

The femoral head may protrude into the pelvis for varying distances depending upon the intensity of the driving force.

Generally the superior dome of the acetabulum remains intact.

In 40 to 50 per cent of these lesions there are concomitant fractures of the pubic rami and in approximately 15 per cent the sciatic nerve is injured.

Routine x-rays readily demonstrate the fractures.

These fractures are readily treated by closed methods; rarely is operative intervention indicated.

The most important factor in achieving a satisfactory reduction is restoration of the femoral head to its normal relation with the dome of the acetabulum; whether or not the fragments of the inner wall are reduced is of no significance in determining the ultimate success of the treatment of the hip.

All these lesions should be reduced as soon as the patient's condition permits; however, in these lesions the interval of time between the injury and the reduction is less significant than in posterior or anterior dislocations of the hip, in which a matter of minutes may make a difference in the ultimate fate of the femoral head.

Prereduction X-Ray

1. Fracture of the inner wall with minimal displacement.

2. Superior dome of the acetabulum is intact.

3. Femoral head and dome are in normal relationship.

Note: This fracture needs no manipulative reduction.

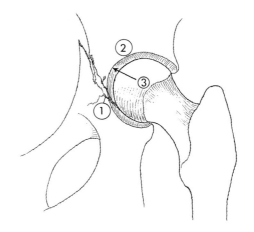

Immobilization

Apply skin traction to the leg in balanced suspension.

1. The extremity is in balanced suspension.
2. Apply 10 to 15 pounds of traction.

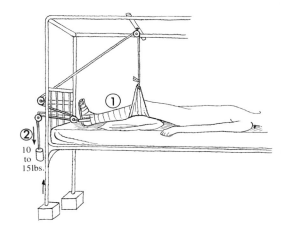

Maintain the traction for eight to ten weeks.

During this period permit active motion at the hip and knee.

Encourage the performing of quadriceps setting exercises.

At the end of eight to ten weeks permit crutch walking without weight bearing on the affected hip.

Permit unprotected weight bearing at the end of 12 weeks.

Return the patient to light activity at the end of four to six months and to full activity at the end of six to eight months.

MANAGEMENT OF INNER WALL FRACTURES WITH MILD OR MODERATE INTRAPELVIC DISPLACEMENT OF THE FEMORAL HEAD

Prereduction X-Ray

1. Fracture of the inner wall with inward displacement.
2. Fracture of the pubic rami.
3. Femoral head is displaced inward.
4. Acetabular dome is intact.

Note: This fracture must be reduced so that the femoral head and the acetabular dome are in normal relationship.

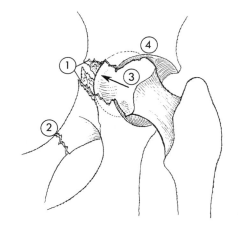

Manipulative Reduction

1. Place the patient on the fracture table.
2. Fasten the unaffected limb to a foot plate.
3. Make longitudinal traction on the limb.
4. Make lateral traction on the upper end of the thigh.

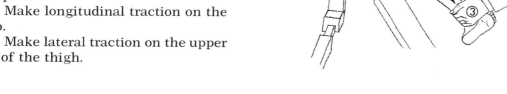

Postreduction X-Ray

1. Displacement of the inner wall is markedly reduced but not completely.
2. The femoral head is seated under the dome in its normal position.

Note: This reduction must be maintained by skeletal traction.

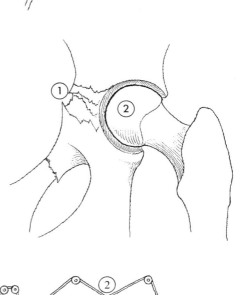

Immobilization

Apply skeletal traction:
1. Insert a threaded wire immediately below the tibial tubercle.
2. Place the limb in a Thomas splint (with a Pearson attachment) balanced from an overhead frame.
3. The hip and knee are slightly flexed.
4. Apply 20 to 25 pounds of weight.

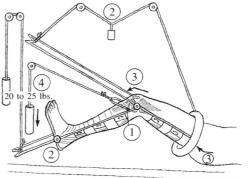

Begin quadriceps setting exercises immediately but do not allow motion at the hip for three weeks.

At the end of three weeks begin gentle hip and knee motion.

Maintain the skeletal traction for eight to ten weeks.

After eight to ten weeks permit crutch walking without weight bearing on the affected limb.

Permit full weight bearing after 12 weeks.

Return the patient to light activity in four to six months and to full activity in six to eight months.

MANAGEMENT OF UNSTABLE FRACTURES OF THE INNER WALL WITH MARKED INTRAPELVIC PROTRUSION OF THE FEMORAL HEAD

Prereduction X-Ray

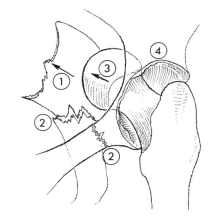

1. Fracture of the inner wall with severe inward displacement.
2. Fracture of both pubic rami.
3. Severe intrapelvic protrusion of the femoral head.
4. The acetabular dome in intact.

Note: This unstable fracture must be reduced and reduction then maintained by longitudinal and lateral traction.

Manipulative Reduction

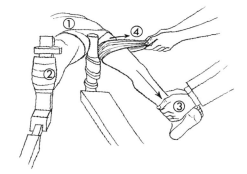

1. Place the patient on the fracture table.
2. Fasten the unaffected limb to the foot plate.
3. Make strong longitudinal traction on the extremity, and at the same time,
4. Make strong lateral traction on the upper end of the thigh.

Postreduction X-Ray

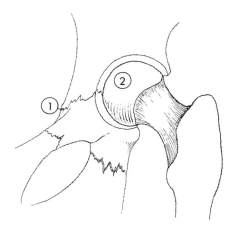

1. The displacement of the inner wall is almost completely reduced.
2. The femoral head is in normal relationship to the acetabular dome.

Immobilization

Apply skeletal traction.

1. Insert a threaded wire below the tibial tubercle.

2. Insert a second threaded wire through the greater trochanter in the vertical plane.

3. Apply a Thomas splint without a perineal ring but with a Pearson attachment.

4. Apply 25 to 40 pounds of traction to the leg, and

5. Apply 10 to 15 pounds to the trochanter.

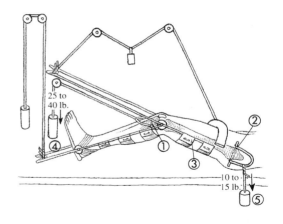

After 10 to 12 days reduce the longitudinal traction to 10 to 15 pounds; don't disturb the lateral traction.

After three weeks discontinue the lateral traction.

During this period institute quadriceps setting exercises but do not allow hip motion.

After three additional weeks allow gentle hip and knee motion and continue with the quadriceps setting exercises.

Maintain longitudinal traction for 10 to 12 weeks, or until there is x-ray evidence of solid body union of the acetabular fractures.

After 12 weeks permit partial weight bearing on the affected limb with crutches, and 16 to 20 weeks after injury permit unprotected weight bearing.

Return the patient to light activity six to eight months after injury and to full activity in 10 to 12 months.

Associated Lesions of Fractures of the Acetabulum

REMARKS

Associated lesions have a direct bearing on the fate of the hip joint from a functional viewpoint; when such lesions are present, management of the acetabular fracture becomes more difficult and the prognosis more guarded. The most important associated lesions are:

Loose bodies in the joint: Usually these are osteochondral fragments derived either from the femoral head or the posterior rim of the acetabulum. Following reduction they may be pulled into the joint, thus preventing concentric reduction of the femoral head. Always consider this possibility when reducing dislocations of the hip, especially posterior dislocations. The presence of loose bodies in the joint is an indication for early operative intervention and extraction of the bodies. Failure to remove the bodies will invariably result in traumatic arthritis of the hip joint.

Injury to the femoral head: This lesion is not uncommon, occurring in 12 to 14 per cent of all fractures of the acetabulum. The injury may result in the extrusion of loose bodies into the joint or in depressed fractures of the femoral head. Damage to the femoral head occurs most frequently in posterior acetabular fractures. Generally the presence of this complication connotes a poor prognosis.

Fracture of the neck of the femur: This is a rare complication but when it occurs it compounds the difficulty of management of the fracture-dislocation of the hip.

It may occur in both anterior and posterior dislocations, and it may be produced during the reduction of a dislocation.

As a rule the head of the femur undergoes aseptic necrosis. This lesion is best treated by excising the femoral head and performing a salvage procedure, the nature of which depends on the age, occupation and functional demands of the patient.

Fractures of the shaft of the femur: Dislocation of the hip may be associated with a fracture of the shaft of the ipsilateral femur or the opposite femur. This associated lesion occurs in approximately 2 to 4 per cent of all dislocations of the hip. When such dislocations occur on the same side as the fracture, the dislocation is frequently overlooked. In every fracture of the femur, x-rays of the hips should be taken to avoid this error.

Sciatic nerve injuries: Implication of the sciatic nerve occurs more frequently appreciated in fracture-dislocations of the hip, the incidence being between 10 and 12 per cent; the majority are found in posterior acetabular fractures and bursting fractures.

MANAGEMENT OF LOOSE BODIES IN THE JOINT (FROM THE RIM OF THE ACETABULUM OR FROM THE FEMORAL HEAD)

When present, the bony fragments prevent concentric reduction of the head of the femur just as does soft tissue, such as the labrum, when pulled into the joint during reduction of a posterior dislocation.

Early removal of the loose bodies is essential in order to prevent the development of traumatic arthritis.

Operative Procedure

The surgical technique and postoperative management for these lesions is described on page 1159.

MANAGEMENT OF OSTEOCHONDRAL FRACTURES OF THE FEMORAL HEAD

REMARKS

An osteochondral fracture of the femoral head may complicate posterior dislocation of the hip joint.

In some instances, replacement of the bony fragment is achieved at the time of reduction of the dislocation.

If anatomic repositioning of the bony fragment is not effected when the dislocation is reduced, the fragment must be excised.

In rare instances, during reduction of the dislocation the bony fragment is displaced into the acetabulum and bars reduction; this situation demands open reduction.

It is most important that the dislocation be reduced within the first 24 hours, and preferably within 12 hours.

The size of the osteochondral fragment varies; if it is more than one-third the size of the head or if it involves the weight-bearing surface of the head, poor results are inevitable as a result of aseptic necrosis of the head, osteoarthritis or both.

In these cases primary arthroplasty, arthrodesis or prosthetic replacement is the procedure of choice.

WHEN THE FRAGMENT IS LESS THAN ONE-THIRD OF THE FEMORAL HEAD

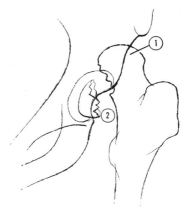

Prereduction X-Ray

1. Posterior dislocation of the femoral head.

2. Marginal fragment detached from the inferior aspect of the femoral head.

Postreduction X-Ray

1. Dislocation is reduced.
2. The marginal fragment is at a distance from the femoral head.

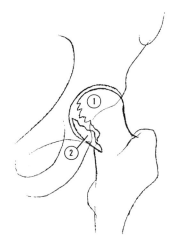

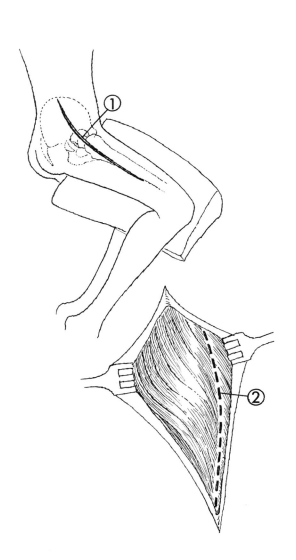

Excision of the Fragment

1. Make a vertical incision on the lateral aspect of the thigh beginning 5 inches below the tip of the greater trochanter, then extend the incision posteriorly for 5 more inches along the anterior margin of the gluteus maximus muscle.
2. Deepen the incision through the deep fascia.

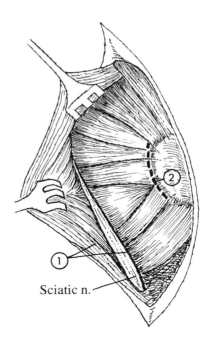

Excision of the Fragment
(Continued)

1. Divide the gluteus maximus along its line of insertion into the fascia lata and displace the muscle mass posteriorly. Visualize the sciatic nerve.

2. Divide the tendons of the piriformis, superior gemellus, internal obturator and inferior gemellus muscles.

3. Retract the detached external rotators of the hip joint posteriorly.

4. Locate the marginal fragment and remove it. (By making traction on the leg it may be possible to distract the fragment without dislocating the hip.)

Note: In case the fragment lies in the joint and is inaccessible, the hip should be dislocated in order to gain access to the fragment in the acetabulum.

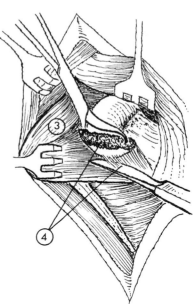

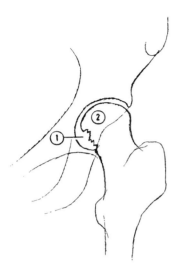

Postoperative X-Ray

1. Defect in the femoral head.
2. The femoral head is well seated in the acetabulum.

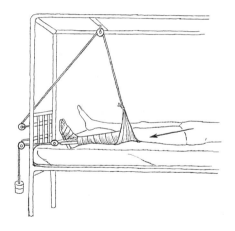

Immobilization

Apply skin traction to the lower leg. The hip is extended and the extremity slightly abducted.

Postoperative Management

Maintain the traction for three weeks. During this period, institute, within a few days after operation, passive and active motion at the hip joint and quadriceps setting exercises.

At the end of three weeks permit crutch walking without weight bearing on the affected extremity.

Permit unprotected weight bearing at the end of 12 to 14 weeks.

Return the patient to light duty in four to six months and to full duty 10 to 12 months after injury.

Follow the patient for two years (every three months); at each examination record the range of motion in the hip and take x-rays to note the presence or absence of aseptic necrosis or traumatic arthritis.

WHEN THE FRAGMENT IS ONE-THIRD OR MORE OF THE FEMORAL HEAD

For young patients perform an arthroplasty or an arthrodesis (see pages 1187, 1195).

For patients over 65 substitute a prosthesis for the femoral head (see page 1203).

MANAGEMENT OF FRACTURE OF THE NECK OF THE FEMUR

REMARKS

This lesion cannot be reduced by closed methods; open operation is necessary because it is impossible to control the head during manipulative reduction.

Replacement of the head on the neck and fixation by some form of internal fixation invariably results in aseptic necrosis of the head; in these cases the blood supply of the head is totally disrupted.

I prefer one of three primary procedures: (1) arthroplasty of the hip, (2) arthrodesis of the hip and (3) replacement of the head by a prosthesis.

ARTHROPLASTY OF THE HIP

This procedure should be performed in young and middle-aged patients possessing good muscles about the hip, and in whom, because of their occupation, a movable hip joint is desirable.

In my hands the arthroplasty about to be described has resulted in better functioning hips by far than any other type of arthroplasty. It is also employed in cases of arthritis following Perthes' disease, slipped capital femoral epiphysis and aseptic necrosis of the head of the femur.

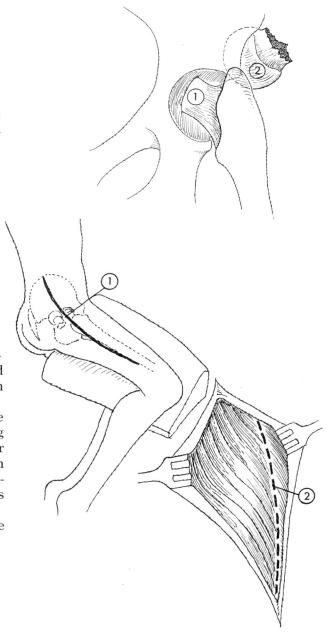

Prereduction X-Ray

1. Stump of the femoral neck is in the acetabulum.
2. Femoral head lies outside of the acetabulum in a superoposterior position in relation to the acetabulum.

Arthroplasty (Technique of DePalma)

Posterior exposure of the hip joint — the patient is in the lateral position and the leg is draped separately with stockinet.

1. Make a vertical incision on the lateral aspect of the thigh beginning 7 inches below the tip of the greater trochanter, then extend the incision posteriorly for 5 inches along the anterior margin of the gluteus maximus muscle.
2. Deepen the incision through the deep fascia.

Page 1187

Arthroplasty (Technique of DePalma) (Continued)

1. Divide the gluteus maximus along its line of insertion into the fascia lata and displace the muscle mass posteriorly.

2. Visualize the sciatic nerve and inspect it for any evidence of injury.

3. Divide the tendons of the piriformis, superior gemellus, internal obturator and inferior gemellus muscles.

4. Retract the external rotator muscles and the sciatic nerve posteriorly.

Note: At this point the femoral head will be visualized outside of the capsule.

5. Dislocated femoral head.

6. Neck of the femur in the acetabulum.

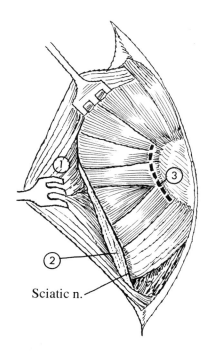

Sciatic n.

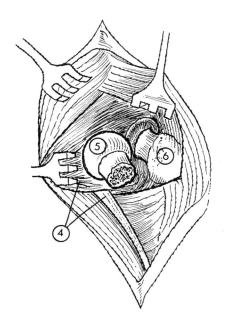

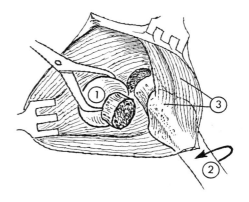

Arthroplasty (Technique of DePalma) (Continued)

1. Grasp the femoral head with a large towel clip and deliver it from the wound.

2. Externally rotate the femur in order to bring into view the lateral aspect of the greater trochanter.

3. Identify the abductors of the hip— the gluteus minimus and the gluteus medius.

4. Begin about ¾ inch below the tip of the greater trochanter; by sharp dissection peel off from the trochanter, in the form of a cuff, the insertion of the gluteus minimus and gluteus medius muscles.

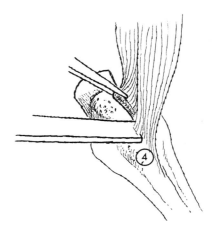

5. Carry the dissection proximally beyond the tip of the trochanter until the posterior portion of the capsule is reached. Peel the muscle mass off the capsule to the line of insertion of the capsule on the rim of the acetabulum.

6. Excise all the accessible capsule close to the acetabulum on one side and to the femur on the other.

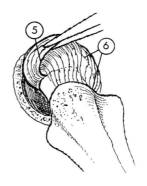

Arthroplasty *(Technique of DePalma) (Continued)*

1. Deliver the upper end of the femur into the wound.

Note: In order to do this, it may be necessary to divide the insertion of the iliopsoas muscle and sever the anterior portion of the capsule at its insertion into the femur.

2. With a sharp, thin osteotome remove the remnants of the femoral neck by cutting through its base close to the femoral shaft.

3. Round off the trochanteric end of the femur with large rongeurs.

4. Choose a vitallium cup that fits loosely (but it must not be overlarge) over the remodeled end of the femur.

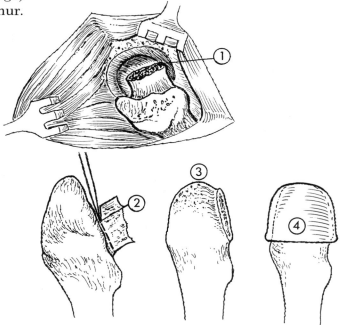

Arthroplasty (Technique of DePalma (Continued)

1. Four inches below the tip of the trochanter split the vastus lateralis down to the bone for an inch in both the proximal and distal directions, and by subperiosteal dissection expose the entire circumference of the shaft of the femur.

2. With an electric saw divide the femur transversely 4 inches below the tip of the trochanter.

3. Deliver the distal end of the proximal fragment into the wound.

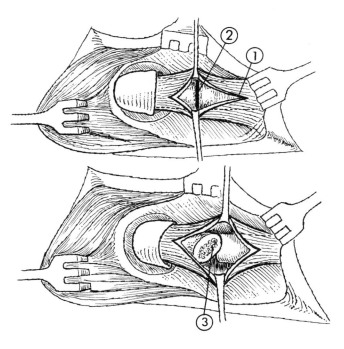

Arthroplasty (Technique of DePalma) (Continued)

1. Insert into the medullary canal of the proximal fragment, a 3½ inch Jewett nail with an angle of 135 degrees. Insert the nail so that the center of the side plate lies directly over the center of the lateral surface of the shaft of the femur.

2. Split the vastus lateralis over the distal fragment for 4 inches and by subperiosteal dissection expose only the lateral surface of the bone.

1. While an assistant holds the leg so that the toes and patella point directly forward (the patient is in the lateral position), the side plate of the nail is secured to the lower fragment with a bone clamp. Adjust the rotation of the upper fragment so that it is in 10 to 15 degrees of anteversion.

2. Anchor the side plate to the femoral shaft with four screws.

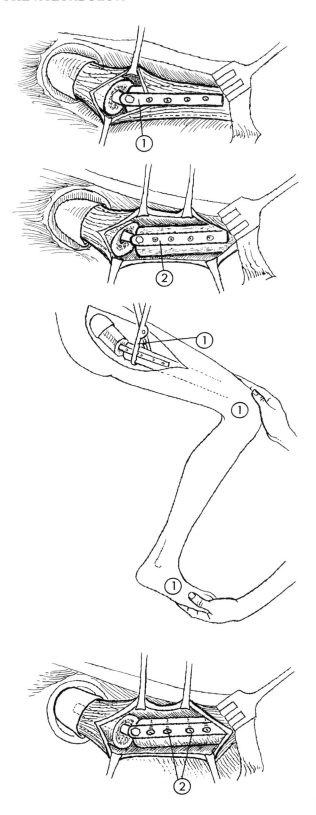

Arthroplasty (Technique of DePalma) (Continued)

1. While an assistant makes traction on the leg the capped upper end of the femur is guided into the acetabulum with a bone skid.

2. Make two drill holes in the lateral aspect of the distal end of the proximal fragment.

3. Attach the abductor cuff to the proximal fragment by stout sutures passing through the drill holes in the bone. This is facilitated by abducting the limb 45 to 60 degrees.

4. Suture the edges of the vastus lateralis over and to the abductor cuff.

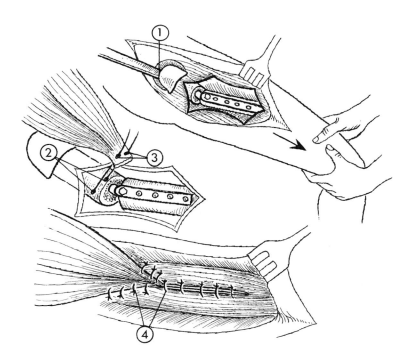

Postoperative X-Ray

1. Upper end of the femur lies in the vitallium cup.
2. The proximal fragment makes an angle of 135 degrees with the distal fragment of the femur.

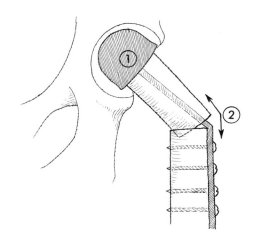

Immobilization

Apply a plaster spica.
1. The leg is abducted 45 to 60 degrees.
2. Knee and hip are slightly flexed.
3. Extremity is slightly internally rotated.

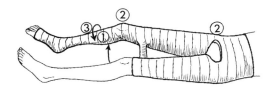

Postoperative Management

At the end of 4 or 5 weeks remove the plaster spica.

Place the limb in balanced suspension.

Institute a regulated program of active exercises for all muscle groups around the hip.

Also institute a program of quadriceps setting exercises.

Keep the patient's limb in balanced suspension two weeks.

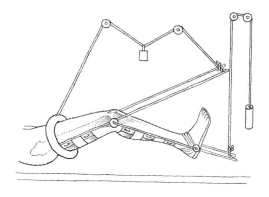

Postoperative Management
(Continued)

At the end of 6 or 7 weeks after operation allow the patient up on crutches with no weight bearing on the affected extremity.

Permit weight bearing with crutches when there is bony union at the osteotomy site (12 to 16 weeks).

With the return of good muscle power and control, the crutches are discarded in favor of a cane.

Note: Development of the muscles of the hip, especially the abductors and the quadriceps muscle, is the most important facet of the postoperative program, which must be carried out faithfully.

ARTHRODESIS OF THE HIP

REMARKS

Arthrodesis of the hip is still a valuable salvage procedure which insures the patient a stable, painless extremity.

It should be employed in young and middle-aged patients whose daily activity demands long hours of standing and walking. Elderly patients have great difficulty in adjusting themselves to a fused hip. In these patients substitution of a prosthesis for the femoral head is the procedure of choice.

The type of arthrodesis about to be described has many advantages over the older conventional types. It assures primary bony union in over 95 per cent of the cases; stiffness of the knee joint due to long periods of immobilization is no longer a problem; the patient is ambulatory during the convalescent period and the hospitalization period is reduced to three weeks.

Arthrodesis of the Hip
(Technique of DePalma)

POSITION OF THE PATIENT

1. Place the patient in the supine position with a small pack under the buttock of the affected hip.

2. Drape the affected leg separately with stockinet to facilitate positioning of the extremity.

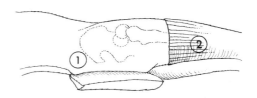

Arthrodesis of the Hip
(Technique of DePalma)
(Continued)

INCISION

1. Begin the skin incision over the iliac crest approximately 3 inches posterior to the anterosuperior spine.

2. Continue the incision over the iliac crest and then downward on the leg in the interval between the tensor fasciae latae and the rectus femoris muscles for a distance of 7 inches.

3. Develop the interval between the tensor fasciae latae and the rectus femoris.

4. Ligate the ascending branch of the lateral femoral circumflex artery and vein found crossing the wound.

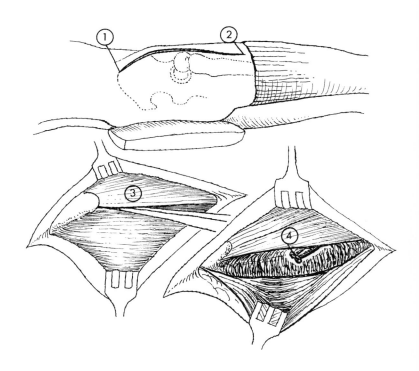

Arthrodesis of the Hip
(Technique of DePalma)
(Continued)

1. Deepen the skin incision on the iliac crest to the bone and by subperiosteal dissection reflect the tensor fasciae latae, the gluteus minimus and gluteus medius from the side of the ilium.

2. Isolate the reflected head of the rectus femoris, separate it from the capsule, divide it and reflect it medially together with the anterior head.

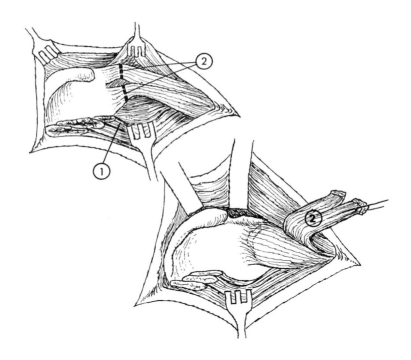

Arthrodesis of the Hip
(Technique of DePalma)
(Continued)

PREPARATION OF THE FEMORAL HEAD AND ACETABULUM

1. By subperiosteal dissection strip the muscles from the inner aspect of the ilium as far as the superior rim of the acetabulum.

Note: At this point the dislocated head is isolated and removed, and the remnant of the neck is rounded to fit up against the roof of the acetabulum.

The subsequent steps of the operation described are for those cases requiring an arthrodesis (as in aseptic necrosis of the femoral head or osteoarthritis of the hip) in which the head and neck are intact and no dislocation exists. These steps are also applicable to achieve an arthrodesis when the hip is dislocated and the femoral neck is fractured.

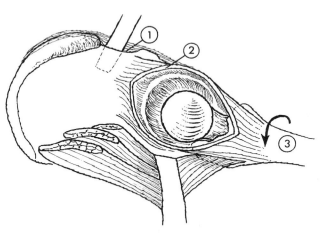

2. Excise as much of the joint capsule as is accessible.

3. Dislocate the femoral head by external rotation of the extremity.

4. With a sharp osteotome remove $3/5$ of the head of the femur and round the remaining portion of the head with a rasp.

5. Denude the acetabulum (particularly the superior articular surface) of all cartilage down to the subchondral bone.

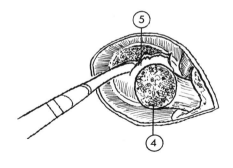

Note: At this point the femoral head is relocated into the acetabulum; do any minor remodeling necessary to insure good contact between the superior surface of the acetabulum and the superior surface of the head. Displace the head centrally into the acetabulum so that the inner surface of the greater trochanter is immediately adjacent to the acetabular rim.

6. Sever the abductors from the greater trochanter. (This facilitates medial displacement of the femur and the insertion of the intramedullary spline.)

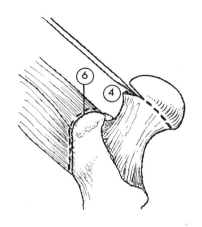

Arthrodesis of the Hip
(Technique of DePalma)
(Continued)

ALIGNING THE INTRAMEDULLARY SPLINE

Note: A specially designed spline is used; it is 10 inches long and ½ inch wide, tapering slightly at the end. On the inner surface of the distal 7 inches of the spline is a centrally placed vertical fin. When driven into the intramedullary canal of the femur the distal end of the spline performs like a triflanged nail and prevents rotation; therefore, the rotational position of the spline must be determined before it is driven into the femur. (See figure of special instruments for this operation.)

1. Remove the pack from under the buttock so that the pelvis is level on the operating table.

2. Reduce the hip and push the trochanter inward so that it abuts the acetabular rim.

3. Rotate the femur to the neutral position so that the patella points straight upward.

4. Place the tip of the spline at the juncture of the greater trochanter and the femoral neck.

5. Rotate the spline so that it is parallel with the surface of the ilium.

6. With the spline held in this position drive it into the medullary canal of the femur so that only ⅛ to ¼ inch of the central fin shows above the superior cortex of the femoral neck.

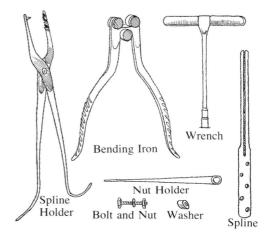

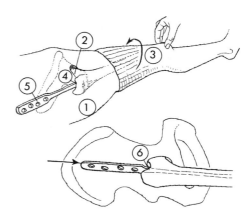

PLACING THE EXTREMITY IN THE DESIRED POSITION OF FLEXION AND ABDUCTION

Note: The desired position of flexion is 10 to 20 degrees. The position of flexion is varied as desired with only a slight change in the position of the spline upward or downward on the ilium.

The degree of abduction is determined by bending the spline to conform to the flare of the ilium with the femur held in the desired position of flexion. I prefer the neutral position; this makes possible a smooth, even gait.

1. Adduct the femur so that the spline falls away from the ilium.

2. Apply the bending iron to the spline and bend the spline to fit the flare of the ilium while the extremity is in the neutral position.

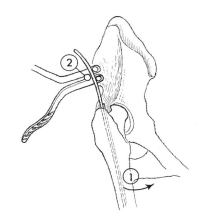

FIXATION OF THE SPLINE

1. Place the extremity in the selected position (preferably 10 to 20 degrees of flexion and in the neutral position).

2. Fix the spline to the side of the ilium by a specially designed clamp.

3. Anchor the spline permanently with three or four bolts which are placed from outside in.

Note: A specially designed beveled washer is fitted over each bolt to conform to the inner surface of the ilium. A specially designed wrench facilitates holding the nut while the bolt is tightened from the outside. In its final position the spline provides rigid fixation between the femur and ilium.

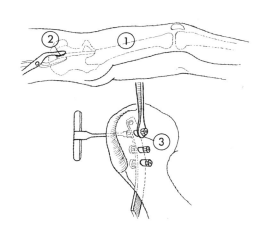

Arthrodesis of the Hip
(Technique of DePalma)
(Continued)

PLACEMENT OF BONE GRAFTS

1. Remove bone slabs from the anterosuperior portion of the ilium.

Note: The slabs are approximately 2 to 3 inches long and the entire thickness of the ilium wide.

2. With a sharp osteotome do a partial osteotomy of the greater trochanter in the vertical plane and parallel to the side of the ilium. Open up the osteotomy site like a book—the base of the trochanter acts like a hinge.

3. Span the interval between the side of the decorticated ilium and the base of the osteotomy site with the bone slabs arranged so that the entire posterior, lateral and anterior aspect of the trochanter now is in continuity with the ilium.

Note: In the event that the head and neck are absent:

1. Remove the lesser trochanter.
2. Perform a subtrochanteric wedge osteotomy with the base of the wedge placed medially.
3. Displace the top of the trochanter under the roof of the acetabulum.
4. Drive the spline through the lateral aspect of the upper portion of the trochanter, through the proximal segment of the femur and into the distal segment.

Note: The remainder of the procedure is identical with the procedure described previously.

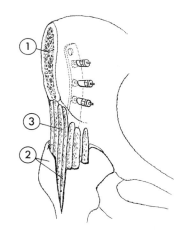

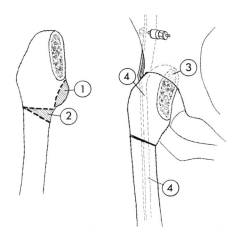

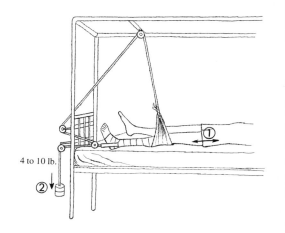

4 to 10 lb.

Immobilization

1. Place the patient in bed with the hip extended.

2. Use 4 to 10 pounds of skin traction on the operated leg.

3. On the tenth postoperative day apply a single, short, above-the-knee plaster spica and allow the patient out of bed using crutches but without weight bearing on the affected limb.

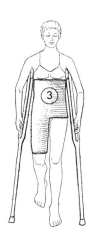

Postoperative Management

After two to three weeks allow the patient to "touch down" on the operated side. (The patient may now be discharged from the hospital.)

At the end of six to eight weeks readmit the patient to the hospital and change the plaster spica; also at this time x-rays are taken to note the state of the fusion.

Solid bony fusion of the hip is usually achieved in 12 to 16 weeks. (Bony fusion should be achieved in 95 per cent of the cases.)

PROSTHETIC REPLACEMENT

REMARKS

This is the procedure of choice for elderly patients (over 65 years of age) with a dislocation of the hip and a fracture through the femoral neck.

This procedure is always employed in properly selected cases of fractures of the femoral neck without dislocation, aseptic necrosis of the femoral head, nonunion and degenerative hip disease in elderly patients.

I employ one of two types of prostheses: (1) the Moore design when a portion of the femoral neck remains which is sufficiently large to provide a seat for the prosthesis and (2) the DePalma prosthesis when the base of the neck is severely comminuted or absorbed.

Always use a medullary prosthesis and never a stem prosthesis.

Operative Technique
(Continued)

The patient is in the lateral position.

1. Make a vertical incision 5 inches long on the lateral aspect of the thigh beginning 5 inches below the tip of the greater trochanter, then extend the incision posteriorly for 5 more inches along the anterior margin of the gluteus maximus muscle.

2. Deepen the incision through the deep fascia.

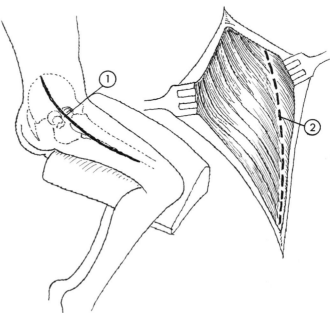

Operative Technique
(Continued)

1. Divide the gluteus maximus along its line of insertion into the fascia lata.

2. Displace the muscle mass posteriorly. Visualize the sciatic nerve.

3. Divide the tendons of the piriformis, superior gemellus, obturator internus and inferior gemellus muscles.

4. Retract the detached external rotators and the sciatic nerve.

5. Isolate the dislocated femoral head which usually lies superior and posterior to the acetabulum and remove it from the wound.

6. The neck of the femur may be in the acetabulum.

Note: The subsequent steps are also employed when a prosthesis is substituted for the femoral head in cases of fractures of the femoral neck without dislocation.

If no dislocation exists, the head is removed from the acetabulum.

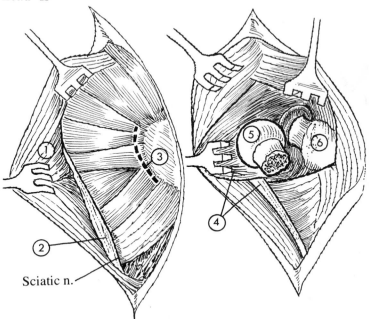

Sciatic n.

At this point inspect the remnant of the neck of the femur. If it is sufficiently large to seat a Moore prosthesis proceed with the subsequent steps; if not use a DePalma prosthesis.

Operative Technique
(Continued)

When the size of the femoral neck will support a prosthesis:

1. Internally rotate the extremity; this brings into full view the stump of the neck.

2. With an electric saw reshape the femoral neck to provide a seat for the Moore prosthesis. Enough of the calcar must remain to provide adequate support to the medial portion of the prosthesis.

3. With a rasp open the medullary canal.

4. Cut out a notch in the greater trochanter with a "starter" which permits easy insertion of the prosthesis.

Note: Choose a prosthesis which is of the same size as the femoral head removed. Also check the size of the prosthesis by placing it directly into the acetabulum before insertion of the stem into the medullary canal.

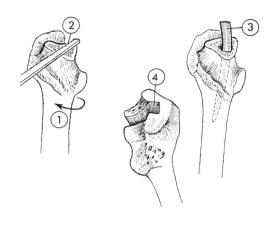

1. Insert the prosthesis by gently tapping an impactor placed over the head of the prosthesis.

Note: Insert the prosthesis so that the head and neck are in normal relation to the acetabulum; there should be no change in the degree of anteversion or retroversion of the prosthesis.

2. Reduce the prosthesis into the acetabulum by making

3. Traction on the extremity and at the same time

4. Rotating the limb externally. Close the capsule.

Caution: An excessive rotatory force must not be employed because a fracture of the femur may result.

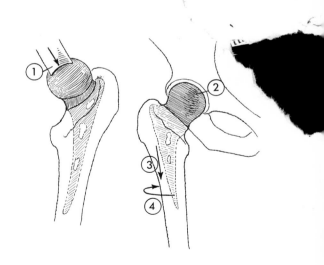

Operative Technique
(Continued)

When the remnant of the femoral neck is severely comminuted or absorbed:

1. Remove the femoral head.

2. Externally rotate the femur to bring into view the lateral aspect of the greater trochanter.

3. Identify the abductors of the hip, the gluteus medius and gluteus minimus muscles.

4. Begin about ¾ inch below the tip of the greater trochanter; by sharp dissection peel off from the trochanter, in the form of a cuff, the insertions of the gluteus medius and gluteus minimus muscles.

5. Carry the dissection proximally beyond the tip of the trochanter until the posterior portion of the capsule is reached. Peel the muscles off the ___ to the line of insertion of the ___ule on the rim of the acetabulum.

6. Excise all the accessible capsule close to the acetabulum on one side and to the femur on the other.

Deliver the upper end of the femur into the wound and internally rotate the leg to bring into view the lesser trochanter. In order to do this it may be necessary to divide the insertion of the iliopsoas muscle and sever the anterior portion of the capsule at its insertion into the femur.

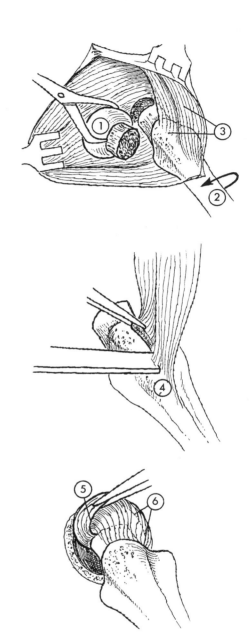

Operative Technique
(Continued)

1. With an electric saw make a vertical cut through the greater trochanter beginning ¼ inch lateral to the inner margin of its tip.

2. Carry the cut distally to a point ¼ to ½ inch distal to the superior margin of the lesser trochanter.

3. Make a second saw cut at right angles to the first at the point of termination of the vertical cut.

4. Remove the detached inner segment of the upper end of the femur.

5. With a rasp open the medullary canal.

6. Insert the prosthesis by tapping an impactor placed over the head of the prosthesis.

7. The flat base of the prosthesis should fit directly on massive dense bone of the lesser trochanter.

Note: The size of the head of the prosthesis should be the same as the femoral head removed. Also check the size by fitting the head directly into the acetabulum before inserting its stem in the medullary canal.

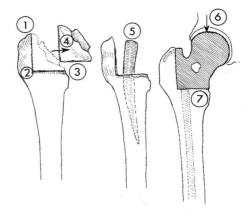

Reduce the prosthesis into the acetabulum by traction and external rotation of the femur.

Caution: Don't apply excessive rotatory force to achieve the reduction; this may produce a fracture of the shaft of the femur.

1. Make several drill holes through the tip of the greater trochanter.

2. Reattach the abductor cuff to the trochanter with stout sutures passing through the drill holes.

Note: In order to facilitate reattachment of the cuff, abduct the femur 30 to 45 degrees.

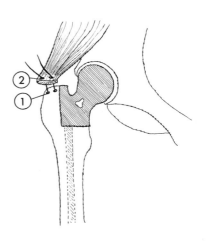

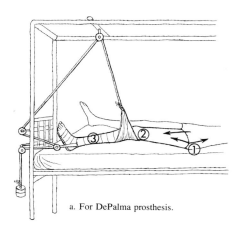

a. For DePalma prosthesis.

Postoperative Management

Place the extremity in balanced suspension.

1. The limb is only slightly flexed at the hip.

2. The limb is abducted 45 degrees.

3. The limb is in the neutral position when a DePalma prosthesis is used (*a*) and in mild external rotation when a Moore prosthesis is used (*b*).

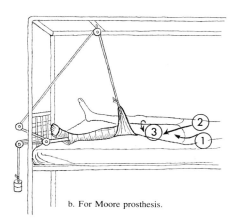

b. For Moore prosthesis.

Encourage early passive and active motion at the hip and knee. When the abductor muscles have been detached, don't permit abduction exercises for three weeks.

Institute a regulated regimen of quadriceps setting exercises. Patients with a Moore prosthesis may start partial weight bearing in parallel bars two weeks after operation. Patients with a DePalma prosthesis begin this activity at the end of five weeks.

Parallel bars are replaced by crutches just as soon as the patient is capable of using crutches.

Crutches are discarded when the muscles of the hip are sufficiently strong to permit unaided full weight bearing.

This may require several more months.

DISLOCATION OF THE HIP JOINT WITH FRACTURE OF THE SHAFT OF THE FEMUR

REMARKS

If at all possible, dislocation of the hip associated with a fracture of the shaft of the femur should be reduced by closed methods. This will give the femoral head a better chance of survival than if an open reduction is done.

Reduction should be achieved just as soon as possible, but it is important to remember that these injuries are usually the result of severe violence and the patient may be in profound shock. The patient's vital functions must be stabilized before attention is directed to the hip. The functional result in these lesions varies with the promptness of diagnosis and treatment.

Fifty to 60 per cent of dislocations of the hip, when associated with fracture of the shaft of the femur, are not recognized; always take an x-ray of the pelvis when there is a fracture of the femur.

Unrecognized dislocations of the hip are frequently associated with nonunion of fractures of the femur.

The type of dislocation usually associated with fracture of the shaft of the femur is the posterior dislocation with or without a fracture of the posterior portion of the acetabulum.

Fragments of the posterior portion of the acetabulum may be displaced in the acetabulum during attempts at closed reduction and thus prevent reduction of the femoral head into the acetabulum. This situation calls for an open reduction (see page 1159). If the fragments are small and do not interfere with reduction they can be disregarded.

METHODS OF CLOSED REDUCTION

Prereduction X-Ray

1. Posterior dislocation of the femoral head.

2. Small fragments off the posterior rim of the acetabulum.

3. Fracture of the shaft of the femur.

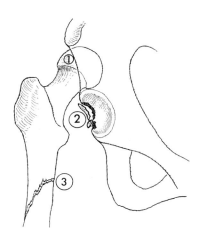

Manipulative Reduction

1. The patient is placed in the supine position on the floor.

2. An assistant makes downward pressure on the anterosuperior spines of the ilium.

3. The operator makes upward traction on the leg with the hip flexed 90 degrees.

4. Another assistant applies direct pressure on the dislocated femoral head in an upward and inward direction.

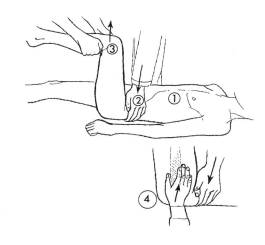

After the head enters the acetabulum:

1. While upward traction is maintained,

2. Lower the thigh to the floor to the extended position.

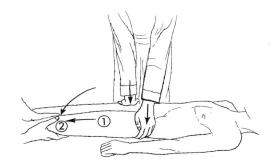

If reduction is not achieved:

1. Drive a Steinmann pin through the trochanter in the anteroposterior plane.

2. Fasten the pin to a traction bow.

3. While an assistant makes upward traction on the flexed leg and another makes downward pressure on the anterosuperior iliac spines,

4. The operator makes upward and inward (adduction) traction on the bow lifting the head into the acetabulum.

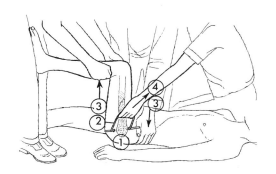

If reduction is still not achieved:

First: Stabilize the femur by use of an intramedullary nail as described on page 1330.

Appearance on X-Ray

1. Femur is reduced and stabilized by an intramedullary nail.

Second: Reduce the posterior dislocation of the hip as just described under *Manipulative Reduction.*

2. Posterior dislocation of the hip is reduced.

Note: All attempts at closed reduction as just described may fail; in this event open reduction of the posterior dislocation is indicated.

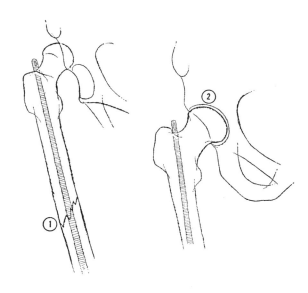

Management of Fracture of the Femur After Closed Reduction of Dislocation

Apply skeletal traction to the affected femur, either with a pin through the lower fragment just above the femoral condyles or through the tibia just below the tibial tubercle.

or

Reduce and stabilize the femoral fracture with an intramedullary nail introduced through a posterolateral incision as described on page 1330. This may be performed at the same time that the hip is reduced if the patient's condition permits it or at a later time.

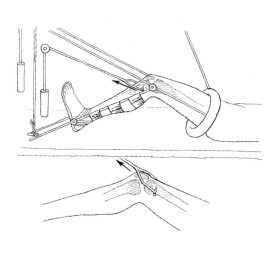

1. Femur is reduced by open reduction and stabilized with an intramedullary nail.

2. Hip dislocation is reduced.

3. Limb is in balanced suspension.

4. Hip is in abduction and only minimal flexion.

5. The limb is in the neutral position as regards internal and external rotation.

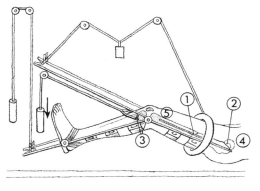

OLD IRREDUCIBLE DISLOCATIONS OF THE HIP

REMARKS

These lesions are rare and when encountered are usually of the posterior type; however, occasionally anterior dislocations of long standing are also encountered.

For up to three weeks an attempt to reduce the dislocation by closed manipulative methods is justifiable; if this fails, open reduction is indicated.

After three weeks aseptic necrosis of the femoral head is a certainty; therefore, if open reduction can be achieved the hip should be fused.

In some instances, open reduction of old dislocations may be impossible or the procedure may be too formidable; in this event, the operation of choice is an angulation osteotomy in order to improve the gait, correct the deformity and provide stability to the pelvis.

For old posterior dislocations, open reduction should be preceded by preliminary skeletal traction.

MANAGEMENT OF OLD IRREDUCIBLE POSTERIOR DISLOCATIONS OF THE HIP

Prereduction X-Ray (Posterior Dislocations of Three Months' Duration)

1. The head and neck of the femur show marked demineralization.

2. The articular surface of the femoral head is irregular, indicative of destruction of the articular cartilage.

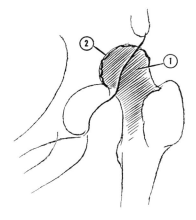

Preliminary Operative Procedure

Stripping of side of ilium.

Freeing of the femoral head and neck.

Removal of fibrous tissue from the acetabulum.

Application of skeletal traction.

Note: In cases of three to six weeks' duration, this procedure may be eliminated and only skeletal traction applied. This may suffice to stretch contracted tissues and allow the head to descend to the level of the acetabulum and facilitate open reduction.

1. Make a skin incision along the iliac crest beginning at its middle and extending to the anterosuperior spine, thence downward on the leg in the interval between the tensor fasciae latae and the rectus femoris for 4 to 6 inches.

2. Divide the deep fascia and develop the interval between the tensor fasciae latae laterally and the sartorius and rectus femoris medially.

3. Deepen the incision along the iliac crest to the bone.

4. Strip subperiosteally from the ilium the tensor fasciae latae, gluteus medius and gluteus minimus muscles.

5. Isolate and ligate the ascending branch of the lateral circumflex artery approximately 2 inches below the joint.

6. Cut the acetabular tendon of the origin of the rectus femoris.

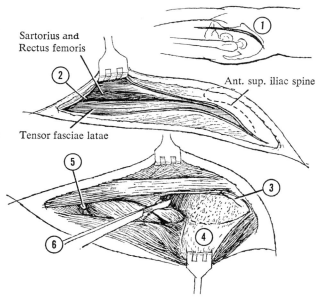

Sartorius and Rectus femoris

Ant. sup. iliac spine

Tensor fasciae latae

Preliminary Operative Procedure (Continued)

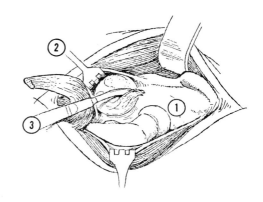

1. Locate the head of the femur on the dorsum of the ilium and dissect it free of scar tissue and degenerated muscle tissue.

2. Incise the ligaments and the capsule and expose the acetabulum.

3. With a large sharp curette, clear the acetabulum of all fibrous tissue.

PATIENT IN SKELETAL TRACTION

1. Close the wound.

2. Pass a stout threaded pin below the tibial tubercle for skeletal traction.

3. Elevate the foot of the bed.

4. The hip and knee are slightly flexed.

5. Apply 25 to 35 pounds of weight.

Note: Take check x-rays every 48 hours to note the position of the femoral head. When the femoral head is opposite the acetabulum or near its superior rim, the patient is ready for the final operative procedure.

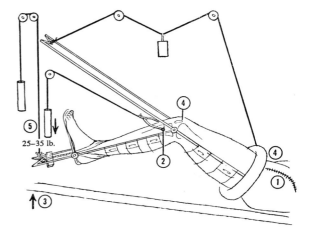

Open Reduction and Fusion of the Hip Joint

Note: This procedure should not be performed before two and one-half to three weeks have elapsed since the first operation. The soft tissues should be given time to recover from the surgical trauma of the first operation.

The femoral head and acetabulum are exposed through the same approach depicted above.

From this point on proceed with the hip arthrodesis operation and postoperative management as described on pages 1195 to 1202.

Angulation Osteotomy for Old Irreducible Posterior Dislocation of the Hip

REMARKS

This is performed to correct deformity, provide pelvic stability and to gain length of the extremity.

If properly performed and a spline is used to fix the fragments in the desired position, no external plaster fixation is required.

I prefer a modification of the Hass osteotomy; essentially it comprises an osteotomy below the lesser trochanter and displacement of the upper fragment medially so that the lesser trochanter is displaced into the acetabulum and is now in position to bear most of the weight.

Before the osteotomy is performed, the desired angle of the osteotomy is calculated from tracings of x-rays of the hip. On paper cutouts of the femur cut the femur just below the lesser trochanter and place the upper segment along the pelvis so that the lesser trochanter is in the acetabulum; now line up the distal segment with the proximal one so that it is directed straight downward. Finally, measure the angle made by the two segments and adjust the angle of the spline to correspond to it.

Operative Technique

The patient is in the lateral position, lying on the unaffected side. Drape the leg separately with stockinet.

1. Begin the skin incision approximately 2 inches proximal and anterior to the greater trochanter; curve the incision distally and posteriorly over the posterolateral aspect of the trochanter; then continue it distally on the lateral aspect of the thigh parallel to the femur.

2. Deepen the incision to the fascia lata.

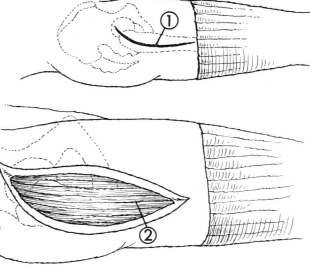

Operative Technique
(Continued)

1. Just posterior to the tensor fasciae latae muscle divide the fascia lata and then split the fascia distally in line with the skin incision.

2. Spread the edges of the fascia lata and bring into view the vastus lateralis muscle.

3. Divide transversely the vastus lateralis muscle at its site of origin along the inferior border of the greater trochanter.

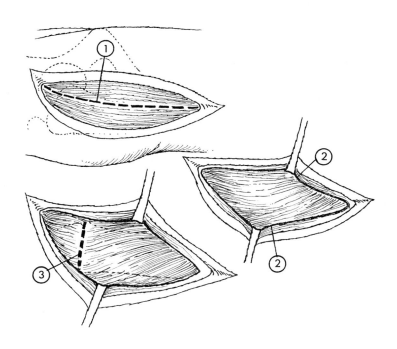

Operative Technique
(Continued)

1. Displace the vastus lateralis muscle anteriorly and

2. Divide it longitudinally on its posterolateral surface about ¼ inch from its line of attachment to the linea aspera.

Note: As the muscle is divided be prepared to encounter the perforating arteries; clamp and ligate these vessels as you proceed distally.

3. By sharp subperiosteal dissection elevate the muscle from the anterior and anterolateral surfaces of the femur.

4. Continue this dissection proximally until the intertrochanteric area of the femur is exposed.

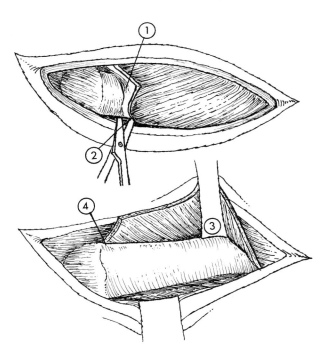

1. Just inferior to the lesser trochanter divide the femur transversely with an electric saw.

2. Displace the distal segment medially and

3. Insert the spline (preadjusted) into the medullary canal of the proximal segment of the femur.

Note: The direction of the spline should be such that the proximal and distal segments will angulate posteriorly a few degrees.

4. With a bone clamp secure the distal segment of the femur to the plate of the spline.

5. Rotate the distal segment so that the patella points straight forward.

6. Fix the plate to the lower segment with screws.

7. Pack the open interval between the two fragments with cancellous bone chips. (These are obtained from the iliac crest through a small separate incision directly over the crest.)

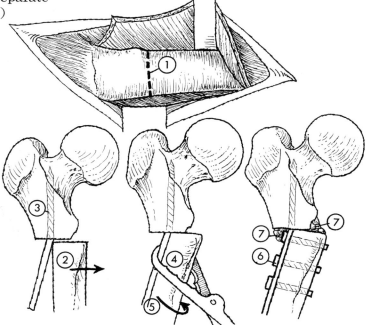

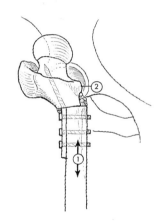

Postoperative X-Ray

1. The distal fragment is in good weight-bearing position.
2. The lesser trochanter lies in the acetabulum.

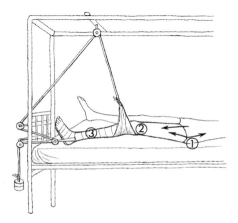

Immobilization

Place the limb in balanced suspension.
1. The hip is slightly flexed.
2. The knee is flexed.
3. The leg is slightly abducted.

Postoperative Management

Institute active motion at the hip and knee as soon as pain subsides, usually within three or four days.

Institute quadriceps setting exercises.

After three weeks ambulate the patient on crutches without weight bearing on the operated extremity.

Permit full weight bearing only after there is x-ray evidence of solid bony union at the osteotomy site.

MANAGEMENT OF OLD IRREDUCIBLE ANTERIOR DISLOCATIONS OF THE HIP

This patient exhibits a severe deformity of the extremity and trunk.

1. The lumbar lordosis is exaggerated with scoliosis toward the affected side.

2. Pelvis on the affected side is lower and rolled anteriorly.

3. Limb is abducted and laterally rotated.

4. Hip and knee are flexed.

5. Apparent lengthening of the limb. (There is actually some true lengthening.)

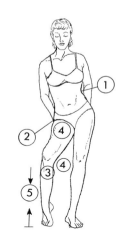

Preoperative X-Ray

1. Acetabulum is empty.

2. Head of the femur is dislocated anteriorly in the obturator position.

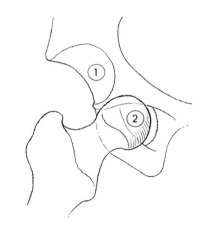

Operative Reduction

The patient is in the supine position with a pack under the affected hip. The leg is draped separately with stockinet.

1. Begin the incision over the iliac crest 3 inches posterior to the antero-superior spine.

2. Continue the incision over the iliac crest and then downward on the leg in the interval between the tensor fasciae latae and the rectus femoris.

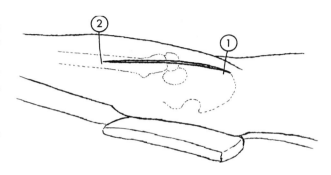

Page 1220

Operative Reduction
(Continued)

3. Ligate the ascending branch of the lateral femoral circumflex artery and accompanying vein found crossing the wound.

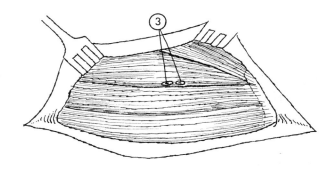

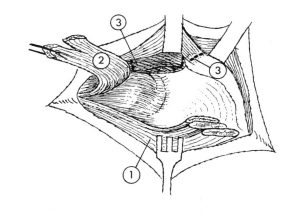

1. Deepen the incision on the iliac crest to the bone and by subperiosteal dissection reflect the tensor fasciae latae and the gluteus medius and gluteus minimus from the side of the ilium.

2. Isolate and detach the reflected head and the straight head of the rectus femoris.

3. Detach the tendon of the sartorius and the iliopsoas.

4. Displace all these muscles medially.

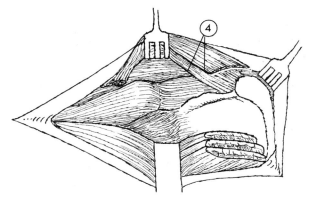

Operative Reduction
(Continued)

1. Palpate the femoral head under the pectineus and adductor longus muscles.

2. With a sharp curette excise all fibrous tissue and adherent capsule from the acetabulum.

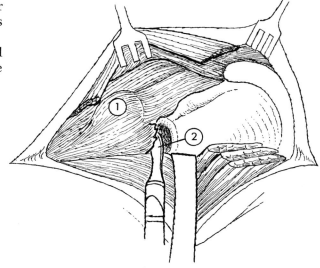

1. Retract medially the pectineus together with the femoral vessels and nerve.

2. Excise all fibrous tissue surrounding and binding the femoral head until the head is freely mobilized.

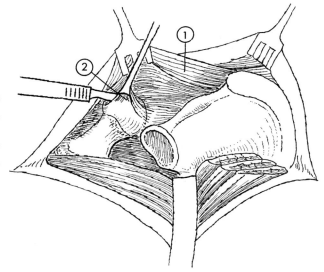

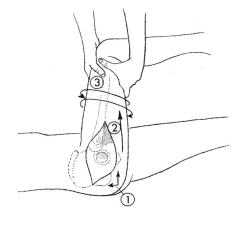

Operative Reduction
(Continued)

Mobilize the femur further by:

1. Flexing the hip to 90 degrees.

2. Apply traction with the extremity slightly adducted.

3. Internally and externally rotate the femur.

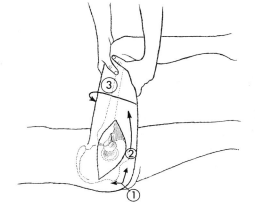

Reduce the dislocation by:

1. Flexing the hip to 90 degrees.

2. Apply traction to the adducted extremity.

3. While traction is maintained, internally rotate the extremity.

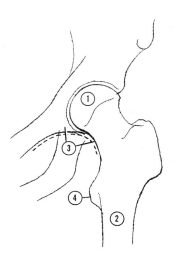

Postreduction X-Ray

1. Head of the femur is seated in the acetabulum.

Arthrodesis of the Hip Joint

From this point on proceed with the hip arthrodesis operation and postoperative management as described on pages 1195 to 1202.

OSTEOTOMY FOR OLD IRREDUCIBLE ANTERIOR DISLOCATION OF THE HIP

REMARKS

This is performed to correct the deformity of the extremity and trunk, to provide stability to the pelvis and to improve the gait.

Also it is performed when it is impossible to reduce the hip or when open reduction is considered too formidable a procedure for the patient.

Preoperative X-Ray

1. The head is dislocated anteriorly in the obturator position.
2. Shaft of the femur is abducted,
3. Flexed and
4. Externally rotated.

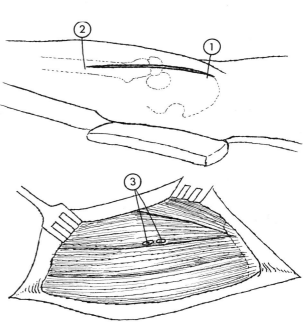

Operative Technique

The patient is in the supine position with a pack under the affected hip. The extremity is draped separately with a stockinet.

1. Begin the incision over the iliac crest 3 inches posterior to the antero-superior spine.
2. Continue the incision over the iliac crest and on the leg in the interval between the rectus femoris and the tensor fasciae latae.
3. Ligate the ascending branch of the circumflex artery and accompanying vein found crossing the wound.

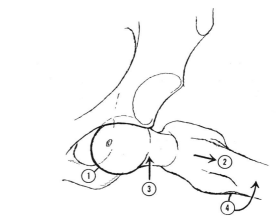

Operative Technique
(Continued)

1. Deepen the incision on the iliac crest to the bone and by sharp subperiosteal dissection reflect the tensor fasciae latae, the gluteus medius and the gluteus minimus from the side of the ilium.

2. Isolate and detach the reflected and straight heads of the rectus femoris.

3. Detach the tendon of the sartorius and iliopsoas.

4. Displace all these muscles medially.

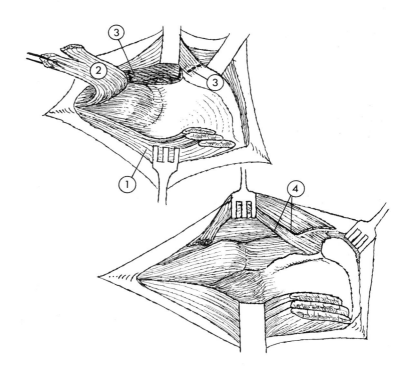

Operative Technique
(Continued)

Palpate the head of the femur under the pectineus and adductor longus muscles.

1. Retract the pectineus together with the femoral vessels and nerve medially.

2. Excise all fibrous tissue surrounding and binding the femoral head and neck of the femur.

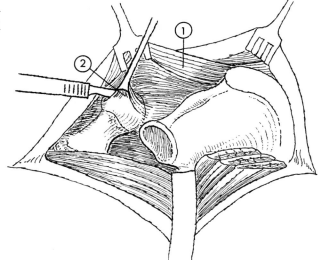

1. With a sharp thin osteotome, osteotomize the femur at the base of the neck from above downward and medially.

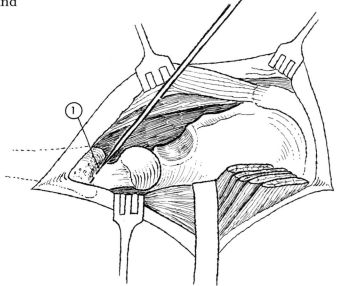

Operative Technique
(Continued)

After the osteotomy is completed, the limb is:
1. Slightly adducted,
2. Extended, and
3. Internally rotated.

Note: Now the extremity is in the neutral position with the patella pointing forward.

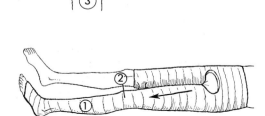

Postoperative X-Ray

1. Femoral head is still dislocated.
2. Site of osteotomy.
3. Distal fragment is in the neutral position.
4. Proximal fragment is in the position of varus.

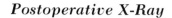

Immobilization

Apply a plaster spica.
1. Extremity is in the neutral position.
2. Patella points forward.

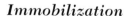

Postoperative Management

Union at the osteotomy site is achieved in 12 to 16 weeks.

When bony union is achieved, as evidenced by x-rays, remove the plaster spica.

Allow crutch walking with partial weight bearing at first and then full weight bearing.

At this time institute a program of muscle exercises for the hip and knee.

Crutches are discarded as soon as the patient no longer needs them for support.

LATE COMPLICATIONS OF DISLOCATIONS OF THE HIP AND FRACTURES OF THE ACETABULUM

REMARKS

Late complications that may occur are aseptic necrosis of the femoral head, traumatic arthritis and myositis ossificans; all these connote a guarded prognosis.

ASEPTIC NECROSIS OF THE FEMORAL HEAD

This complication is definitely related to the time interval the head remains in a dislocated position and to the severity of the initial violence. The longer the head is dislocated and the greater the violence producing the lesion the higher will be the incidence of aseptic necrosis. Although most of the cases of aseptic necrosis occur in posterior dislocations and posterior fracture-dislocations, the lesion may occur in anterior dislocations; the incidence is 8 to 10 per cent for all anterior dislocations.

Varying gradations of aseptic necrosis are encountered varying from mild to severe. Invariably this complication is responsible for varying degrees of arthritis of the hip joint. Arthritis is responsible for many clinical failures and like aseptic necrosis is definitely related to the intensity of the initial violence; it is responsible for the high incidence of poor results encountered in superior dome and bursting fractures of the acetabulum. However, the changes noted on x-rays are not comparable to the clinical findings. Many patients with a good clinical result exhibit advanced alterations of the hip on x-rays.

Together, aseptic necrosis and traumatic arthritis occur in approximately 25 per cent of all dislocations of the hip and fractures of the acetabulum. X-ray evidence of these complications is usually apparent within one year after the injury; only rarely is this evidence seen for the first time after one year.

MANAGEMENT OF ASEPTIC NECROSIS AND ARTHRITIS OF THE HIP

REMARKS

The type of treatment is governed by the age of the patient, his occupation and the intensity of the clinical manifestations.

When surgical intervention is indicated, one of three procedures are available—arthrodesis, arthroplasty and prosthetic replacement.

The indications and surgical techniques for these procedures are described on pages 1187 to 1208.

MYOSITIS OSSIFICANS

This complication occurs in approximately 15 per cent of the cases. It is more frequently encountered in affected hips treated by open reduction than by closed methods, in a ratio of 7 to 1.

It is also encountered more frequently in patients treated without immobilization or immobilized for only short periods of time.

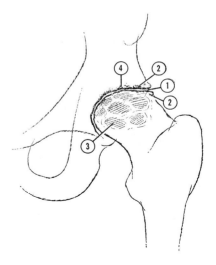

Appearance on X-Ray—Traumatic Arthritis

Traumatic arthritis following posterior dislocation of the hip joint.
1. Narrowed joint space.
2. Marginal osteophytes of the acetabulum and femoral head.
3. Cystic areas in the femoral head.
4. Flattening of the femoral head.

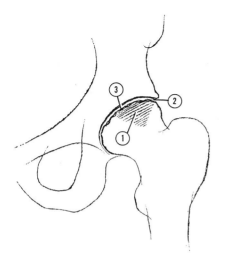

Appearance on X-Ray—Aseptic Necrosis

Aseptic necrosis of the femoral head.
1. Triangular area of increased density.
2. Collapse and flattening of the femoral head.
3. Irregularity of the articular surface of the femoral head.

Page 1229

Appearance on X-Ray — Myositis Ossificans

Myositis ossificans and calcification of the capsule. This x-ray was taken ten weeks after the injury.

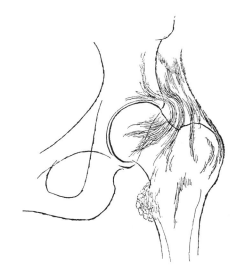

Appearance on X-Ray — Old Unreduced Dislocation

Old unreduced dislocation in a boy 14 years old. This lesion is three months old.

1. The head and neck of the femur show marked demineralization.

2. The articular surface of the femoral head is irregular, indicative of destruction of the articular cartilage.

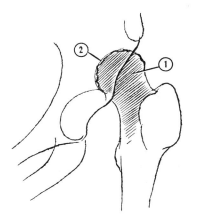

TRAUMATIC DISLOCATION OF THE HIP IN CHILDREN

REMARKS

This lesion is not common but neither is it rare; it may occur in any age group between two and 15 years of age. Cases in children under two years of age have been reported.

It occurs more frequently in boys than in girls, the ratio being 2 to 1.

In younger children, under six years of age, dislocation may be produced by trivial injuries; in older children more violence is usually required to produce the lesion.

Most dislocations in children are of the posterior type, although anterior and central dislocations may occur.

Although rare, the dislocation may be complicated by fracture of the acetabulum; in these cases the prognosis is poor.

When the lesion is the result of major violence, associated injuries may obscure the dislocation; this is particularly true when the associated lesion is a fracture of the ipsilateral femur. It is not uncommon with this combination not to recognize the dislocation for two to four months after injury.

Always take x-rays of the pelvis when there is a fracture of the femur.

Most dislocations are readily reduced by closed methods under general anesthesia. However, a few cannot be reduced by closed methods and require open reduction. The usual causes are buttonholing of the femoral head through the capsule or interposition of soft tissue in front of the head during reduction.

The methods of closed and open reduction of dislocation of the hip in children are the same as those employed for adults (see pages 1113 to 1153).

In older children failure of closed reduction is more common than in children under six years of age.

All dislocations, conditions permitting, should be reduced immediately, and certainly within 24 hours after injury.

The longer the delay in reduction the higher the incidence of aseptic necrosis of the femoral head and of degenerative changes of the hip joint; incidence is approximately 10 per cent of all dislocations.

Aseptic necrosis invariably follows in hips reduced after 24 hours, except in very young children.

The incidence of complications is greater following open reduction than closed reduction.

Aseptic necrosis may be evident in x-rays within a few months after injury; however, degenerative changes of the hip may not occur for several years. These patients should be followed carefully for several years after the injury.

Page 1231

It is doubtful that the time of weight bearing has any relation to the development of aseptic necrosis; however, there is evidence that the time of weight bearing does relate to the gradation of the lesion. Weight bearing in young children is permissible in four to six weeks; in older children in three to four months.

MANAGEMENT

Always use general anesthesia.
Perform the reduction with the utmost gentleness.
Usually simple upward traction on the flexed femur is sufficient to reduce all types of dislocations.

Reduction (For Both Anterior and Posterior Dislocation)

The child is under general anesthesia.
1. While an assistant presses downward on the anterosuperior spine of the pelvis,
2. Flex the hip to 90 degrees.
3. Make gentle traction upward and inward.

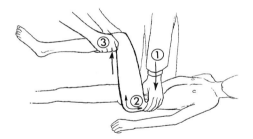

Postreduction X-Ray

1. Femoral head is seated in the acetabulum.

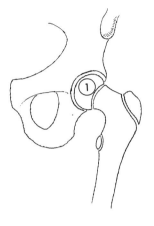

Postreduction Management

For children under six years of age:

IMMOBILIZATION

Apply a plaster spica.
1. The hip is extended.
2. The extremity is slightly abducted.

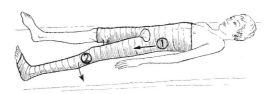

Maintain the patient in plaster four to six weeks.
After four to six weeks allow full weight bearing and normal activity;
these children need no physical therapy.

For children over six years of age:

IMMOBILIZATION

Apply a plaster spica.
1. The hip is extended.
2. The extremity is slightly abducted.

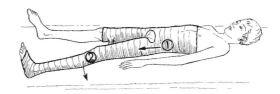

or

Apply skin traction to the leg.
1. The hip is extended.
2. Use 4 to 10 pounds at traction,
depending on the size of the child.

After six weeks permit ambulation
on crutches with no weight bearing on
the affected extremity.

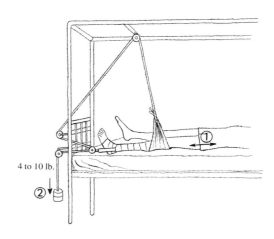

Postreduction Management
(Continued)

1. The affected limb is suspended by a hip sling.

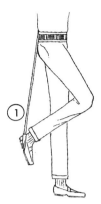

Protect the hip from weight bearing for three months from the time of injury.

After three months permit partial weight bearing on crutches and then full weight bearing.

Crutches are discarded as soon as the patient feels he has no further need of them.

CAUTION

Check the patient carefully; if he begins to complain of stiffness or pain without x-ray evidence of changes in the femoral head protect the hip from weight bearing for four to six additional weeks.

Follow these patients for several years (every three or four months). At each examination check and record the arcs of motion of the hip and take x-rays to determine the presence or absence of aseptic necrosis of the femoral head or other degenerative alterations in the hip joint.

FRACTURES OF THE FEMUR

FRACTURES OF THE UPPER END OF THE FEMUR

REMARKS

Fractures of the upper end of the femur include:
  Fractures of the greater trochanter;
  Fractures of the lesser trochanter;
  Trochanteric fractures (extracapsular fractures);
  Fractures of the neck of the femur (intracapsular fractures).

Fractures of the Greater Trochanter

REMARKS

Generally, a fracture of the greater trochanter occurs as the result of a direct blow on this bony prominence; occasionally the greater trochanter is avulsed by muscular action.

In adolescents the separation usually occurs at the epiphyseal line.

Displacement of the distal fragments upward and inward is rarely marked.

Prereduction X-Ray

1. Communited fracture of the greater trochanter.

2. The fragments are displaced upward and inward.

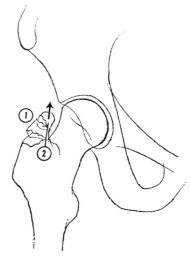

Reduction and Immobilization

1. Full abduction of the limb. (This position usually effects approximation of the upper end of the shaft of the femur and the avulsed trochanter.)

2. Maintain abduction of the limb with a plaster spica.

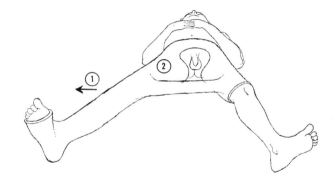

Postreduction X-Ray

The upper end of the shaft of the femur is in apposition with the avulsed greater trochanter.

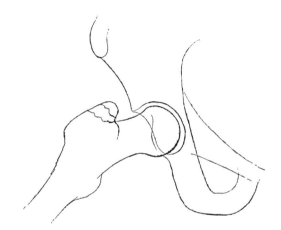

Postreduction Management

Remove the plaster cast at the end of six weeks.

Allow the patient up on crutches.

After one week, discard the crutches for a cane.

Discard the cane just as soon as the patient is able to tolerate full weight bearing on the affected limb.

Fractures of the Lesser Trochanter

REMARKS

This fracture, a common associated lesion in comminuted intertrochanteric fractures of the femur, may be ignored because it in no way materially affects the ultimate result.

In some instances the epiphysis of the lesser trochanter is avulsed by the iliopsoas muscle; the same mechanism may pull off the lesser trochanter in adults.

Prereduction X-Ray

Avulsion of the lesser trochanter.
1. The fragment is displaced upward by the iliopsoas muscle.

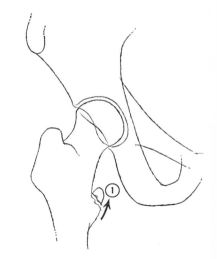

Reduction and Immobilization

1. Reduction is achieved by flexion of the hip to 90 degrees.
2. The position is maintained by placing the limb on pillows.

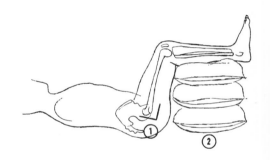

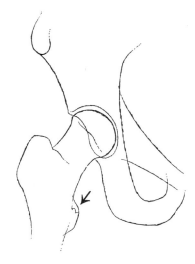

Postreduction X-Ray

The upper end of the shaft of the femur is in apposition with the avulsed fragment.

Postreduction Management

Keep the limb flexed 90 degrees on pillows for four weeks.
Then allow the patient up on crutches.
Discard the crutches at the end of one week and allow use of a cane.
Discard the cane when full weight bearing on the affected limb is tolerated.
Prevent forceful abduction and hyperextension movements of the hip for several months.

Trochanteric Fractures

REMARKS

Trochanteric fractures include all extracapsular fractures in the trochanteric region of the femur to a point 2 inches below the lesser trochanter.

The lesions occur in elderly people whose average age (75 years) is roughly five years older than that of persons sustaining intracapsular fractures.

These fractures may be produced by a violent external rotational force applied to the extremity, such as twisting the body away from the affected limb while the limb is firmly fixed, or they may result from direct violence to the hip in addition to twisting of the body.

Of these lesions 80 per cent occur in people over 60 years of age and the great majority occur in women, the ratio being 2 to 1. The high incidence encountered in women may be due to two factors: (1) After 60 years the life expectancy of women is greater than that of men by five years and (2) in these age groups, senile osteoporosis is by far more prevalent in women.

If these fractures are adequately reduced and fixed, aseptic necrosis or nonunion rarely are complications; on the other hand, the fractures are often complicated by other serious problems: (1) The mortality and morbidity rates are high; almost 20 per cent of these patients die within six months from causes related to the injury. (2) Shortening of the limb and varus deformity are common sequels, occurring in 70 to 75 per cent of the severely comminuted fractures.

Early operative reduction and internal fixation have reduced the mortality and morbidity rates by almost 50 per cent; nevertheless, trochanteric fractures are the result of major violence often associated with much soft tissue disruption; in addition, the surgery to achieve adequate internal fixation is extensive and formidable. These factors contribute to the high mortality and morbidity rates.

All trochanteric fractures should be treated surgically; the only contra-indications are: (1) in a moribund patient, (2) in advanced osteoporosis associated with severe comminution of the bone and (3) in uncontrolled diabetes. (Sepsis frequently complicates the postoperative course of a diabetic patient with fracture of the hip).

If closed methods must be used, apply skeletal traction by means of a stout threaded wire passed just below the tibial tubercle; support the limb in a balanced suspension apparatus. These patients will not tolerate skin traction for prolonged periods of time. Patients in traction require adequate nursing care and proper management in bed.

Although rare, trochanteric fractures may occur in children.

After fracture the limb assumes a complete external rotation deformity (90 degrees) with the foot resting on its outer edge; this deformity is in contrast to that of the patient with an intracapsular fracture, whose limb, because the capsule is intact, rotates externally no more than 45 degrees.

CLASSIFICATION OF TROCHANTERIC FRACTURES

Many varieties of fractures are encountered in the trochanteric region; however, they do fall into certain types. Some types can be treated with little difficulty while others present major problems. Moreover, the morbidity is greater in some than in others.

TYPE I

This type is characterized by a fracture line traversing the intertrochanteric line; the fracture is extracapsular and, as a rule, the greater and lesser trochanters are not implicated. Depending upon the intensity of the force the proximal and distal fragments may or may not be displaced.

When displacement is marked the proximal fragment may exhibit a varus deformity of 90 degrees in relation to the distal fragment, and the distal fragment may assume a position of extreme external rotation.

Reduction and fixation for this lesion presents no difficulty and the prognosis as to morbidity is good.

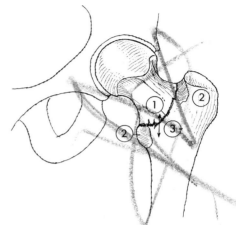

1. Fracture line extends along the intertrochanteric line.

2. The trochanters are not involved.

3. The proximal and distal fragments are in normal anatomical alignment.

Type II

In this lesion the main fracture line extends along the intertrochanteric line but there is considerable comminution of the proximal fragment. The proximal fragment shows varying degrees of varus deformity; in some instances the base of the femoral neck, which is shaped like a sharp spike, digs deeply into the cancellous bone of the intertrochanteric area; the distal fragment is adducted and externally rotated. Both trochanters may be implicated and in some instances the greater trochanter may be split in the vertical plane and pulled posteriorly by the external rotator muscles of the femur while the lesser trochanter is avulsed and displaced medially.

This is the commonest trochanteric fracture; reduction and fixation of this fracture is difficult and the prognosis as to morbidity is not as good as in Type I fractures.

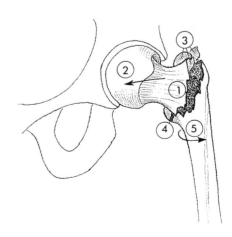

1. Fracture through the intertrochanteric line.

2. Varus deformity of the proximal fragment.

3. Comminution of the greater trochanter.

4. Fracture into the lesser tuberosity.

5. External rotation of the distal fragment.

1. Fracture through the intertro-chanteric line and into the greater trochanter.

2. Varus deformity of the proximal fragment.

3. Comminution of the greater tro-chanter.

4. Vertical split of the greater tro-chanter.

5. Avulsion and medial displace-ment of the lesser trochanter.

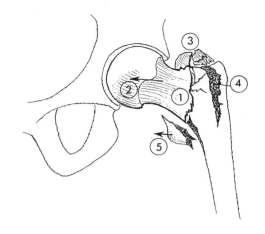

TYPE III

This lesion is primarily characterized by a fracture line passing through the subtrochanteric area.

Both trochanters may be involved; the greater trochanter may be split vertically and the lesser trochanter avulsed and displaced medially. The end of the subtrochanteric fragment may present a conical configuration. These fractures occur in all age groups, but chiefly in young, active individuals, as the result of severe trauma. These are very unstable fractures; they are difficult to reduce and fix and they carry a high mor-bidity rate. Fortunately these fractures are not very common (10 per cent of all trochanteric fractures).

1. Fracture of the greater trochanter.

2. Avulsion and medial displace-ment of the lesser trochanter.

3. Varus deformity of the proximal fragment.

4. Conical subtrochanteric frag-ment.

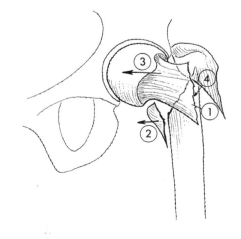

TYPE IV

The main features of this lesion are fractures in the pretrochanteric region and fractures of the proximal end of the femur in several planes. The fracture planes through the upper end of the femoral fragment may be vertical, oblique or spiral, and a triangular fragment may be completely separated from the shaft of the femur.

These are difficult fractures to assemble and require fixation in two or more planes. Fortunately they are not common lesions; together with Type III fractures they comprise about 30 per cent of all trochanteric fractures.

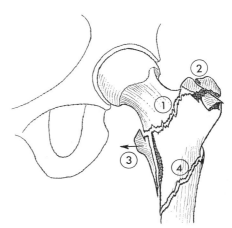

1. Fracture through the intertrochanteric region.
2. Comminution of the greater tuberosity.
3. Avulsion and medial displacement of the lesser tuberosity.
4. Spiral fracture of the upper end of the femoral shaft.

MANAGEMENT OF TROCHANTERIC FRACTURES

REMARKS

Immediate Management:
Take x-rays of the hip in the anteroposterior and lateral planes.

Apply some form of traction to the extremity, preferably Russell's traction.

Evaluate the medical condition of the patient.

Make the necessary preparations for reduction and internal fixation of the fracture.

Remember that surgical management may be a life-saving procedure for elderly patients.

Surgery is contraindicated only if the patient is moribund, if the fracture implicates osteoporotic bone and is so comminuted that reassembly of the fragments is impossible, and if uncontrolled diabetes exists. Diabetes renders these patients vulnerable to postoperative sepsis.

Don't delay the operation; it should be done in the first 12 hours and not later than 24 hours after injury.

Don't disturb the patient; the operative area should be cleansed and prepared in the operating room.

Page 1243

Russell Traction

1. Foam rubber straps.
2. Sling (padded with foam rubber) under the knee and provided with a spreader to prevent pressure against the head of the fibula and compression of the popliteal vessels.
3. The knee is flexed.
4. The hip is flexed.
5. Pillow supports the leg.
6. The foot of the bed is elevated.
7. Apply 5 to 10 pounds of weight; this should be sufficient to prevent shortening.

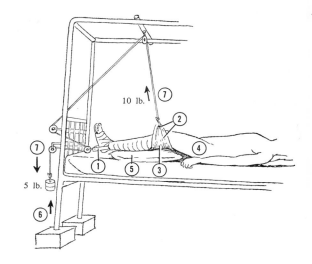

Note: Excessive weight may cause the skin to break down; if heavy weight is necessary (over 12 pounds) make traction through a threaded Kirschner wire inserted just below the tibial tubercle.

SURGICAL CONSIDERATIONS

Always employ general anesthesia; elderly people tolerate general anesthesia very well.

Do the operation on a fracture table with the feet fastened to the foot pieces; this insures good control of the extremity and reduces the number of assistants required.

Study the x-rays very carefully and decide upon the type of internal fixation best suited for the patient.

Be prepared to change your plans, because certain features of these fractures are detected only by direct visualization and may not be revealed in the x-ray films.

The goal in the management of these fractures is to return the patient to the level of activity enjoyed prior to the injury, in the shortest time possible. Long periods of convalescence expose these patients to many medical complications which may end fatally.

Ideally the patients should be ambulating with protection within a few days after operation. Many fractures, if properly managed, lend themselves to this form of treatment; these are Type I and many Type II fractures. If in these lesions the anteromedial cortex is not comminuted and can be assembled, the patients can bear weight with protection. A high angle nail-plate, such as the Jewett or the Sarmiento nail-plate, makes possible the necessary fixation that permits early weight bearing.

Some severely comminuted fractures such as may occur in Types II and III, in which there is marked instability because of destruction of the anteromedial cortex of the neck of the femur, are best treated by medial displacement of the proximal fragment; at times an osteotomy may be necessary to achieve this.

In Type IV fractures fixation of the femoral fragments in different planes may be necessary before the main proximal and distal fragments are fixed by a nail-plate.

Operative Procedure

POSITION OF PATIENT

1. Patient is on a fracture table with a cassette holder under the buttocks; the affected hip is well over the side of the table (this facilitates insertion of the nail if the fracture must be fixed in a position of external rotation).

2. The unaffected extremity is fastened to the foot plate.

3. Make traction on the affected extremity in the position of the deformity (external rotation and moderate abduction).

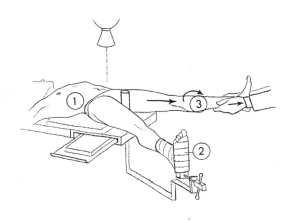

1. Internally rotate the extremity.
2. The hip is in neutral flexion and extension.

Note: Do not forcefully manipulate the limb, because a simple trochanteric fracture may be converted into a type very difficult to manage.

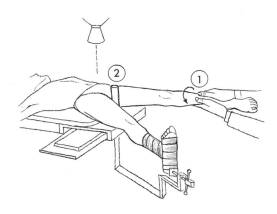

1. Now fasten the affected limb to the foot piece.

2. Apply sufficient traction to restore length and the normal neck-shaft angle.

3. Abduct the limb to 20 to 30 degrees. (Further abduction may cause angulation at the site of fracture.)

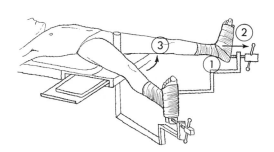

Operative Procedure (Continued)

EXPOSURE

Note: In my opinion all components of the upper end of the femur should be visualized in order to appreciate the extent of the fracture and to attain adequate reduction and fixation of the fracture; this includes visualization of the neck of the femur.

1. The skin incision begins 1 inch distal and lateral to the anterosuperior spine; it continues downward over the posterior aspect of the greater trochanter and the lateral aspect of the femur for a distance of 6 inches below the base of the greater trochanter.

2. Divide the fascia lata the length of the skin incision.

3. Develop the interval between the gluteus medius and the tensor fasciae latae and divide the reflection of the fascia lata beneath the tensor fasciae latae; retract the tensor fasciae latae medially.

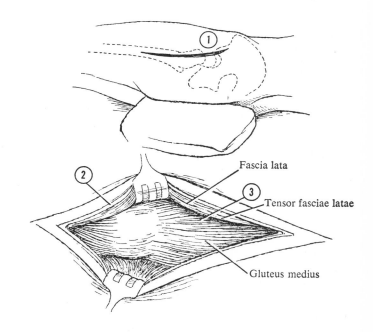

Fascia lata

Tensor fasciae latae

Gluteus medius

1. Displace the gluteus medius posteriorly to expose the anterolateral aspect of the capsule of the hip joint.

2. Divide the capsule with a T-shaped incision, exposing the femoral head and neck.

3. Displace the muscle mass of the vastus lateralis anteriorly and by sharp dissection divide it longitudinally ½ to 1 inch anterior to the linea aspera; proximally in the subtrochanteric region continue the incision forward into the tendinous origin of the muscle.

Note: While splitting the fibers of the vastus lateralis, branches of the large perforating arteries are encountered and, if severed, may cause much bleeding; therefore, proceed slowly and as the vessels are encountered clamp and ligate them.

4. By sharp subperiosteal dissection elevate the vastus lateralis from the femur and retract it anteriorly and toward the midline; this exposes the entire upper end of the femur and the trochanter region.

5. Maintain the exposure by hooking the edges of two Bennett retractors around the shaft of the femur.

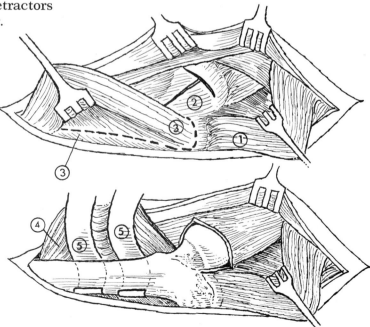

ANALYSIS OF THE FRACTURE

At this point of the operation make a detailed inspection of the fracture site and determine (1) the type of fracture and (2) the best method of internal fixation for the fracture encountered.

WHEN THE ANTEROMEDIAL CORTEX IS NOT COMMINUTED

Most Type I fractures (the main fracture extends along the inter-trochanteric line) and many Type II fractures fall into this classification.

A high angle nail-plate (150 degrees, Jewett or Sarmiento nail-plate) if properly inserted will permit early protected weight bearing.

REDUCTION OF THE FRACTURE

REMARKS

Reduction is achieved by traction, rotation and abduction.

Traction should be sufficient to restore the length of the extremity and the normal neck-shaft angle.

Rotation is employed to approximate the proximal and distal fragments; too much internal rotation may close the fracture line on the anterior aspect of the trochanteric region but open it posteriorly. At times, because of the plane of the fracture, external rotation of the distal fragment may be necessary to approximate it to the proximal fragment, which may be displaced posteriorly and rotated externally by the short external rotators of the femur.

If rotation of the femoral fragment fails to attain anatomic apposition of the two main fragments or if reduction can be attained but cannot be held, insert a Steinmann pin through the greater trochanter and the femoral neck at right angles to the shaft of the femur and use it to lever the proximal fragment into the desired position.

ABDUCTION

Generally 20 to 30 degrees of abduction suffices to approximate the distal and proximal fragments; the amount of abduction required can readily be determined by direct visualization of the fracture.

FINAL REDUCTION

While an assistant at the foot of the table carries out the preceding maneuvers as directed by the operator, the operator, under direct vision, makes the necessary final adjustments of the fragments to restore anatomic alignment.

Before Reduction

1. The proximal fragment is in varus.

2. The distal fragment is externally rotated.

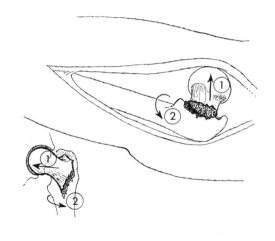

Reduction

1. Traction restores the normal neck-shaft angle.

2. Internal rotation of the distal fragment approximates the two fragments.

3. Moderate abduction of the femoral fragment.

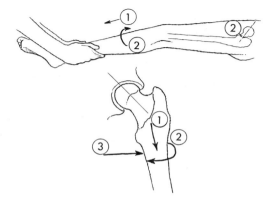

Postreduction X-Rays

These are necessary at this time to check the reduction in two planes.

ANTEROPOSTERIOR VIEW

1. Fragments are in anatomic position.

2. Neck-shaft angle is restored.

LATERAL VIEW

3. Head,

4. Neck and

5. Greater trochanter lie in a horizontal plane.

Note: This is the position to strive for before inserting the nail-plate.

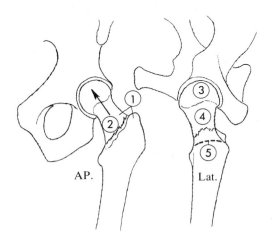

INSERTION OF GUIDE PIN

REMARKS

Since the neck of the femur and the trochanteric region are clearly visualized, the use of the guide pin may appear superfluous; hence, some surgeons endowed with great technical skill may insert the nail without the use of a guide pin.

However, the use of the guide pin has many advantages: (1) If the nail is not in the desired position its removal and repeated insertions cause much destruction of bone in the femoral neck and head. This will not occur if a guide pin is used. (2) The guide pin when properly inserted assures the correct position of the nail in the neck and head, establishes the exact length of the nail and permits placing the nail at the same angle to the shaft as the fixed angle of the nail-plate. Finally, in a measure, the guide pin provides some stability to the fracture when the nail is inserted.

The pin should be inserted in such a manner as to guide a high angle nail-plate (150 degrees) into the desired position; the nail should abut directly against the inferior cortex of the neck and penetrate deeply into the femoral head; also it should be placed anteriorly at the level of the fracture so that it rests against the anterior cortex. This prevents antero-posterior displacement of the fragments.

To attain this position the nail should be so placed that it traverses the neck obliquely and the end of the nail penetrates the posterior quadrant of the head.

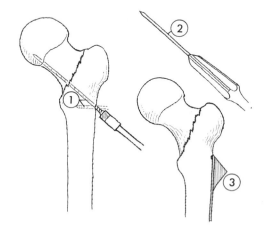

1. With a ³⁄₁₆ inch drill make a hole on the lateral side of the shaft of the femur midway between the anterior and posterior cortices and 1⅞ to 2 inches below the flare of the greater trochanter. First direct the drill at a right angle to the shaft and then upward at an angle of 45 degrees.

2. Place a guide pin in the drill leaving 4 inches protruding beyond the drill.

3. Place an angle guide, set at 150 degrees, opposite the drill hole.

4. Directing the pin parallel and close to the anterior cortex of the neck, insert it into the trochanter, neck and head until the end of the drill abuts the cortex.

Note: At this point remove the drill and angle guide and take anteroposterior and lateral x-ray views. If the pin is in the desired position proceed with insertion of the nail-plate; if not, reinsert the pin until it is in the desired site.

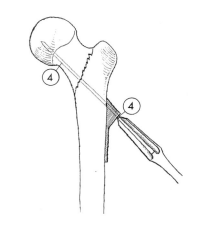

Postreduction X-Rays

ANTEROPOSTERIOR VIEWS

1. The fragments are in normal alignment.
2. Normal neck-shaft angle is restored.
3. Guide pin lies close to the inferior cortex.
4. Guide pin penetrates deeply into the femoral head.

LATERAL VIEW

5. Guide pin traverses the anterior portion of the neck.
6. The end of the pin penetrates the posterior quadrant of the femoral head.

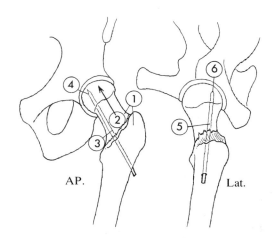

Insertion of Nail-plate

1. With a cannulated reamer (or any other electric drill) enlarge the hole in the lateral cortex to accommodate the nail. (Failure to do this may result in splintering of the lateral cortex when the nail is inserted.)

2. Insert the nail over the guide pin. (I prefer the high-angle nail-plate designed by Sarmiento.)

3. Hold the plate of the nail parallel to the shaft. When seated the plate should be flush and in complete contact with the shaft.

4. Now drive the nail across the fracture site and into the femoral head.

Note: Since the length of the pin traversing the fracture site is known (4 inches), by studying the x-rays the exact length of the nail desired is readily determined; don't choose a nail that is too long because, with settling of the fragments, the end of the nail may protrude out of the head.

1. While the desired position is maintained, hold the plate to the shaft with a bone forceps.

2. Secure the plate to the shaft of the femur with four screws.

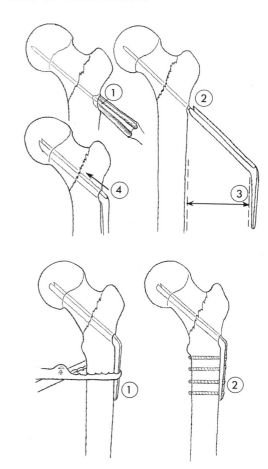

Postreduction X-Rays

ANTEROPOSTERIOR VIEW

1. Normal neck-shaft angle is restored.

2. The nail lies close to the inferior cortex.

3. The nail penetrates deeply into the femoral head.

LATERAL VIEW

4. The nail lies against the anterior cortex.

5. The end of the nail penetrates the posterior quadrant of the femoral head.

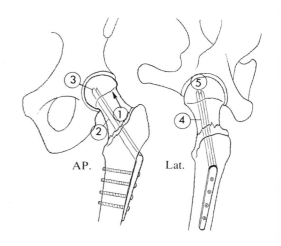

AP.   Lat.

Page 1252

Postoperative Management

Allow the patient out of bed in a chair on the second day.

Institute a program of active exercises for the hips and knees just as soon as soreness from the operation subsides.

This program should include exercises to strengthen the quadriceps, glutei and muscles of the upper extremities.

If the fracture is properly reduced and the nail is in proper position allow the patient to use a walker. Also, permit protected weight bearing on the operated extremity; later the walker is replaced by one cane.

Although protected weight bearing is allowed as soon as the patient has the desire to ambulate, do not allow unprotected weight bearing until there is x-ray evidence of healing at the fracture site, usually at the end of 12 to 16 weeks.

Don't insist that elderly patients learn the use of crutches. This is a difficult feat for the aged and gives rise to fear and apprehension.

Check the progress of healing by x-ray at six-week intervals.

WHEN THE ANTEROMEDIAL CORTEX IS COMMINUTED (OR WHEN THERE IS A SUBTROCHANTERIC FRACTURE WITH COMMINUTION OF THE PROXIMAL FRAGMENT)

REMARKS

These fractures comprise some of the fractures of Type II and some of the fractures of Type III in which there is comminution of the medial cortex or posterior aspect of the proximal fragment.

These are not rare lesions; they comprise about 40 to 45 per cent of all trochanteric fractures and carry a high incidence of morbidity.

In these fractures the outstanding feature is instability due to severe comminution of the anteromedial aspect of the neck or of a large posterior fragment or of both. When this situation is confronted, medial displacement of the distal fragment, followed by impaction and internal fixation, produces excellent functional results and lowers the morbidity rate.

In the presence of comminution of the medial cortex or if a posterior fragment is present, internal fixation of the proximal and distal fragments in correct anatomic position will not withstand the stress placed on the fracture by muscle action. The adductors pull the distal fragment medially, and with weight bearing the fracture collapses because of the lack of bony support.

This gives rise to the complications encountered with these lesions: (1) The nail bends or breaks, or (2) the nail cuts through the head and neck as the fracture settles in a position of varus, or (3) the nail penetrates the head and acetabulum as the distal fragment migrates medially or (4) the plate is pulled away from the shaft.

In Type III fractures, if there is no comminution of the medial cortex, internal fixation with a high angle nail-plate will provide adequate stability; however, if there is severe comminution of the trochanters and of the medial cortex, then primary medial displacement of the distal fragment should be done.

Preoperative X-Rays

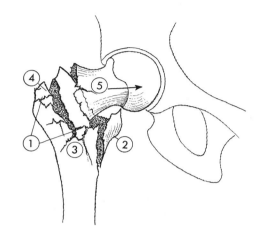

1. Severe comminution of the greater trochanter.
2. The lesser trochanter is avulsed from the shaft.
3. Comminution of the medial cortex.
4. Posterior trochanter fragment.
5. Head and neck fragment are in varus.

Operative Procedure

The patient is placed on a fracture table, the fracture is reduced and the fracture site is exposed, as described on page 1249.

Appearance of Fracture Site after Reduction

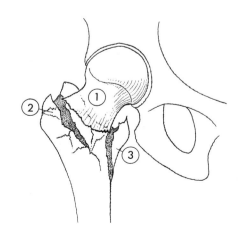

1. Head and neck fragment in normal alignment with the shaft.
2. Posterior trochanteric fragment.
3. Lesser tuberosity displaced medially.

Appearance of Fracture Site after Reduction *(Continued)*

1. With an osteotome divide the greater trochanter at its base.

2. Insert a guide pin parallel to the inferior surface of the neck and parallel to the anterior surface of the neck.

Note: At this point take anteroposterior and lateral x-rays to check the position of the guide pin.

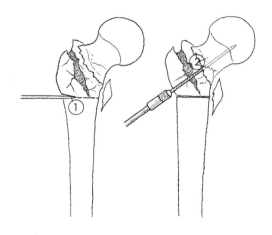

ANTEROPOSTERIOR VIEW

1. The guide pin is parallel to the inferior cortex of the femoral neck and penetrates deep into the head.

LATERAL VIEW

2. The guide pin is parallel to the anterior cortex of the neck and penetrates the posterior quadrant of the head.

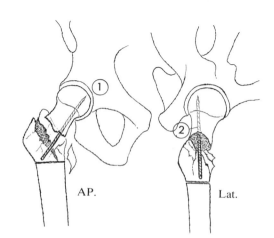

AP.   Lat.

1. Displace the distal fragment medially under the head and neck.

2. By measuring the pin protruding from the neck, determine the length of the nail (usually the measurement will be 2 to 2½ inches); use a high angle nail (150 degrees); this will give a valgus neck-shaft angle.

3. Pass a nail of the desired length over the wire and drive it into the head and neck.

4. Release the traction to allow impaction of the fragments.

5. Secure the plate to the shaft of the femur with four screws.

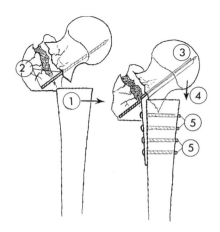

Page 1255

Postreduction X-Ray

1. A valgus neck-shaft angle is present.

2. The medial cortex of the neck is in apposition to the lateral cortex of the distal fragment.

3. The distal fragment is displaced medially.

4. The nail penetrates deeply into the head.

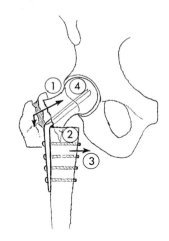

WHEN THERE IS SEVERE COMMINUTION OF THE GREATER TROCHANTER AND A HIGH SUBTROCHANTERIC FRACTURE (TYPE III)

These lesions are best treated by medial displacement of the shaft fragment so that the medial cortex of the neck impinges on the lateral cortex of the shaft fragment.

An osteotomy may not be necessary and is done only if some spicules of bone on the femoral fragment prevent its medial displacement.

Use a high angle nail to attain a valgus position. The technique for the insertion of the nail is the same as that described on page 1255.

Preoperative X-Ray

1. Severe comminution of the greater trochanter.

2. Comminuted subtrochanteric fracture.

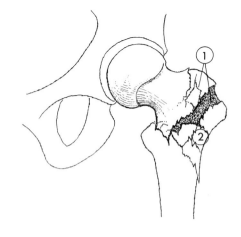

Postoperative X-Ray

1. Medial displacement of the shaft fragment.

2. Medial cortex of proximal fragment abuts against the lateral cortex of the femoral fragment.

3. Valgus position of proximal fragment attained with a high angle nail.

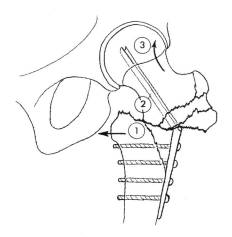

WHEN THERE IS COMMINUTION OF THE PRETROCHANTER REGION, A SUBTROCHANTERIC FRACTURE AND A FRACTURE OF THE FEMORAL SHAFT

REMARKS

The fracture in the femoral shaft may be vertical, oblique or spiral.

Do not try to secure all these fragments at one time to a nail-plate.

These lesions are best managed by first assembling the femoral fragments and fixing them with as many screws as necessary; then reduce and fix the two main fragments with a nail-plate.

Once the femoral fragments are assembled the management of the two main fragments is the same as that described for Type III fractures. (See pages 1255 and 1256.)

Preoperative X-Ray

1. Comminuted fracture of the pretrochanteric region.

2. Comminution of the greater trochanter.

3. Vertical fracture of the femoral fragment.

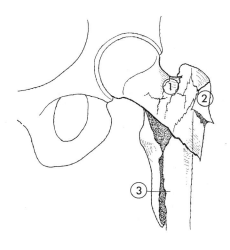

Plan of Management

1. Assemble the femoral fragments.
2. Fix the fragments with screws.
3. Reduce the two main fragments.
4. Fix them with a long Jewett nail-plate (135 degrees).

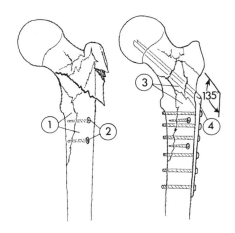

WHEN THERE IS A LOW SUBTROCHANTERIC FRACTURE WITH LITTLE OR NO COMMINUTION OF THE PROXIMAL FRAGMENT

REMARKS

As a rule the proximal fragment exhibits little or no comminution.

The main fracture line is transverse or oblique at a distance from the base of the lesser trochanter, 1½ to 2 inches.

These fractures readily lend themselves to intramedullary fixation.

Prereduction X-Ray

1. Low subtrochanteric fracture.
2. The proximal fragment is intact.
3. There is slight comminution of the upper end of the distal fragment.
4. The proximal fragment is abducted, producing a coxa vara deformity.

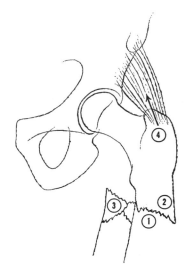

Operative Reduction and Fixation

1. The patient is in the full lateral position lying on the unaffected side.

2. Begin the incision 2 inches behind the anterior superior spine and extend it downward to a point 2 to 3 inches below the level of the fracture site; the incision is centered over the lateral aspect of the greater trochanter.

3. Divide the fascia lata along the line of the skin incision.

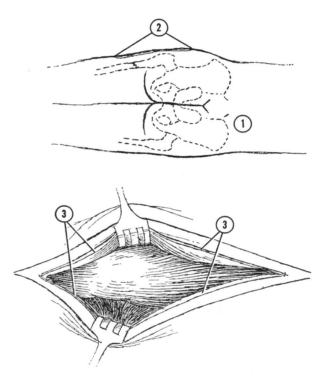

Operative Reduction and Fixation
(Continued)

1. Develop the interval between the tensor fasciae latae and gluteus muscles and reflect the former medially, exposing the tip of the trochanter and the insertion of the gluteus medius.

2. Displace the vastus lateralis anteriorly and by sharp dissection divide it longitudinally ½ to 1 inch anterior to the linea aspera; proximally in the subtrochanteric region continue the incision forward into the tendinous origin of the muscle.

3. By subperiosteal dissection, elevate the muscle from the femur and retract it anteriorly and toward the midline. This exposes the entire upper end of the femur.

4. Maintain the exposure by hooking the edges of two Bennett retractors around the shaft of the distal fragment of the femur.

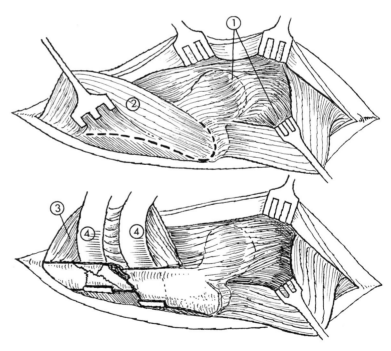

Operative Reduction and Fixation (*Continued*)

1. Elevate the distal fragment into the wound.

2. Determine the exact diameter of the medullary canal by passing long-handled drills of varying sizes into the distal fragment until the one having the correct diameter is found; it should fit snugly in the canal but not tightly.

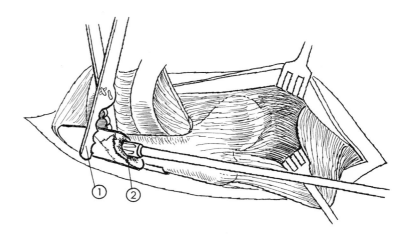

1. Then pass the drill into the medullary canal of the proximal fragment. If the canal is small, ream it out until it accommodates a nail at least 10 mm. in diameter.

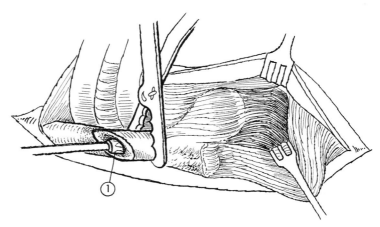

Operative Reduction and Fixation *(Continued)*

1. Now determine the correct length of the nail to be used. Pass a guide wire of known length down the medullary canal of the distal fragment until resistance of subchondral bone is encountered; note the length of the distal fragment.

2. Then pass the guide wire up the medullary canal of the proximal fragment until it abuts against cortical bone of the trochanter. Determine this length; the total of the two measurements minus 1 inch will give the correct length of the nail.

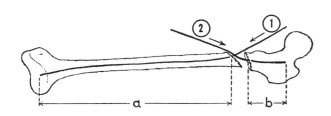

1. Make a small incision in the insertion of the gluteus medius muscle over the tip of the greater trochanter.

2. Insert a Kuntscher nail at the junction of the neck and trochanter through the medullary canal of the proximal fragment into the canal of the distal fragment. Place the open side of the nail on the convex side of the angulation.

3. Leave 2 to 2.5 cm. of the nail protruding above the tip of the greater trochanter.

Note: During insertion of the nail be sure that the alignment is maintained at all times as the nail is being driven through the canal of the distal fragment.

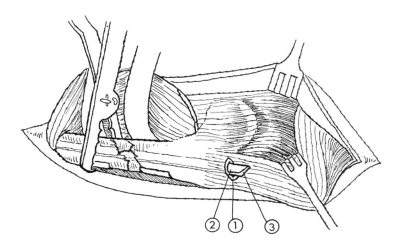

Postoperative Management

Place the extremity in balanced suspension for seven to ten days.

During this period encourage active flexion and extension of the knee just as soon as postoperative reaction permits. Take the leg out of the apparatus when the patient can actively raise the extended leg off the bed.

Warn the patient against the feeling of security provided by the nail.

Allow the patient out of bed on crutches without weight bearing on the leg at the end of the third week.

At the end of six weeks allow the patient weight bearing with crutches, keeping the knee stiff.

Crutches are not discarded until there is x-ray evidence of consolidation of the callus in the vicinity of the fracture, about 12 to 16 weeks.

Caution: Do not be fooled by the presence of exuberant callus, which does not enter into the union of the fragments and is eventually absorbed.

Healing may be slow and it may take months before consolidation is complete and union firm enough to permit unprotected weight bearing.

Extract the nail only when x-rays show complete obliteration of the fracture site. This rarely occurs under one year.

Progressive intensive exercises of the thigh, leg and foot muscles and graduated exercises at the knee joint must continue during the entire convalescent period.

Never manipulate the joint forcefully to increase its range of motion.

Alternate Method for Trochanteric Fractures

REMARKS

A conservative nonoperative method may be employed in those who refuse surgery or when surgery is contraindicated.

1. Place the limb in a Thomas splint with

2. Pearson attachment.

3. The limb and splint are in 45 degrees abduction.

4. The hip is flexed 30 degrees.

5. The limb and splint are supported by cords and weights a, b, c in such a manner that the limb is nicely balanced.

6. Traction grip on the leg is made by a threaded wire through the upper end of the tibia.

7. The foot of the bed is elevated for counter traction.

8. Foot strap supporting foot at 90 degrees dorsiflexion.

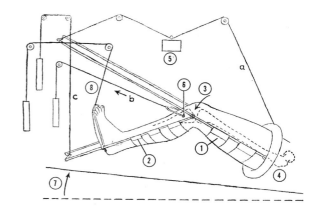

Postreduction Management

Traction is maintained until the fracture is united — 10 to 12 weeks. The apparatus should be checked several times daily.

Meticulous nursing care and bed management must be instituted during the traction period.

Insist on daily exercises of the ankle and knee on the affected side and general body exercises which can be executed in bed.

After union is solid as noted by x-ray, allow the patient up on crutches with protected weight bearing on the affected limb.

The patient should use crutches for three or four weeks.

Trochanteric Fractures in Children

REMARKS

Although rare, these lesions do occur in children and are occasionally complicated by avascular necrosis of the capital epiphysis.

No loss of neck angle can be accepted in children with trochanteric fractures because this is a permanent deformity; it does not correct itself with growth.

In children, a residual coxa vara deformity must be corrected by an angulation osteotomy.

Prereduction X-Ray

1. Intertrochanteric fracture.
2. The normal angle of the neck is decreased (coxa vara).

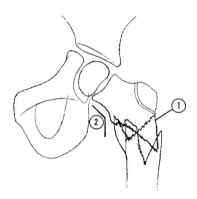

Reduction and Immobilization

1. Wide abduction will restore the normal neck-shaft angle.
2. Apply a plaster hip spica with the leg in wide abduction.

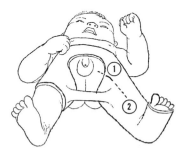

Management

Healing is usually complete at the fracture site in eight to ten weeks; now remove the plaster spica.

No special postimmobilization treatment is necessary except to allow the child free use of the limb.

Intertrochanteric Fractures in Children

REMARKS

Be sure that the coxa vara deformity, if present in the intertrochanteric fractures, is eliminated.

Generally, wide abduction of the limb will correct the deformity; if not, open reduction and fixation with a blade plate such as described for intertrochanteric fractures in adults is indicated.

Although rare, these lesions may be complicated by development of avascular necrosis of the caput or late osteochondral changes simulating coxa plana of the hip joint.

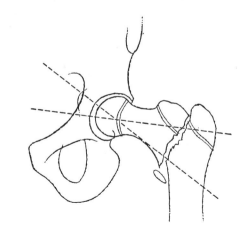

Prereduction X-Ray
(Intertrochanteric Fracture)

Intertrochanteric fracture with displacement and coxa vara deformity.

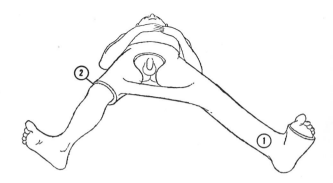

Reduction and Immobilization

Apply a bilateral leg plaster spica.
1. The affected limb is in wide abduction.
2. The plaster extends to just above the knee on the unaffected side.

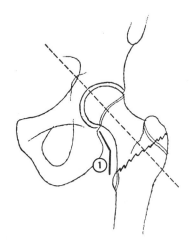

Postreduction X-Ray
(Intertrochanteric Fracture)

1. Coxa vara deformity is corrected.

Postreduction Management

Remove the cast after 10 to 12 weeks.
Check x-rays should show adequate union at the fracture site.
Allow protected weight bearing for two weeks on crutches.
Take check x-rays every three months and look for evidence of avascular necrosis of the caput and delayed osteochondral changes.

Subtrochanteric Fractures in Children

REMARKS

Subtrochanteric fractures may occur in very young and older children.

In young children slight angulation in the anteroposterior plane is acceptable because it straightens out with growth.

Coxa vara deformities resulting from trochanteric and subtrochanteric fractures do not disappear with growth; this deformity can and must be prevented by the initial treatment.

Overriding of fragments (bayonet apposition) is acceptable and even desirable provided alignment is good and no angulation exists.

Young children are best treated by double overhead traction.

Older children (over five or six years) are treated by Russell traction with acute flexion of the hip and knee and abduction of the limb.

Open reduction is never indicated in children.

Coxa vara deformity can be corrected only by a subtrochanteric osteotomy.

Reduction and Immobilization in Young Children (Under Five or Six Years)

1. Apply overhead traction to both limbs. Use a strip of foam rubber instead of adhesive plaster.
2. Use pulleys and weights but not fixed traction.
3. Weight should be sufficient to elevate the sacrum from the bed.
4. Always use a restraint.
5. Keep the legs well abducted.

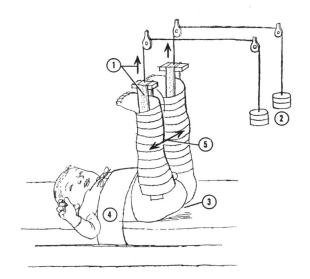

CAUTION

Make traction on the legs with strips of foam rubber secured by an elastic cotton bandage.

Don't apply the bandages too tightly because circulatory embarrassment may result.

Check the circulatory status of both limbs several times daily.

Cyanosis or pallor of the toes and swelling and pain indicate circulatory embarrassment. Take off the bandages immediately and inspect the leg.

Failure to observe these warnings may result in sloughs or ischemic necrosis, a tragic complication.

Management

Make frequent inspections of the limbs. Check for evidence of circulatory embarrassment.

If the circular bandages slip, rewrap the legs.

Maintain traction until callus is no longer tender—four to six weeks.

Then remove traction and keep the child in bed for another seven to ten days.

Now allow the child up on crutches (if of walking age), permitting partial weight bearing.

The crutches will be discarded voluntarily just as soon as the child is able to bear full weight on the affected limb with confidence.

No physical therapy is necessary.

Reduction and Immobilization
in Older Children
(Over Five or Six Years)

RUSSELL TRACTION
(MODIFIED BLOUNT)

1. Make continuous skin traction on the lower leg.

2. The knee is supported in a canvas sling lined with a sheet of foam rubber and suspended from an overhead beam.

3. Pulley system A makes traction in the line of the femur; pulley system B flexes the hip more acutely, which is essential in order to align the distal with the proximal fragment, which is held in flexion by the iliopsoas muscle.

4. The pillows should be high enough to hold the leg almost horizontal.

5. Generally 3 to 6 pounds of weight is sufficient (the pull distalward is twice the upward pull and the resultant pull is approximately in the line of the femur).

6. Abduct the leg 45 to 60 degrees.

7. Elevate the foot of the bed for counter traction.

8. The foot plate prevents rotation.

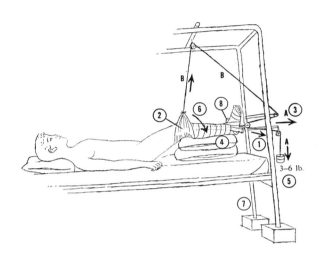

Management

Observe the same precautions relative to skin traction recorded on page 1268.

Check the traction apparatus several times daily and make necessary adjustments.

Check constantly for evidence of circulatory embarrassment.

Maintain the limb in traction until callus is no longer tender — six to eight weeks.

Now take the traction apparatus off and keep the child in bed one more week.

Allow the child up on crutches, permitting partial weight bearing.

Crutches will be discarded voluntarily just as soon as full weight can be borne on the limb with confidence.

No physical therapy is necessary.

Fractures of the Neck of the Femur

EPIDEMIOLOGY

The incidence of fractures of the neck of the femur increases as age increases; the highest incidence is between the ages of 70 and 80 years.

These lesions occur more frequently in women than in men, the ratio being approximately five to one. This is because there are more women in the aged population and also because alteration in the architecture of the upper end of the femur due to osteoporosis is more prevalent in women than in men. These lesions rarely occur in hips with osteoarthritis.

The average age of patients with these lesions is 72 years and that of patients with trochanteric fractures is 76 years.

Age is definitely related to the type of fracture sustained; fractures of the neck of the femur occur in the younger age group, whereas trochanteric fractures occur in the older; also, since more violence is needed to produce a fracture in the younger age group, these lesions are more frequently encountered in men.

Since the advent of internal fixation, the mortality rate of 60 to 85 per cent has been reduced to 8 to 10 per cent; however, the morbidity rate has climbed precipitously to 30 per cent, indicating that internal fixation is a lifesaving procedure.

Death is rarely caused by the fracture per se, but is the result of the many medical disorders which affect people in this advanced age group, such as cardiac disorders, pulmonary diseases, diabetes mellitus, cerebral thrombosis, hypertension and senile dementia.

The mortality rate over 60 years of age increases in each successive decade, reaching its peak in the ninth and tenth decades.

The prognosis is definitely better in men than in women; the highest incidence of failure occurs in women over 65 years of age.

The morbidity rate is closely related to the type of fracture; it is lower in Stage I and II fractures than in Stage III and IV fractures.

REMARKS

Conventional internal fixation has definitely increased the rate of union in impacted and undisplaced fractures (Stages I and II), but it has not significantly altered the results in displaced fractures (Stages III and IV).

For all fractures of the neck of the femur, the current methods of treatment yield a rate of union of 80 to 85 per cent; however, this does not convey the true picture because, if adequately fixed, nonunion rarely occurs in undisplaced and impacted fractures; in displaced fractures union is rarely achieved.

Treat all fractures of the neck of the femur by reduction and internal fixation; the poorer the general condition of the patient, the more urgent is early surgical intervention. This is a lifesaving procedure.

If the medical condition of the patient permits, perform the operative procedure immediately (under 12 hours from the time of injury). If for medical reasons the operation is contraindicated, every effort should be made to stabilize the patient within 24 hours. There is little to gain by delaying surgery longer.

By delaying the operation beyond 24 hours, greater comminution occurs at the fracture site and the damaged circulation of the femoral head is further compromised.

The incidence of union for fractures treated within the first 24 hours is far greater (80 per cent) than that for fractures treated after 48 hours (50 per cent).

All impacted valgus fractures should be fixed without disturbing the position of the fragments, providing the valgus deformity is not excessive; excessive valgus frequently results in aseptic necrosis of the head fragment. Although some impacted fractures heal without internal fixation, others fall apart, converting a relatively simple problem to a catastrophic one.

True transcervical fractures are indeed rare; neck fractures are usually of the subcapital type.

MECHANISM OF SUBCAPITAL FRACTURES OF THE NECK OF THE FEMUR

REMARKS

In the elderly and particularly in women, certain structural alterations occur in the upper end of the femur predisposing these persons to fractures of the neck of the femur. Because of loss of muscle tone and changes in the sense of balance, which are associated with aging, these persons are forced to change the pattern of their gait.

Change of gait is responsible for the rearrangement of the weight-bearing bony trabeculae of the upper end of the femur along the new lines of stress. This process together with senile osteoporosis produce weakening of the neck of the femur, which may result in dissolution of some of the bony trabeculae, in a line more or less perpendicular to the long axis of the neck starting superiorly at the junction of the head and neck; this is comparable to a fatigue or stress fracture.

If, as the result of vertical loading or a minor twist, the incomplete fracture becomes a complete fracture extending through the inferior cortex, the patient falls because of loss of support at the hip. He does not sustain the fracture because of the fall; the fracture comes first and next the fall.

Fractures may be produced by subjecting the weakened neck to vertical and rotational stresses acting simultaneously, such as when the extremity rotates externally and the body rotates in the opposite direction. In this mechanism the posterior aspect of the neck impinges on the rim of the acetabulum as it rotates posteriorly; the acetabulum now acts as a fulcrum. In young people this same mechanism is produced by major violence, fracturing the neck.

The obliquity of the fracture line as seen in anteroposterior x-rays of reduced fractures is essentially the same in all subcapital fractures; only rarely does this obliquity change. It begins on the superior aspect of the neck at the juncture of the head and neck and extends downward and outward until it encounters the inferior cortex of the neck. The difference noted in x-rays in the nature of the plane of the fracture is due to varying degrees of displacement of the fragments; such displacement primarily is caused by lateral rotation of the distal fragment.

Obliquity of the Fracture Line in Subcapital Fractures

1. Fracture line begins at the superior cervico-capital junction.

2. Fracture line extends obliquely through the neck to the inferior cortex.

3. Beak of the neck attached to the proximal fragment.

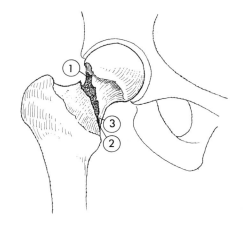

Note: Pauwels classified subcapital fractures according to the obliquity of the fracture line as noted in the anteroposterior x-rays of reduced fractures, as Types I, II and III. However, all these types can be produced in the same fracture by placing the distal fragment in varying degrees of lateral rotation; Types II and III correspond to marked increases in the amount of lateral rotation.

Occasionally a fall on the trochanter causes an impacted subcapital fracture; however, this mechanism usually produces trochanteric fractures.

The Role of Lateral Rotation of the Extremity in the Mechanism of Subcapital Fractures of the Neck of the Femur

1. The extremity rotates laterally.
2. The pelvis rotates in the opposite direction.
3. Tension force is applied at the anterior aspect of the neck as
4. Compression force is applied at the posterior aspect of the neck.
5. Incomplete fracture occurs perpendicular to the long axis of the neck.
6. The capital fragment is in slight valgus.

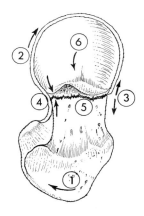

As the forces continue:
1. The fracture is completed and
2. The capital fragment is in normal position with the distal fragment.
3. The posterior neck is not comminuted.
4. The posterior retinaculum (retinaculum of Westbrecht) is intact.

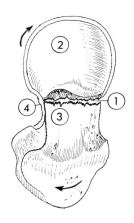

With further external rotation of the extremity:
1. The femoral head rotates medially and in abduction.
2. The extremity rotates laterally.
3. The fracture line opens anteriorly.
4. The posterior cortex is compressed at the fracture line but not collapsed.
5. The posterior retinaculum is still intact and the fragments are not detached.

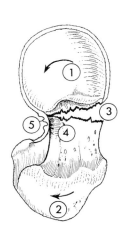

Page 1273

The Role of Lateral Rotation of the Extremity in the Mechanism of Subcapital Fractures of the Neck of the Femur (Continued)

With further external rotation of the extremity and complete displacement and detachment of the fragments:

1. The extremity is in full external rotation.

2. The distal fragment is displaced upward by muscular action.

3. The head returns to its normal position in the acetabulum and assumes a varus position in relation to the neck.

4. The neck fragment lies anterior to the head.

5. Complete collapse of the posterior cortex with separation of a large triangular fragment from the postero-inferior cortex adjacent to the head.

6. The posterior retinaculum is disrupted, permitting complete detachment of the fragments.

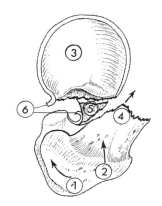

CLASSIFICATION OF SUBCAPITAL FRACTURES OF THE NECK OF THE FEMUR

Garden has provided us with a simple and logical classification based on the varying stages of displacement as noted on x-rays before reduction. There are four stages of fracture, from I to IV. This classification also provides information concerning the degree of disruption of the posterior and inferior cortex and whether or not the posterior retinaculum is intact (in this structure are situated the main blood vessels going to the femoral head) and is helpful in the assessment of the prognosis of the different fractures.

Stage I (Incomplete Subcapital Fracture)

1. Incomplete fracture of the neck.
2. External rotation of the distal fragment.
3. The proximal fragment is in valgus.
4. The medial bony trabeculae of the head make an angle greater than 180 degrees with the medial cortex of the femur.

Note: This anteroposterior x-ray view gives the impression that the fracture is impacted; this is not true – lateral rotation of the distal fragment produces this radiographic illusion. If this fracture is not fixed in this position it may become a complete fracture and assume the features of the fractures of Stage II, III or IV, depending upon the degree of external rotation of the distal fragment.

This is a stable fracture with a good prognosis.

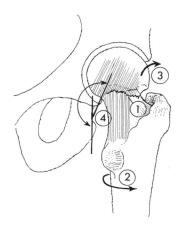

Stage II (Complete Subcapital Fracture Without Displacement)

1. Complete oblique fracture through the neck.
2. The capital fragment is not displaced.
3. The distal fragment is in normal alignment with the proximal fragment.
4. The medial trabeculae of the head make an angle of approximately 160 degrees with the medial femoral cortex.

Note: Lateral rotation of the distal fragment may cause displacement of the fragments, thus producing a fracture of Stage III or IV.

The posterior cortex of the femur is still not collapsed and the posterior retinaculum is intact.

This is a stable fracture with a good prognosis.

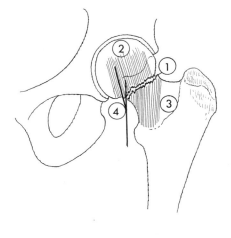

Stage III (Complete Subcapital Fracture with Partial Displacement)

1. The distal fragment is rotated laterally.

2. The proximal fragment is tilted into varus and rotated medially.

3. The medial trabeculae of the head are not in alignment with those of the pelvis.

Note: The posterior cortex of the neck is not collapsed; the posterior retinaculum is still intact holding the fragments together, but this may be injured.

Further lateral rotation of the distal fragment will convert this lesion to a Stage IV fracture.

This fracture, if properly reduced, can be converted to a stable fracture with a good prognosis.

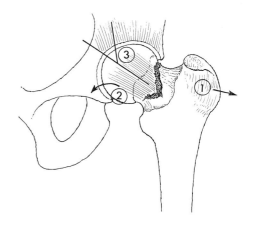

Stage IV (Complete Subcapital Fracture with Full Displacement)

1. The capital fragment is completely detached from the distal fragment and has returned to its normal position in the acetabulum; its medial trabeculae now are in alignment with those of the pelvis.

2. The distal fragment is rotated laterally.

3. The distal fragment is displaced upward and anterior to the proximal fragment.

Note: The posterior cortex of the neck has collapsed and the posterior retinaculum is stripped or torn from the posterior aspect of the neck.

This fracture is difficult to reduce perfectly; and even if the reduction is achieved, the defect in the posterior cortex renders it unstable. The prognosis is poor.

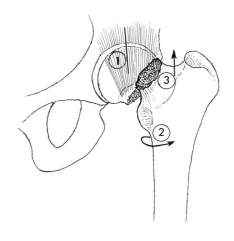

Page 1276

PERTINENT ANATOMIC FEATURES OF THE HEAD AND NECK OF THE FEMUR

REMARKS

The anterior surface of the femoral neck is convex and the head of the femur overhangs the posteroinferior portion of the neck.

In elderly people the flared posteroinferior juncture of the head and neck is thin and friable. When subjected to compression forces it readily crumbles. However, the type of lesion produced is fairly constant: a triangular piece of bone separates from the posteroinferior surface of the neck at its point of union with the head producing a collapse of the posterior cortex.

This defect in the posterior and inferior cortices is responsible for the instability of subcapital fractures in the Stage IV category. This fracture is difficult to reduce and, even if anatomic reduction is achieved, the defect in the posterior cortex still persists, rendering the reduced fracture unstable.

In fractures of the neck of the femur in the Stage IV category, anatomic reduction does not mean that the fracture is stable.

Lateral View of the Upper End of the Femur

1. Anterior convexity of the neck of the femur.
2. Overhang of the femoral head over the posteroinferior cortex of the neck.

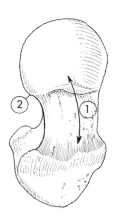

Collapse of the Posteroinferior Cortex of the Neck in Stage IV Fracture

1. The distal fragment is in full lateral rotation.
2. Compression of the posterior cortex results in comminution of the cortex with separation of a triangular piece of bone.

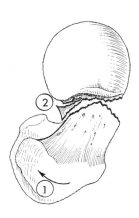

Page 1277

The weight-bearing trabeculae of the head, neck and pelvis lie in line with the pathways of stress.

In subcapital fractures a change in the relationship of the weight-bearing trabeculae in the pelvis, head and neck indicates fairly accurately the relationship of the proximal fragment to the distal fragment.

In the anteroposterior view the medial trabeculae of the head make an angle of approximately 160 degrees with the medial cortex of the femur.

In the lateral view the medial and lateral trabeculae of the head converge and intersect on a straight line running through the center of the neck. Hence, the normal anteroposterior-lateral arrangement of the weight-bearing trabeculae of the head and neck can be expressed as 160/180 (Garden).

Clinical experience reveals that the acceptable limits of malposition, with regard to both union and avascular necrosis, lie between an alignment index of 155/180 in the anteroposterior view and 180/155 in the lateral x-ray view.

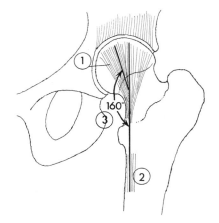

Anteroposterior X-Ray — Normal Anteroposterior Alignment

1. Medial trabeculae of the head.
2. Medial cortex of the femur.
3. These make an angle of approximately 160 degrees.

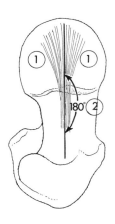

Lateral X-Ray — Normal Lateral Alignment

1. Medial and lateral trabeculae intersect on
2. A straight line running through the center of the neck — 180 degrees.

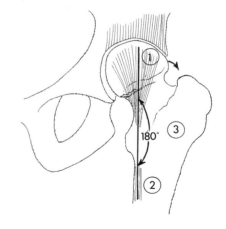

Capital Fragment in Valgus

1. Medial trabeculae of the head.
2. Medial cortex of the femur.
3. These make an angle of 180 degrees.

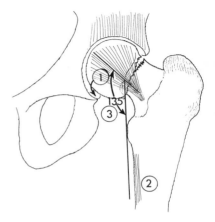

Capital Fragment in Varus

1. Medial trabeculae of the head.
2. Medial cortex of the femur.
3. These make an angle of 135 degrees.

CIRCULATION OF THE HEAD OF THE FEMUR

REMARKS

The main circulation of the femoral head is derived from three sources:

1. The lateral epiphyseal vessels, which are branches of the posterolateral retinacular vessels. These supply the greater portion of the head; it is estimated that they are the most constant and supply approximately two-thirds of the head. They are found on the posterosuperior aspect of the neck and enter the bone just distal to its articular surface at an angle of 45 degrees. These are in a most vulnerable position and probably are injured or ruptured in most displaced subcapital fractures.

2. The inferior metaphyseal vessels. These are branches of the posteromedial retinacular arteries. They supply that portion of the head derived from the metaphysis. Like the lateral epiphyseal arteries, they most likely are severed in fully displaced subcapital fractures.

3. Artery of the ligamentum teres, a branch of the obturator artery. It penetrates the head at the fovea capitis. This source is not very significant in the total blood supply of the head; in some instances it may be absent. When present, except in rare instances, it does not freely anastomose with the lateral epiphyseal and inferior metaphyseal vessels, but rather it is confined to a small area of bone immediately adjacent to the fovea capitis comprising approximately 10 per cent of volume of the head. Although this source of blood supply is insignificant under normal conditions, its role gains in importance when the head is rendered ischemic following subcapital fractures. This source is the only hope for revascularization of the head.

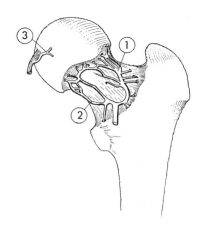

Blood Supply of the Femoral Head

1. Lateral epiphyseal arteries.
2. Inferior metaphyseal arteries.
3. Artery of the ligamentum teres.

PATHOLOGY OF SUBCAPITAL FRACTURES

REMARKS

Following subcapital fracture, the fate of the head depends in a large measure upon the extent to which its circulation is impaired. The degree of displacement of the fragments decides the severity of the impairment.

In undisplaced fractures it can be assumed that the circulation is intact; in partially displaced fractures the posterolateral retinacular vessels are preserved in most instances, but in fully displaced fractures these vessels are ruptured and, depending upon the adequacy of the foveal vessels, ischemia of the femoral head ensues in varying degrees.

X-ray evidence is unreliable for determination of the presence of avascular necrosis of the head until there is redisplacement of the fracture following fixation or the development of segmental collapse of the weight-bearing surface of the head.

Histologic examination indicates that partial or total ischemic necrosis of the head occurs in approximately two-thirds of the displaced fractures (Cato).

Although a valgus position of the head insures stability of subcapital fractures, extreme valgus (over 180 degrees) causes torsion and obliteration of the foveal vessels, destroying, in displaced fractures, the only remaining blood supply to the head.

Rotation of the femoral head in any plane (vertical, coronal or sagittal) may similarly affect the foveal vessels.

Revascularization of the head in displaced fractures depends upon patent foveal vessels (if present) and occasionally upon some of the inferior metaphyseal vessels which may be spared.

The contribution that the neck makes toward revascularization of the head is negligible.

Other factors may comprise the circulation of the head:
1. Unwise and forceful manipulative maneuvers may sever the remaining intact vessels.
2. Long delays before reduction may cause thrombosis of kinked vessels or allow a nondisplaced or partially displaced fracture to become a fully displaced fracture, thereby rupturing the remaining intact posterior retinacular vessels. Displaced fractures treated in the first 24 hours have a higher incidence of union than fractures treated after 48 hours. If possible, the fracture should be reduced and fixed within 12 hours after injury.
3. The foveal vessels may be injured by appliances (nails, pins and screws) penetrating the fovea capitis.

Avascular necrosis is not a deterrent to bony union, providing the fracture is adequately reduced and stabilized by rigid fixation.

In displaced fractures, total ischemic necrosis is sure to occur if the foveal vessels are not capable of revascularizing the head. Nevertheless, with adequate reduction and fixation bony union does occur; but revascularization across the fracture line from the neck is slow and often comes to a stop long before complete revascularization of the head can occur. Late segmental collapse occurs in approximately one-third of these cases and is caused by collapse of the necrotic trabeculae in the weight-bearing sector of the head; this sequela may not occur for two to three years after the injury but may occur earlier.

Nonunion definitely increases the incidence of avascular necrosis; it occurs in approximately 60 per cent of the cases of nonunion.

The incidence of nonunion and ischemic necrosis is directly related to the degree of the original displacement, not withstanding the type of treatment instituted; in both, the dominant factor is the impairment of the blood supply to the head.

Although in some cases ischemic necrosis may not become evident by x-ray for two to three years, its presence can often be detected long before this period by visible flattening of the head in its weight-bearing sector.

Flattening of Head (Forerunner of Segmental Collapse)

1. Fracture line.
2. Flattening of weight-bearing area of the head (seen as early as six months).

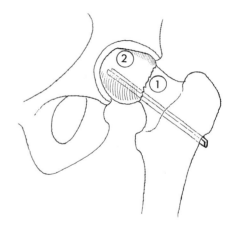

Segmental Collapse

1. Fracture line almost obliterated.
2. Segmental collapse (may occur as late as three years).

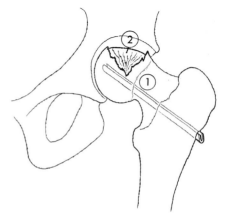

NATURE OF THE FRACTURE

In displaced fractures comminution and collapse of the posterior wall occurs in approximately 60 per cent.

An intact posterior wall, such as seen in Stage I and II fractures, prevents redisplacement of the femoral head after reduction because it functions as a buttress against posterior rotation of the head.

In fully displaced fractures a posterior buttress is absent; only the anterior fracture surfaces are in contact. Therefore, the head can, and in many instances does, rotate posteriorly as the distal fragment rotates laterally. This occurs even when the reduction and internal fixation are adequate; it occurs in one-third of the cases.

Traction and marked internal rotation may restore anatomic alignment; but, just as soon as traction is released, the fracture collapses because of the lack of a posterior bridge.

Adequate realignment of the fragments may be perfect, but this does not provide stability. Reduction does not mean stability in fully displaced fractures (Stage IV).

On the other hand, fixation of an unreduced fracture invariably results in nonunion.

There are some methods available to us which will provide stability in some undisplaced fractures, but no one method has as yet evolved which is applicable to all displaced fractures.

Each displaced fracture must be studied individually and that method of treatment should be chosen which will meet the challenge of the particular fracture.

Some displaced fractures defy all methods of conventional treatment; this is especially true when there is complete disruption of the posterior bridge and the head is rotated. Traction and manipulative maneuvers of the distal fragment are unable to derotate the head into a normal position. There may be interpositioning of the capsule between the fragments, or a spike of bone on the head may pierce the capsule preventing reduction, or there may be so much comminution of the neck that anatomic reduction is impossible.

Traction Applied to a Displaced Fracture

1. Traction and
2. Internal rotation realigns the fragments.
3. Posterior wall is defective and provides no stability.
4. Fracture surfaces are apposed only on the anterior aspect of the neck.

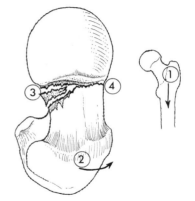

When Traction is Released

1. Traction is released.
2. Capital fragment rolls posteriorly off the neck.
3. Collapse of the posterior wall.

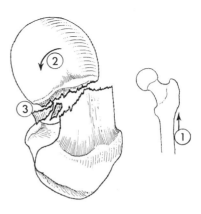

When a Displaced Fracture is Reduced and Fixed

1. Nail holds the fragments in alignment.

2. Only the surfaces on the anterior aspect are in contact.

3. Collapse of the posterior wall.

Note: This is an unstable fracture in spite of adequate reduction and fixation. The natural tendency for the limb to go into a position of lateral rotation will eventually cause redisplacement of the fragments.

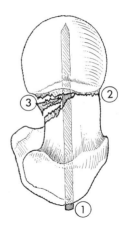

4. The distal fragment rotates laterally.

5. The proximal fragment rotates posteriorly.

6. Tip of nail cuts through the head.

7. The posterior wall collapses.

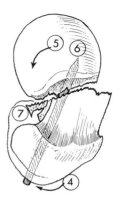

MECHANICAL CONSIDERATIONS IN THE TREATMENT OF SUBCAPITAL FRACTURES

REMARKS

Fractures in the Stage I and II categories are stable and offer no difficulty in management; any of the conventional methods of internal fixation will provide adequate splintage until bony union is achieved. This is also true of fractures in Stage III, providing the posterior wall has not collapsed and the posterior hinge (the posterior retinaculum) is intact.

Stage IV fractures in which there is a tear of the posterior retinaculum and a collapse of the posterior wall demand special consideration because reduction in most instances can be obtained, but it is difficult to maintain with most of the conventional appliances in use today.

The severity of the obliquity of the plane of the fracture in these lesions (which corresponds to Pauwels' Type II and Type III and to Garden's Stage III and Stage IV) is not the basic reason for failure. If these fractures can be reduced, and if the fixation is rigid enough to resist the gravitational and muscular forces pulling the extremity into lateral rotation, and if the appliance has a firm grip on both fragments, bony union will result as readily as in the Pauwels' Type I or Garden's Stage I and II fractures.

When the fragments are adequately reduced and rigidly fixed, no absorption takes place at the fracture line during healing.

So called absorption at the fracture line and settling of the proximal fragment indicate motion and instability; they are caused by further collapse of the posterior cortex and redisplacement of the fragments.

The amount of comminution of the posterior surface of the neck varies and, in some fractures, precludes accurate reduction with stability. The greater the amount of comminution, the higher is the incidence of nonunion.

Following accurate reduction and internal fixation, settling of the head without tilting may be desirable, providing there is no comminution, because it permits the head to find and to settle in a more stable position on the neck. This is possible only if the appliance has a firm grip on the proximal fragment and will allow the head to settle. Some appliances, such as the sliding nail, are designed to perform this function; the Smith-Petersen nail and multiple pins, if placed parallel, also permit settling of the head by backing out of the neck. On the other hand, screws and fixed angle nail-plates will hold the fragments apart.

Failure in unstable fractures is caused by inadequate reduction and lack of rigid internal fixation.

Stability may be restored in some fractures by one of the following procedures: (1) telescoping the neck into the head, (2) taking a small wedge of bone from the anterosuperior part of the neck, thereby permitting the head to settle on the broad surface of the neck, and (3) placing the nail or pins in the posteroinferior quadrant of the head so that the forces of lateral rotation are resisted by the large number of bony trabeculae lying in front of the nail.

Impacted fractures in the position of valgus will heal readily regardless of the type of internal fixation employed; however, if the valgus position of the head is excessive (when the medial trabeculae of the head make an angle of over 180 degrees with the medial cortex of the femur) avascular necrosis will develop in 80 per cent of the cases. This is caused by impairment of the blood supply. An excessive valgus position or a rotational deformity of the head obliterates the foveal vessels in the ligamentum teres. A rotational deformity is difficult to detect on x-ray; if it occurs together with a valgus deformity of the head, avascular necrosis ensues in the majority of the cases.

Impaction of the head in a position of varus is a rare lesion; when it occurs the deformity must be corrected or nonunion or avascular necrosis is sure to occur.

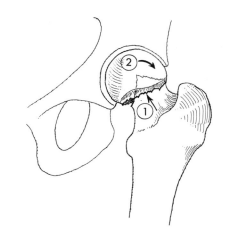

Method to Stabilize the Head on the Neck

1. Telescope the neck into the head.
2. Head should be in only slight valgus.

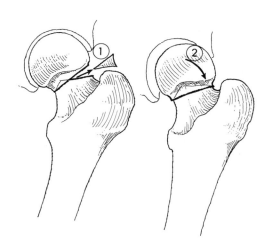

1. Remove a small wedge from the anterosuperior portion of the neck.
2. Place the head in slight valgus.

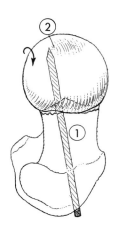

1. Insert a low nail so that it lies in the cortex of the calcar.
2. The end of the nail is in the posteroinferior quadrant.

METHODS OF INTERNAL FIXATION

REMARKS

The goal of internal fixation is to fix and hold rigidly both fragments until bony union is achieved.

The appliance used should be capable of resisting all forces directed to the fracture site; these include bending, torsional and shearing forces. The greatest force is that of lateral rotation: the natural tendency of the extremity is to roll out into lateral rotation.

Any form of fixation which permits a change of position of the fragments, such as settling of the head, fails to provide rigid fixation; any evidence of a change in the relation of the head and neck indicates instability and is the forerunner of nonunion.

The Smith-Petersen nail used in the conventional manner fails to provide rigid fixation in displaced fractures. It does prevent lateral rotation of the head on the long axis of the neck, but it fails to prevent lateral rotation of the head in the more vertical mechanical axis of the femur. It has only a two-point fixation, one in the center of the head and the other in the thin friable cortex immediately below the greater trochanter, and it lies in the cancellous bone of the neck. It is not capable of resisting the forces of lateral rotation acting at the fracture; therefore, the head may roll off the neck and the nail may cut through the head or it may extrude.

The low angle nail provides better fixation than the Smith-Petersen nail; it has a three-point fixation, one in the thick lamellar cortex on the lateral aspect of the femur, one in the dense cortex of the calcar and one deep in the posteroinferior quadrant of the head, if so placed. In this low position the nail lies in the pathway of longitudinal loading and hence takes less stress. Its position in the posteroinferior quadrant of the head places a maximum number of bony trabeculae in front of the nail to oppose the forces of lateral rotation. Fixation may be further enhanced by the use of a side plate. However, a side plate will prevent settling of the head and, if used, one must assume that fixation of the fragments is so rigid that no motion whatever will occur at the fracture site during the healing process.

A sliding nail with a side plate will allow the head to settle but, if used, one must admit that the fixation is not rigid and allows motion at the fracture site. In some uncomminuted fractures, this feature of the sliding nail is advantageous because it permits the head to find a more stable position on the neck.

Multiple pins may also be used in the same manner that the low nail is employed. If the displaced fracture has been converted to a stable fracture, such as when the neck is telescoped into the head or if a small wedge is removed from the anterosuperior portion of the neck, the pins will provide maximum rigid fixation.

Absorption at the fracture site is really, in most instances, an x-ray illusion caused by displacement of the fragments; it can be detected in the anteroposterior x-rays by telescoping of the neck into the head, providing the head is in the valgus position, or by a varus position of the head and external rotation of the femur.

In the lateral views it is indicated by redisplacement of the fragments and shortening of the posterior surface of the neck and extrusion of the nail (or the nail may be cut through the head or penetrate the joint if a side plate is used).

MANAGEMENT OF FRACTURES OF THE NECK OF THE FEMUR

Immediate Management

Treatment of fractures of the neck of the femur begins just as soon as possible following the injury.

Protect the limb from all motion; this is most essential because unwise handling of the patient may convert a simple undisplaced fracture to a complicated displaced fracture.

Take x-rays in the anteroposterior and lateral views; while this is being done, an assistant should make gentle traction on the limb to prevent further trauma to the fracture site.

The x-rays must be of excellent quality in order to properly evaluate the nature of the fracture.

Apply some form of skin traction to the extremity.

Evaluate the medical condition of the patient.

Make the necessary arrangements for reduction and fixation of the fracture.

Correct all medical deficiencies; reduction and internal fixation in some of these elderly people may be a lifesaving procedure.

During this preliminary period don't disturb the limb; prepare the operative area in the operating room.

If at all possible, perform the reduction and fixation of the fracture within the first 12 hours and not later than 24 hours; remember that the incidence of nonunion is definitely lower in patients operated on in the first 12 hours than in those operated on after 48 hours.

MANAGEMENT OF IMPACTED ABDUCTION FRACTURES AND UNDISPLACED SUBCAPITAL AND TRANSCERVICAL FRACTURES

REMARKS

All impacted abduction fractures should be fixed; it is true that some impacted fractures heal without internal fixation, but it is also true that some fall apart. If the valgus deformity is severe (over 180 degrees) the impaction should be broken up and the fragments realigned.

Handle undisplaced fractures with great care in order to prevent displacement of the fragments.

If these fractures are adequately fixed, bony union should be achieved in 100 per cent of the cases. For these fractures I prefer the use of three Knowles pins, two of which lie in the thick lamellar bone of the calcar.

Preoperative X-Ray of Impacted Valgus Fracture

1. Fracture line.
2. Head is in slight valgus. (The angle that the medial trabeculae of the head makes with the lateral cortex of the femur must not exceed 180 degrees.)
3. Head sits squarely on the neck in the lateral view.

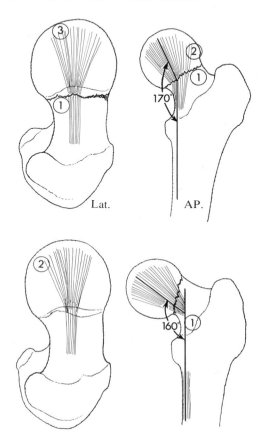

Preoperative X-Ray of Undisplaced Fracture

ANTEROPOSTERIOR VIEW

1. The medial trabeculae of the head make an angle of 160 degrees with the lateral cortex of the femur.
2. Head sits squarely on the neck in the lateral view.

Procedure—Internal Fixation

1. Place the patient on a fracture table in the supine position.
2. Secure the unaffected limb to the foot stirrup in 45 degrees of abduction and neutral rotation.
3. Secure the foot of the affected leg to the foot stirrup with the leg in 20 degrees abduction, neutral flexion and extension and the patella pointing directly upward.

Now take anteroposterior and lateral views to determine whether or not any displacement of the fragment has occurred. If not, continue with the following procedure.

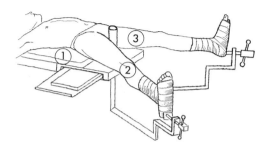

Insertion of Guide Pins

1. Make a 4 inch incision on the lateral aspect of the thigh just below the greater trochanter and centered on the shaft of the femur.

2. Deepen the incision to the bone and by subperiosteal dissection expose the base of the trochanter and the upper end of the femur for approximately 3 inches.

3. Three-quarters to 1 inch below the bony ridge at the lower margin of the greater trochanter and midway between the anterior and posterior cortices of the femur in the lateral cortex, drill a hole 3/16 of an inch in diameter and directed at an angle of approximately 45 degrees with the lateral cortex.

4. Pass a guide pin, 2.5 mm. in diameter, into the neck and head. The pin is directed at an angle of 45 degrees with the shaft and parallel to the floor. Insert the pin gently and slowly until resistance of the subchondral bone of the femoral head is encountered (usually a distance of 3¾ to 4 inches).

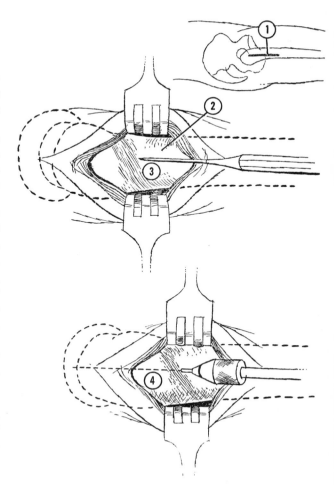

CAUTION

Only minimal resistance is felt as the pin traverses the femoral neck. Undue resistance means that the pin is striking one of the cortices of the neck. The pin should be placed so that it lies in the center of the head and neck of the femur.

Now measure the length of the pin protruding from the shaft and subtract this from a pin of equal length (9 inches); this will determine the amount in the neck and head of the femur.

Note: The purpose of introducing a guide pin across the fracture site before inserting the Knowles pins is two-fold: (1) to determine the exact length of the pins needed and (2) to determine the correct neck-shaft angle at which to insert the pins. The pins should be long enough to engage the subchondral bone of the head (⅛ to ¼ inch from the articular surface).

X-Ray

(Take both anteroposterior and lateral views.)

1. Pin lies in the center of the neck and head.

2. Pin makes an angle of 45 degrees with the shaft. This is the desired angle.

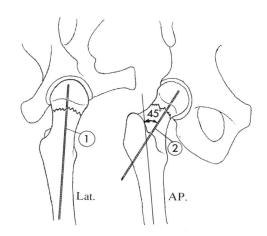

Insertion of Knowles Pins

After extracting the guide pin and determining the exact length of the pin required:

1. Insert the first Knowles pin. Insert the pin slowly and follow the track made by the guide pin.

2. Select two points on the lateral aspect of the femur 1⅞ to 2 inches below the bony ridge at the lower margin of the greater trochanter and just inside the anterior and posterior surfaces of the neck. At each point drill a ³/₁₆ inch hole partly through the lateral cortex of the femur and directed obliquely upward.

3. Place an angle guide, set at 150 degrees, opposite the drill holes and make a drill channel at the set angle for 2 to 3 inches up the neck of the femur.

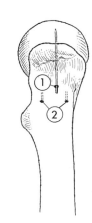

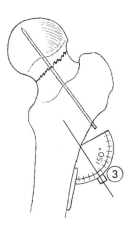

Insertion of Knowles Pins
(Continued)

4. Remove the angle guide and insert Knowles pins following the drill channels.

Note: The length of the second and third Knowles pin is readily determined by studying the x-rays made after the insertion of the guide pin; as a rule, the length is ¾ inch more than the length of the first Knowles pin inserted.

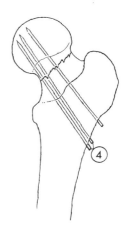

Postoperative X-Rays

ANTEROPOSTERIOR VIEW

1. The two lower pins lie close to the calcar and are directed at an angle of 150 degrees.
2. The upper pin lies in the center of the head and neck.

LATERAL VIEW

3. Each pin is inserted at one angle of a triangle.
4. The lower pins are close to the anterior and posterior surfaces of the neck.

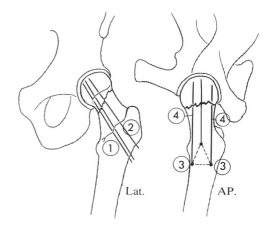

Lat.   AP.

Postreduction Management

Allow the patient out of bed in a wheel chair on the second day.

Insist on frequent changes in position.

Institute active exercises of the hip and knee just as soon as pain and soreness of the limb subside. Particular attention should be given to the quadriceps of both limbs.

On the affected side, the patient should be able to raise the extended leg off the bed unassisted.

The patient must avoid extremes of motion in adduction and abduction.

When possible, teach the patient to walk with the aid of a walker and then on crutches without weight bearing on the affected limb.

If this is not possible, insist that the patient get into a wheel chair and get about unassisted in it.

Check the prognosis of healing by x-ray at six week intervals.

Weight bearing with crutches is allowed when definite evidence of bony union is present, usually at the end of 12 to 16 weeks.

Usually at the end of six months union is sufficiently strong to permit unprotected weight bearing.

Never remove the pins unless there is a definite indication such as protrusion into the acetabulum, extrusion of the pins or if the pin heads irritate the trochanteric area.

Never remove pins until there is x-ray evidence of bony union, and this cannot be determined for certainty under one year.

MANAGEMENT OF PARTIALLY DISPLACED (STAGE III) AND FULLY DISPLACED (STAGE IV) FRACTURES

REMARKS

Whereas bony union is the rule after internal fixation of impacted abduction and undisplaced fractures, failure of union is a common sequela of displaced fractures. Failure of union is also far more common in the fully displaced fracture (Stage IV) than in the partially displaced fracture (Stage III).

Nonunion is caused by failure to achieve adequate reduction and rigid fixation of the displaced fracture.

Anatomic reduction is not adequate or desirable in displaced fractures because it does not produce stability.

When the posteroinferior wall of the neck has collapsed, the forces of external rotation are unopposed and redisplacement of the fragments occurs.

If stability can be achieved, then these fractures should heal as readily as undisplaced fractures.

In order to restore stability the defect on the posteroinferior cortex must be neutralized. This may be accomplished by placing the proximal fragment in a position of slight valgus and telescoping the neck into the proximal fragment, thereby obliterating the defect. Now the forces acting on the fracture site are in equilibrium.

This same effect may be achieved by removing a small wedge of bone from the anterosuperior portion of the neck and allowing the head to sit squarely on the neck in slight valgus. Both these procedures shorten the neck of the femur but this is a small price to pay for bony union of a displaced fracture.

Many appliances have been designed to provide rigid internal fixation and to resist the forces leading to redisplacement. However, critical analysis of these appliances reveals that the only ones that are really effective are those which utilize the principles of low angle fixation plus impaction of the fragments at the time of operation. This applies to multiple pin fixation and to sliding nails.

One must admit that there are some displaced fractures that resist all methods to produce stability at the fracture site.

I prefer to treat all displaced fractures by open operation.

This affords the opportunity to study the nature of the fracture and institute those measures which will reestablish stability of the fragments. My preferences are, first, placing the head in slight valgus and telescoping the neck into the head, and second, removing a wedge of bone from the anterosuperior surface of the neck.

My other reasons for preferring open operation to blind fixation are:

1. In many instances it is impossible to seat the capital fragment in the optimum position in relation to the distal fragment by manipulative maneuvers; this has been observed many times at open operation.

2. Forceful and repeated attempts at reduction cause further comminution of the neck.

3. The interposition of portions of the fibrous capsule between the fragments, preventing reduction, is more frequent than generally appreciated.

4. Visualization of the fracture site through a longitudinal incision in the anterior portion of the capsule does not cause further impairment of the blood supply to the femoral head.

Preoperative X-Ray—Partially Displaced Fracture

1. The capital fragment is in a position of varus.

2. The distal fragment is rotated laterally.

3. The medial trabeculae of the head make an angle of 135 degrees with the medial surface of the femur.

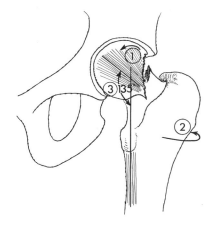

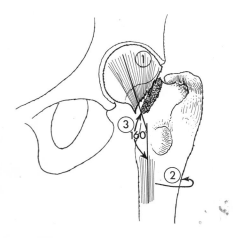

Preoperative X-Ray—Fully Displaced Fracture

1. The capital fragment is in its normal position in the acetabulum.

2. The distal fragment is fully rotated laterally.

3. The medial trabeculae of the head make an angle of 160 degrees with the medial cortex of the femur.

Open Reduction and Internal Fixation

1. The patient is in the supine position and the affected limb is draped separately.

2. Place a sandbag under the affected hip.

3. Beginning at the anterosuperior spine, make a 5 inch incision in the interval between the tensor fasciae latae and the sartorius muscles; then the incision curves sharply posteriorly over the lateral aspect of the femur. Divide the deep fascia in the line of the incision.

4. Incise the fascia lata between the tensor fasciae latae and the sartorius muscles and develop the interval between the two muscles.

5. In line with the horizontal limb of the skin incision, divide transversely the tensor fasciae latae muscle and reflect it laterally. This exposes the subtrochanteric area.

6. In the midportion of the wound, expose the ascending branch of the lateral femoral circumflex artery; cut it between forceps and ligate it.

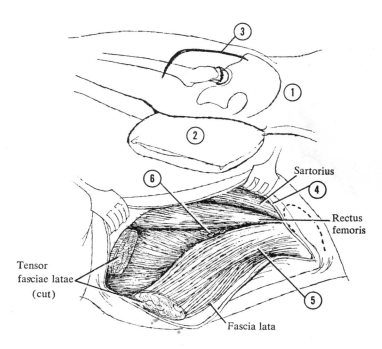

Sartorius

Rectus femoris

Tensor fasciae latae (cut)

Fascia lata

Page 1295

Open Reduction and Internal Fixation (Continued)

1. Divide the reflected head of the rectus muscle and displace it medially.

2. Clear away the fatty layer in front of the hip joint; this exposes the anterior aspect of the capsule.

3. Make a T-shaped incision in the capsule.

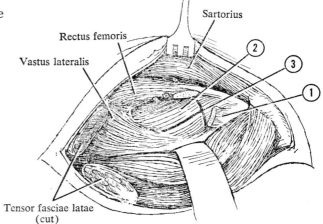

Sartorius

Rectus femoris

Vastus lateralis

② ③ ①

Tensor fasciae latae (cut)

1. Retract the edges of the capsule and visualize the fracture.

Note: At this point determine whether or not the posterior cortex is crushed. In fractures with only partial displacement, the posterior retinaculum is intact (Stage III) and the fracture is a clean break through the neck without comminution. This fracture can readily be converted into a stable fracture by internal rotation of the limb.

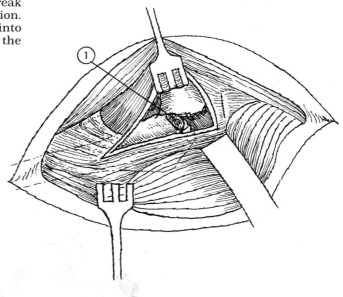

WHEN THERE IS ONLY PARTIAL DISPLACEMENT OF THE FRAGMENTS (STAGE III)

1. With the patient's hip and knee extended, an assistant steadies the limb but makes no traction on the leg.

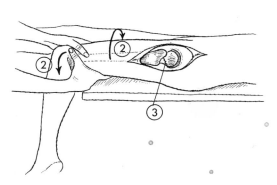

Next
2. Assistant rotates the extremity internally and flexes the knee to 90 degrees. Now
3. The fragments are in normal relation to one another and the fracture is now stable.

Note: Don't perform unnecessary forceful maneuvers. This may cause a collapse of the posterior wall and a tear in the posterior retinaculum.

If on the fractured surfaces there are some serrations which prevent internal rotation, gently lever the fragments into position with a small curette.

A few degrees of valgus of the head will increase the stability of the fracture. This is achieved by:

4. Making moderate traction on the extended, externally rotated and adducted leg while some inward pressure is made over the greater trochanter. Follow this by
5. Abduction of the limb and then release of the traction on the limb with flexion of the knee to 90 degrees.

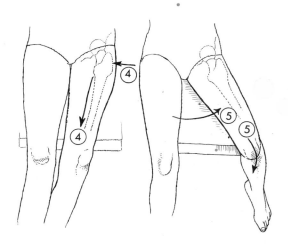

While an assistant holds the leg in slight abduction and internal rotation:

1. Make a 3 inch vertical incision in the vastus lateralis muscle immediately below the base of the greater trochanter and by subperiosteal dissection expose the lateral cortex of the femur.

2. About ¾ to 1 inch below the bony ridge at the lower margin of the greater trochanter and about ⅜ inch on either side of the midline of the lateral cortex, drill two holes in the lateral cortex ³/₁₆ inch in diameter and directed upward at an angle of approximately 45 degrees with the lateral cortex.

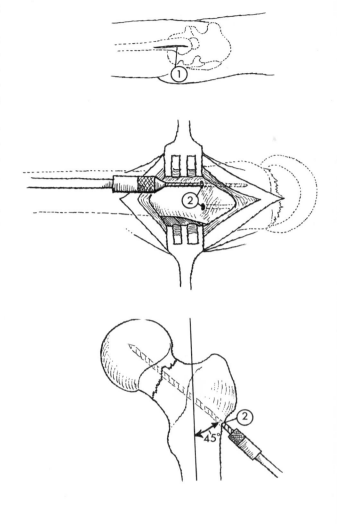

3. Pass guide pins, 2.5 mm. in diameter, into the neck and head. The pins are directed at 45 degrees with the shaft of the femur, parallel to the floor and parallel to one another. Insert the pins slowly until the subcortical bone of the head is encountered. Now determine the desired length of the pins by subtracting the length of the pin protruding from the shaft from a pin of equal length (9 inches).

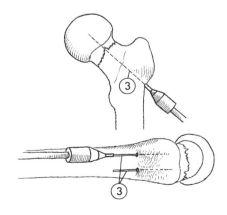

Check position of pins with x-rays. (Both anteroposterior and lateral views are required.)

1. Pins lie in the neck and head and reach the subcortical bone.

2. Pins make an angle of 45 degrees with the shaft and are parallel to each other.

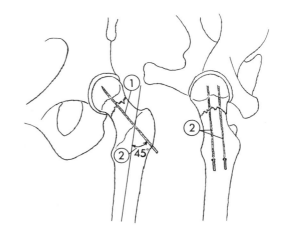

Insertion of Knowles Pins

After extracting the guide pins:

1. Insert the Knowles pins slowly and follow the tracks made by the guide pins.

2. Now impact the fragments by placing a driver against the trochanter and tapping it with a mallet.

3. Select two points on the lateral aspect of the femur 1⅞ to 2 inches below the bony ridge on the lower margin of the greater trochanter just inside the anterior and posterior surfaces of the neck. At each point drill a ³/₁₆ inch hole through the lateral cortex and directed obliquely upward.

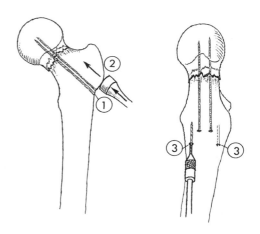

4. Place an angle guide set at 150 degrees opposite the drill holes and make parallel drill channels at the set angle for a distance of 2 to 3 inches up the neck.

5. Remove the angle guide and insert Knowles pins parallel to each other and following the drill channels.

Note: The length of the last two Knowles pins is readily determined by studying the x-rays taken after the insertion of the guide pins; usually the length is ¾ inch more than that of the first two Knowles pins.

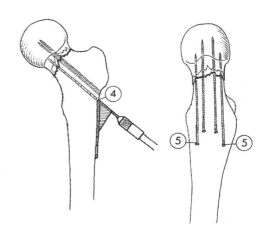

Postoperative X-Ray

ANTEROPOSTERIOR VIEW

1. The two lower pins lie close to the calcar and are directed at an angle of 150 degrees.

2. The head is in slight valgus.

LATERAL VIEW

1. The lower pins are close to the anterior and posterior surfaces of the neck.

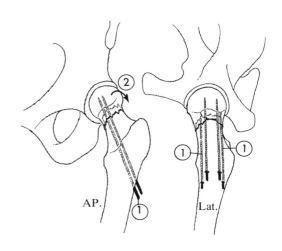

WHEN THERE IS FULL DISPLACEMENT OF THE FRAGMENTS (STAGE IV)

Study the nature of the fracture and note the amount of collapse of the posterior and inferior surfaces of the neck. This is a very unstable fracture and stability can only be restored by compensating for the defect in the neck of the femur. This can be accomplished by:

Telescoping the Femoral Neck into the Capital Fragment

1. An assistant makes steady traction on the leg with the limb extended and in slight external rotation. Traction is continued until the fragments separate.

2. Now internally rotate and abduct the leg widely while some inward pressure is made in the region of the greater trochanter.

3. Gently release the traction and allow the fragments to come in contact with the head in a position of slight abduction.

4. Flex the knee to 90 degrees (this locks the fragments in position). (With the fracture in view, finer adjustments can be made to attain the desired position of the fragments.)

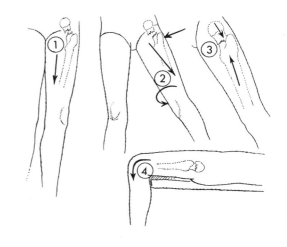

Page 1300

Telescoping the Femoral Neck into the Capital Fragment
(Continued)

1. About ¾ to 1 inch below the bony ridge at the lower margin of the greater trochanter and about ⅜ inch on either side of the midline of the lateral cortex, drill two holes ³⁄₁₆ inch in diameter, directed upward at an angle of 45 degrees.

2. Pass guide pins, 2.5 mm. in diameter, into the neck and head. (The pins are directed at an angle of 45 degrees with the shaft, parallel to the floor and parallel to one another.)

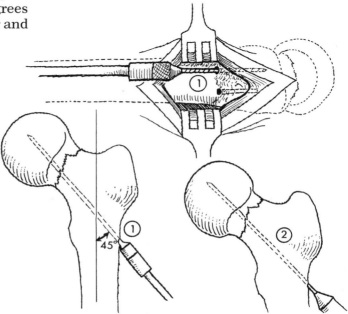

Check Position of Pins by X-Ray

1. Pins lie in neck and head and reach the subcortical bone of the head.

2. Pins make an angle of 45 degrees.

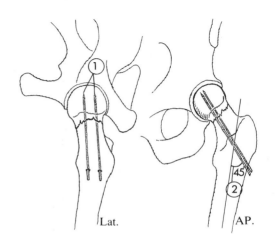

Insertion of Knowles Pins
After Extracting the Guide Pins

1. Insert the Knowles pins slowly and follow the tracks made by the guide pins.

2. Under vision, firmly impact the fragments by tapping a driver placed against the lateral cortex of the femur with a mallet.

Note: (1) The proximal end of the neck should be telescoped into the head; (2) the posterior defect should be closed; (3) the head should be in valgus, and (4) its inferior cortex lying inside the inferior margin of the neck.

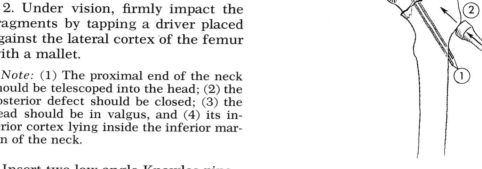

Insert two low angle Knowles pins.

This is performed in the same manner described earlier for partially displaced fractures (see page 1299).

Postoperative X-Rays

ANTEROPOSTERIOR VIEW

1. The two lower pins lie close to the calcar and are directed upward at an angle of 150 degrees.

2. The head is in slight valgus.

3. The neck is telescoped into the head.

4. The inferior margin of the head is inside that of the neck.

LATERAL VIEW

1. The pins are parallel.

2. The lower pins lie close to the anterior and posterior surfaces of the neck.

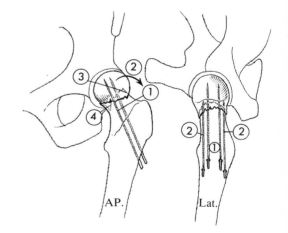

REMOVING A WEDGE FROM THE ANTEROSUPERIOR ASPECT OF THE NECK

REMARKS

This is a valuable procedure and in many instances readily converts a very unstable fracture to a stable one.

The base of the wedge of bone removed is about ¼ to ⅜ inch.

Don't remove an unduly large wedge because it may be difficult to approximate the two fragments.

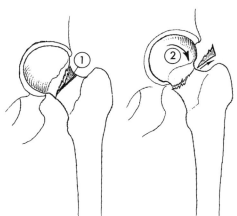

1. Remove a small wedge ¼ to ⅜ inch from the anterosuperior aspect of the neck.

2. Tilt the head into slight valgus. (This seats the head squarely on the neck.)

Fixation of Fragments

Fix the fragments with four Knowles pins as described previously for partially displaced fractures (see page 1299).

Postoperative X-Rays

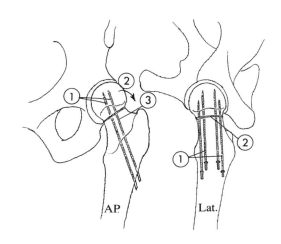

ANTEROPOSTERIOR VIEW

1. The two lower pins lie close to the calcar and are directed upward at an angle of 150 degrees.

2. The head is in slight valgus and sits squarely on the neck.

3. The neck is shortened.

LATERAL VIEW

1. The pins are parallel.

2. The defect in the posterior wall is obliterated.

Postoperative Management

The postoperative management is the same as that described for un-displaced fractures (see page 1292).

Basilar Fracture of the Neck of the Femur

REMARKS

This lesion is encountered less frequently than subcapital or trans-cervical fractures.

Internal fixation by means of a blade plate is more effective than the simple three-flanged nail or Knowles pins.

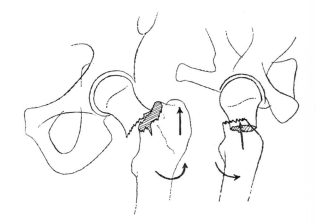

Prereduction X-Ray

Low cervical fracture with displacement.

Open Reduction and Internal Fixation

The patient is in the supine position with a sandbag under the affected hip.

1. The skin incision begins 1 inch distal and lateral to the anterosuperior spine; it continues downward over the posterior aspect of the greater trochanter and the lateral aspect of the femur for a distance of 5 to 6 inches below the base of the greater trochanter.

2. Divide the fascia lata the length of the skin incision.

3. Develop the interval between the gluteus medius and the tensor fasciae latae and divide the reflection of the fascia lata beneath the tensor fasciae latae; retract the tensor fasciae latae medially.

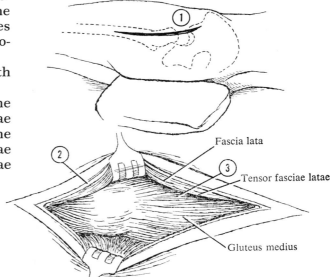

4. Displace the gluteus medius posteriorly to expose the anterolateral aspect of the capsule of the hip joint.

5. Divide the capsule with a T-shaped incision, exposing the femoral head and neck and the fracture site.

6. Make a 5 inch incision in the vastus lateralis centered over the lateral aspect of the femur and beginning just below the base of the greater trochanter.

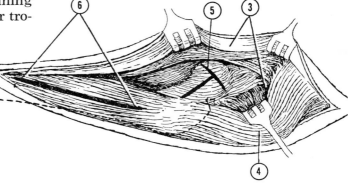

Page 1305

Open Reduction and Internal Fixation (*Continued*)

1. Expose, subperiosteally, the upper end of the shaft of the femur.

2. An assistant makes steady downward traction on the leg until length is restored and then turns the limb inward to the neutral position.

3. If necessary, the surgeon levers the fragments into accurate apposition with a fine curette.

While the desired position is maintained by an assistant:

4. Three-quarters to 1 inch below the bony ridge at the base of the greater trochanter and midway between the anterior and posterior cortices of the femur, drill a hole in the lateral cortex, ³⁄₁₆ inch in diameter and directed at an angle of approximately 45 degrees with the lateral cortex.

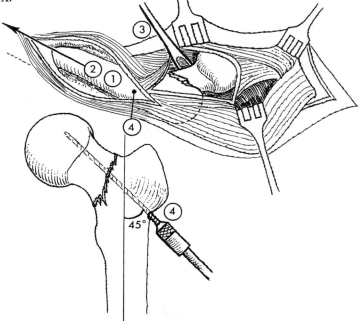

Open Reduction and Internal Fixation (Continued)

1. Center the pin guide at the hole; set the guide at 135 degrees.

2. Insert the guide pin into the drill leaving 3¾ inches protruding beyond the drill. Now insert the pin holding the drill parallel to the floor until the tip of the drill touches the cortex. Now take x-rays.

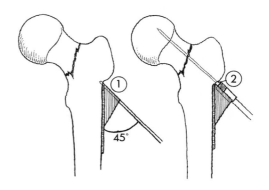

X-Rays

Anteroposterior view

1. Pin is in the center of the neck and head.

2. Pin lies at an angle of 135 degrees with the lateral cortex.

Lateral view

1. Pin is well centered in the neck and head.

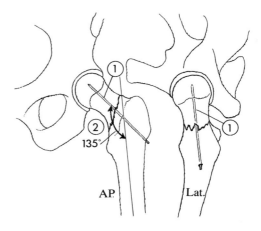

Insertion of the Nail

First determine the length of the nail required by studying the x-rays.

1. Place a cannulated reamer over the guide pin and drill a hole slightly smaller than the diameter of the nail.

2. Place the nail over the guide pin and drive it through the neck and into the head. While driving the nail,

3. Hold the plate of the nail parallel to the femoral shaft at all times; the plate should be flush with the shaft after the nail is seated.

4. Fix the plate to the shaft with three or four screws.

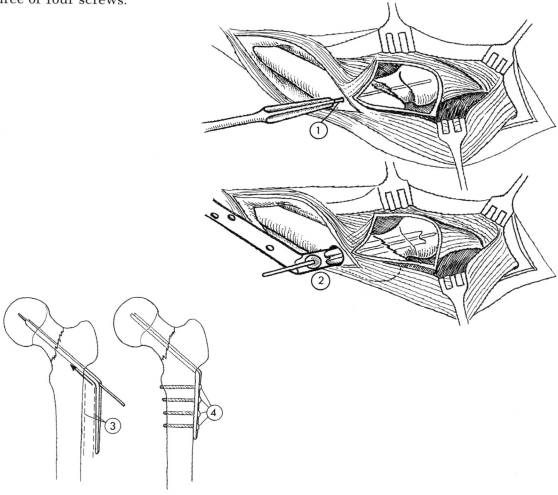

Postreduction X-Ray

The fragments are in normal alignment and fixed by a Jewett nail.

1. The nail is accurately centered in the head and neck of the femur.

2. The blade is flush with the shaft of the femur.

3. The screws barely penetrate the inner cortex of the femur.

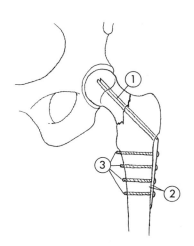

Postoperative Management

Allow the patient out of bed in a wheel chair on the second day.

Insist on frequent changes in position.

Institute active exercises of the hip and knee just as soon as pain and soreness of the limb subside. Particular attention should be given to the quadriceps of both limbs. On the affected side, the patient should be able to raise the extended leg off the bed unassisted.

Avoid extremes of motion in adduction and abduction.

When possible, teach the patient to walk with the aid of a walker and then on crutches, without weight bearing on the affected limb.

If this is not possible, insist that the patient get into a wheel chair and get about unassisted in it.

Check the prognosis of healing by x-ray at six week intervals.

Weight bearing with crutches is allowed when definite evidence of bony union is present, usually at the end of 12 to 16 weeks.

Usually at the end of six months union is sufficiently strong to permit unprotected weight bearing.

Fractures of the Neck of the Femur in Children

REMARKS

Although rare, these lesions are frequently followed by serious complications such as avascular necrosis of the femoral head, nonunion, deformity, growth disturbances, and delayed osteochondral changes simulating coxa plana.

Complications are most frequently encountered in transepiphyseal fractures with and without dislocations.

Transepiphyseal fractures with and without dislocations should be reduced under vision and the fracture fixed by two or three Knowles pins. No weight bearing for at least three months should be recommended.

In these lesions, if avascular necrosis does not occur early, late osteochondral changes similar to coxa plana may develop. In this event, weight bearing must be prohibited until revascularization of the capital epiphysis has occurred – 18 to 24 months.

Basal neck fractures are the most common.

As a rule in intertrochanteric fractures the results are good; but even here avascular necrosis of the caput occasionally is seen.

In intertrochanteric fractures, try to prevent healing with a coxa vara deformity because this does not correct itself with growth and will require an osteotomy to restore the normal neck angle.

TRANSEPIPHYSEAL, TRANSCERVICAL AND BASAL FRACTURES OF THE FEMORAL NECK WITH DISPLACEMENT

REMARKS

These fractures are best managed by reduction under direct vision and fixed by two or three Knowles pins.

Do not use a three-flanged nail to fix these fractures.

Prereduction X-Rays
(Transepiphyseal Fracture)

1. Complete traumatic separation of the proximal femoral epiphysis.
2. The femoral shaft is externally rotated and displaced upward.

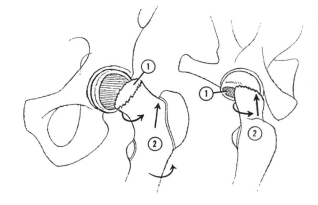

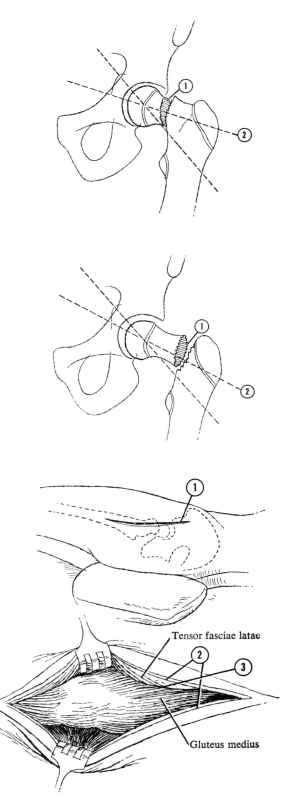

Prereduction X-Ray (Transcervical Fracture)

1. Transcervical fracture with
2. Coxa vara deformity.

Prereduction X-Ray (Basal Fracture)

1. Fracture through the cervico-trochanteric area.
2. Severe diminution of the femoral neck angle.

Open Reduction and Internal Fixation

1. The skin incision begins 1 inch distal and lateral to the anterosuperior spine; it continues over the posterior aspect of the greater trochanter and lateral aspect of the femur for a distance of 2 to 3 inches below the base of the greater trochanter.

2. Divide the fascia lata the length of the skin incision.

3. Develop the interval between the gluteus medius and the tensor fasciae latae and divide the reflection of the fascia lata beneath the tensor fasciae latae; retract this muscle medially.

Tensor fasciae latae

Gluteus medius

Open Reduction and Internal Fixation (*Continued*)

1. Displace the gluteus medius posteriorly, exposing the anterolateral aspect of the capsule.

2. Divide the capsule with a T-shaped incision, exposing the fracture site.

3. An assistant makes steady downward traction on the leg to restore normal length, then turns it to the neutral position; the patella is now in the upright position.

4. The limb is held in slight abduction—30 degrees—to lock the fragments.

5. If necessary, the surgeon levers fragments into accurate apposition with a fine curette.

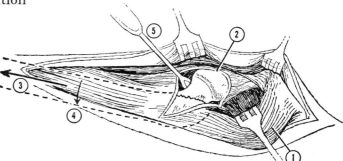

1. While the limb is held in the desired position by one assistant, make a small 1½ to 2 inch vertical incision centered on the lateral aspect of the femur just below the base of the greater trochanter.

2. Insert two or three Knowles pins through the lateral cortex, through the femoral neck, across the fracture line and into the caput. The pins must be parallel to each other.

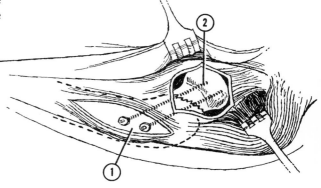

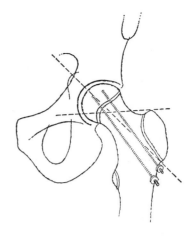

Postreduction X-Ray
(Transepiphyseal Fracture)

The caput is accurately reduced and fixed to the neck by two Knowles pins.

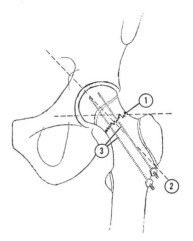

Postreduction X-Ray
(Transcervical Fracture)

1. The fragments are in accurate apposition.
2. The coxa vara deformity is corrected.
3. The fracture is traversed by two Knowles pins parallel to each other.

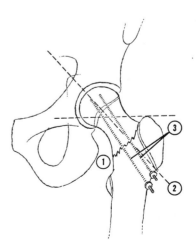

Postreduction X-Ray
(Basal Fracture)

1. The fracture is accurately reduced.
2. The normal angle of the neck is restored.
3. The fracture is stabilized by two Knowles pins.

Postoperative Management

Allow the child out of bed on the second or third day.

Encourage active motion at the hip and knee during the first postoperative week.

Permit walking with crutches after ten or 14 days without weight bearing on the operated limb.

Take check x-rays every four to six weeks to determine the state of healing at the fracture site.

Weight bearing on the affected limb is allowed only when x-rays show evidence of good bony healing, in 12 to 16 weeks.

The pins are removed any time after adequate, mature bony union is manifested at the fracture site, usually from six to 12 months.

Take check x-rays every three months for two years; look for avascular necrosis of the caput and osteochondral changes.

Complications of Fractures of the Neck of the Femur

REMARKS

Most complications of this lesion result from technical errors or poor surgical judgment.

However, even with efficient treatment, some complications occur because of embarrassment of the blood supply of the femoral head at the time of the initial injury or during the surgical procedure.

The most common complications are:

1. Nonunion. This occurs in approximately one third of the cases, the chief causes being (a) inadequate blood supply to the femoral head with subsequent avascular necrosis and (b) incomplete immobilization.

2. Osteoarthritis. This may occur with or without union of the fracture and is caused by (a) mechanical damage to the articular cartilage at the time of injury or by the operative procedure, (b) impairment of the blood supply to the basal layer of cartilage cells or (c) incongruity of the articular surfaces.

In general, the viability of the femoral head can be determined by x-ray studies; however, this method is not infallible.

Increased density of the femoral head in contrast to the surrounding bony structures indicates loss of blood supply and death of the head.

A mottled appearance of the head in cases of long standing indicates replacement of some of the necrotic areas by viable bone (creeping substitution).

In poorly treated or nontreated cases, absorption of the femoral neck may progress so that after six weeks these lesions should be treated as cases of nonunion.

In most instances radiographic and clinical features of nonunion are manifested within six months and frequently even earlier.

As a rule, establishment of definite bony union requires at least one year, and then two or three years must elapse to determine the fate of the femoral head.

The earlier the status of nonunion is established and treated, the higher the incidence of good results.

Many methods of treatment have been devised for nonunion of the femoral neck. In the following pages, only those methods which have given the best results in the hands of the author are depicted.

MANAGEMENT OF UNTREATED FRACTURE OF THE FEMORAL NECK FOUR TO SIX WEEKS OLD

REMARKS

Generally the head is viable and there is minimal absorption of the femoral neck.

Treat this lesion as a fresh fracture.

If there is moderate absorption of the neck, treat this lesion by an osteotomy.

Don't choose to replace the head with a prosthesis except as a last resort.

Prereduction X-Ray (Fully Displaced Fracture)

1. The normal angle of the femoral neck to the capital fragment is reduced; the head is in a varus position.

2. The distal fragment is rotated laterally.

3. The shaft of the femur is displaced upward.

4. The distal fragment lies anterior to the proximal fragment.

5. The plane of fracture is just distal to the femoral head.

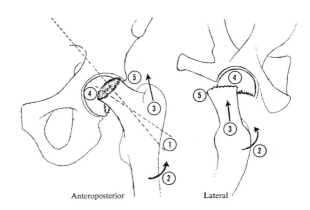

Anteroposterior   Lateral

Postoperative X-Ray

1. The head is in slight valgus.
2. The neck is telescoped into the head.
3. The fragments are fixed by two high angle and two low angle Knowles pins.

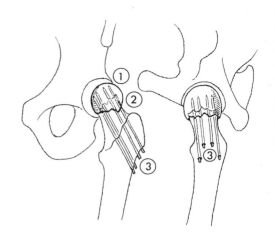

NONUNION OF THE FEMORAL NECK WITH A VIABLE HEAD AND ONLY MINIMAL ABSORPTION OF THE FEMORAL NECK

REMARKS

This lesion is best treated by an osteotomy.

The goal of the osteotomy should be to attain bony union; nonunion of a femoral neck fracture following an osteotomy results in a painful hip.

Also, following an osteotomy all motion at the fracture site should be eliminated; if motion is present absorption of the neck ensues, and the appliances used to stabilize the fracture will penetrate the head. Don't choose a prosthesis to replace the head except as a last resort.

Prereduction X-Ray

1. Only minimal absorption of the femoral neck exists.
2. The plane of fracture is almost vertical.
3. The femoral head is adducted in relation to the femoral neck.

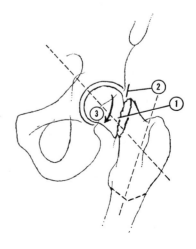

Postoperative X-Ray (Following Angulation Osteotomy)

1. The plane of fracture is now almost horizontal. (On weight bearing, stress is now a compressing force at the fracture site rather than a shearing force.)

2. The axis of the femoral shaft lies immediately beneath the femoral head, reducing leverage stresses on the hip joint.

3. The osteotomy site is immediately below the lesser trochanter.

4. The proximal end of the blade engages but does not penetrate the head too far.

5. Two Knowles pins are inserted parallel to one another across the fracture site before the blade plate is introduced (Blount blade plate).

6. The blade plate is bent at a proper angle (as predetermined on roentgenograms) to place the head and neck in at least 155 degrees of valgus.

7. The most proximal screw engages the proximal fragment.

Note: No external fixation is necessary.

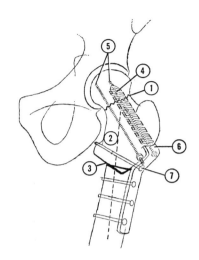

This lesion can also be treated by a high cervical trochanteric osteotomy as described on page 1319; in my hands, this osteotomy has produced more good results than any other type.

NONUNION WITH A VIABLE FEMORAL HEAD AND MARKED OR COMPLETE ABSORPTION OF THE FEMORAL NECK

REMARKS

Every effort should be made to achieve bony union and preserve the femoral head; if successful, the resulting hip is far superior to the result obtained by an arthroplasty (such as the Colonna operation) or to the result obtained by replacing the head with a prosthesis.

A displacement osteotomy is the best procedure to salvage the hip; it should be employed even when the fate of the head is in doubt.

Although x-ray examination provides valuable information in determining the viability of the head, it offers no assurance that avascular necrosis will not develop in the ensuing months.

The salvage procedure of my preference for this lesion is a high cervical trochanteric osteotomy as described later.

Another useful osteotomy is the McMurray osteotomy.

McMurray Osteotomy

Preoperative X-Ray

1. There is marked absorption of the femoral neck.

2. The plane of fracture is almost in the vertical plane.

3. The density of the femoral head is the same as that of the surrounding bone structures, indicating viability of the head.

4. The femoral head is in marked adduction in relation to the shaft.

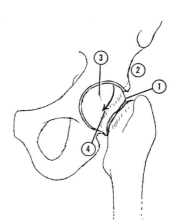

Postoperative X-Ray (McMurray Osteotomy)

1. Osteotomy is performed immediately below the lower margin of the head of the femur; it is directed slightly inward and upward.

2. The shaft fragment is displaced medially; now its axis lies immediately beneath the femoral head, hence lessening the stresses on the hip joint during weight bearing.

3. The position of the fragments is maintained by a spline which penetrates the proximal fragment and is screwed to the shaft fragment; the angle of the blade plate is 150 to 155 degrees.

Note: No external fixation is needed; generally after eight weeks protected weight bearing on crutches is permitted.

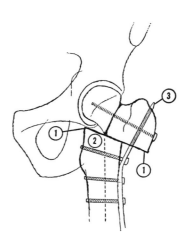

Page 1318

Cervical Trochanteric Osteotomy (Reich)

Preoperative X-Ray

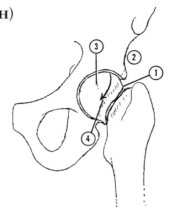

1. There is marked absorption of the neck.

2. The plane between the head and base of the neck is almost vertical.

3. The density of the femoral head is the same as that of the surrounding bony structures, indicating that the head is viable.

4. The femoral head is in marked adduction in relation to the shaft.

Operative Procedure

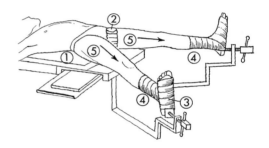

1. Place the patient on a fracture table.

2. Peroneal post is heavily padded.

3. Anchor both feet to foot stirrups; be sure the dorsum of each foot is well padded.

4. Both extremities are in the neutral position and abducted about 30 degrees.

5. Make steady, strong traction on both legs until the length of the affected limb is restored.

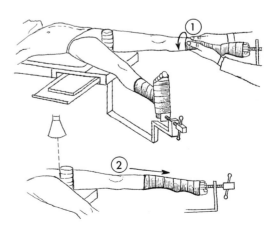

1. Internally rotate the affected limb until the bony axis of the foot is parallel with the floor.

2. Apply more traction to the affected limb; now take an x-ray in the anteroposterior plane to determine the position of the fragments.

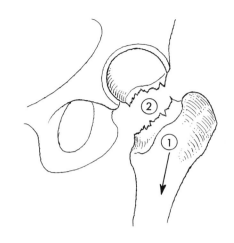

X-Ray

1. The femur is displaced downward.

2. Marked destruction between the head and remnants of the femoral neck.

1. Make a 4 inch incision on the lateral aspect of the thigh just below the greater trochanter and centered on the shaft of the femur.

2. Deepen the incision to bone and, by subperiosteal dissection, expose the base of the trochanter and the upper end of the femur for approximately 3 inches.

3. Three-quarters to 1 inch below the bony ridge at the lower margin of the greater trochanter and midway between the anterior and posterior cortices of the femur insert a Steinmann pin into the neck. The pin is directed at an angle of 45 degrees with the shaft and parallel to the floor.

4. Insert the pin for a distance of 3 inches. Now take another x-ray in the anteroposterior plane. This will show the direction of the pin.

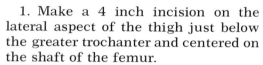

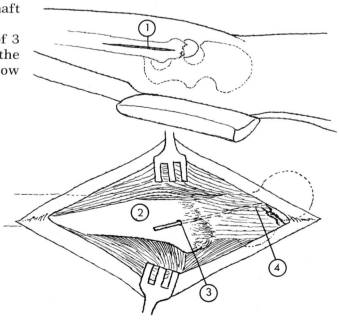

X-Ray

1. Tip of pin penetrates the juncture of the lower and middle thirds of the neck of the femur.

Note: By studying the direction and position of the pin, you can readily determine the direction of the osteotomy. Ideally the pin should be so placed that the osteotome placed on and parallel to the upper surface of the pin can be driven through the neck along the exact plane traversed by the pin.

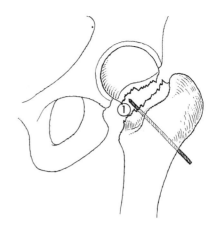

1. Place the osteotome on and parallel to the pin.
2. Perform a complete osteotomy. The osteotome divides the neck at the juncture of its lower and middle thirds.
3. Divide cleanly both the anterior and posterior surfaces of the trochanter region of the femur; now remove the Steinmann pin.
4. Pry the distal fragment away from the proximal fragment so that it lies free of any bony attachment.

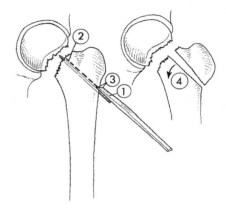

1. Place a wide impactor on the lateral cortex of the distal fragment.
2. With traction maintained, while an assistant widely abducts the leg,
3. With a heavy mallet drive the upper end of the distal fragment inward.

Note: Wide abduction (at least 60 degrees) is essential in order to displace the distal fragment from the proximal fragment and allow the femoral head to roll laterally between the two fragments.

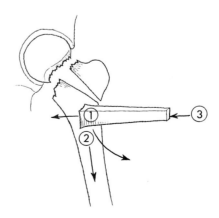

Page 1321

X-Ray *(Continued)*

1. Fix the proximal fragment to the distal fragment with a Steinmann pin.

2. Release the traction on the un-affected side to allow the pelvis to tilt toward the affected side.

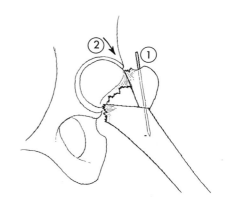

Postoperative X-Ray

1. The proximal fragment is displaced backward and downward.

2. The distal fragment lies under the femoral head.

3. The femoral head lies between the proximal and distal fragment in a position of valgus.

4. Steinmann pin fixes the two fragments.

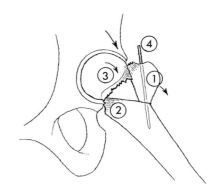

Immobilization

1. Apply a plaster spica with the leg in wide abduction and internal rotation.

2. The Steinmann pin is incorporated in the cast.

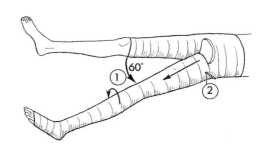

Postoperative Management

These patients need meticulous bed care.

Turn the patient every one or two hours.

Check the skin constantly for early evidence of skin pressure.

Institute deep breathing exercises.

Permit the patient to exercise the upper extremities and to change position by the use of overhead bars.

Remove the cast and the Steinmann pin at the end of six weeks and suspend the limb 3 inches above the bed in balanced traction.

Institute a program to develop all the muscles of the hip and to gain motion at the hip and knee.

At the end of two weeks (eight weeks after surgery) begin partial weight bearing on the affected side, first with a walker.

Complete bony union is achieved in 12 to 16 weeks; now allow full weight bearing on the affected limb.

NONUNION WITH A NONVIABLE FEMORAL HEAD AND MARKED OR COMPLETE ABSORPTION OF THE FEMORAL NECK

REMARKS

In young and middle-aged individuals, every effort should be made to provide a stable, pain-free, movable hip. In this group, the DePalma arthroplasty has proved to be a valuable reconstruction procedure (see page 1187).

In the older person whose general condition is good, one has the choice of a Colonna arthroplasty or replacement of the nonviable head with a metal medullary prosthesis.

In the very old, if any procedure at all is contemplated, replace the femoral head with a metal prosthesis.

At best, replacement arthroplasty is a poor substitute for a normal hip; nevertheless, it has its place as a salvage operation.

SALVAGE OPERATION FOR YOUNG AND MIDDLE-AGED PATIENTS

Preoperative X-Ray (32-year-old Patient)

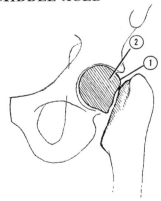

1. Complete absorption of the femoral neck.
2. The femoral head is dense, indicating nonviability.

Postoperative X-Ray
(DePalma Arthroplasty)

1. The femoral head is removed and a Vitallium cup is placed in the acetabulum.

2. A transverse osteotomy is done 3½ inches below the tip of the greater trochanter.

3. The proximal fragment is tilted medially and its proximal end placed in a Vitallium cup.

4. The fragments are fixed by a Neufeld nail at an angle of 135 degrees.

Note: The abductors of the hip are attached to the outer surface of the distal end of the proximal fragment; no external fixation is needed.

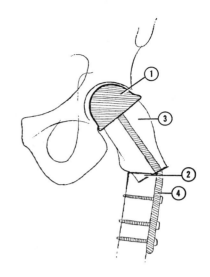

Preoperative X-Ray

1. Complete absorption of the femoral neck.

2. The femoral head is dense and sclerotic.

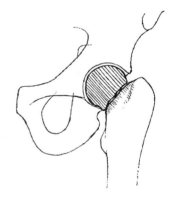

Postoperative X-Ray

1. The femoral head is excised.

2. A wedge of bone is removed from the inner aspect of the greater trochanter and the femoral shaft immediately above the lesser trochanter.

3. A medullary prosthesis (DePalma) sits directly on top of the shaft and abuts against the inner aspect of the greater trochanter.

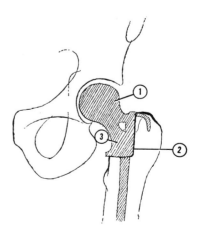

Colonna Arthroplasty

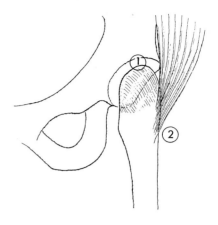

1. The greater trochanter is placed in the acetabulum.

2. The abductors of the hip are transplanted to a lower level on the shaft of the femur.

Note: This procedure is also of value when a prosthetic replacement fails.

FRACTURES OF THE SHAFT OF THE FEMUR

Fractures of the femur are usually the result of severe violence; they occur in all age periods and at any site.

The fracture may be transverse, oblique, spiral or severely comminuted; in children occasionally it is of the greenstick variety.

Generally there is marked displacement of the fragments and usually there are varying degrees of shock resulting from the trauma to the bone and soft tissues and the loss of blood.

Definitive reduction and immobilization of a fractured femur is never an emergency. First treat the patient as a whole; restore lost blood with transfusions, restore fluid and electrolyte balance, relieve pain, and always make a careful search for associated injuries.

If the fracture is an open one, it should be cleaned, débrided and converted to a closed fracture just as soon as the patient's general condition permits.

Most shaft fractures can be adequately treated by the conservative method of reduction by manipulation and skeletal traction.

This conservative method is safe and if correctly executed is accompanied by relatively few complications. It should always be given preference by those who are not yet skillful in the techniques of operative treatment.

In properly selected cases and in the hands of skillful surgeons intramedullary nailing is a very effective method of treatment, but beware! It can be the cause of some catastrophic complications.

CONSERVATIVE METHOD OF TREATING FRACTURES OF THE SHAFT OF THE FEMUR

REMARKS

This is a safe method and is applicable to most fractures of the shaft of the femur.

It is the only method to employ when the fracture is open and when there is potential or actual infection of the fracture site.

It is the method of choice when severe comminution of the femoral shaft exists.

It is the method of choice when severe associated injuries are present precluding further surgical trauma to the patient.

It is the method of choice in adolescent patients and in young women, who do not want to have their legs marred by surgical scars.

This method has the following disadvantages:

1. Immobilization is prolonged.
2. Restoration of normal motion at the knee and of the soft tissues of the thigh is a prolonged process.
3. It necessitates a prolonged hospitalization period.
4. Even when executed by the most experienced surgeon the incidence of malunion and nonunion is greater than that resulting from intramedullary nailing properly done.
5. The incidence of general and local complications, because of the long period of immobilization, is higher than in cases treated by internal fixation.

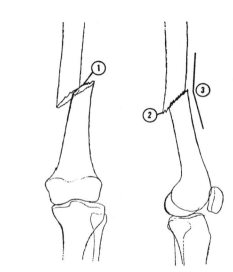

Prereduction X-Ray

1. Slightly oblique fracture through the juncture of the middle and lower thirds of the femur.
2. Moderate overriding.
3. Posterior bowing.

Reduction by Traction and Manipulation

Always make an attempt to obtain some apposition of the bone ends and reasonable alignment before placing the limb in traction and balanced suspension. This is done under general anesthesia in bed.

1. While an assistant makes steady traction on the limb,
2. With aseptic technique pass a threaded wire through the upper end of the tibia just below the tibial tubercle.
3. Clamp the ends of the wire in a U-shaped stirrup.

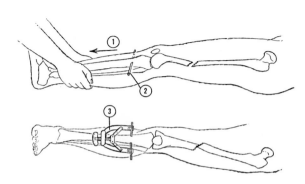

Page 1327

Reduction by Traction and Manipulation *(Continued)*

1. An assistant makes steady downward traction by pulling on the stirrup to restore length correcting any overriding.

2. By pressure and counter pressure the surgeon brings the bones into apposition.

While traction is maintained, pass the Thomas splint with a Pearson attachment over the limb and suspend the limb and apparatus in balanced traction.

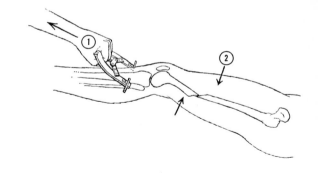

1. The limb is supported in canvas strips stretched between the side bars of the Thomas splint.

2. Regulate the tension of the canvas strips so that two thirds of the thigh is in front and one third behind the side bars.

3. The hip and knee are slightly flexed—15 to 20 degrees.

4. The limb and apparatus are supported by cords and weights *a, b, c* in such a manner that they are nicely balanced.

5. Traction grip is made on the leg by a threaded wire through the upper end of the tibia.

6. Ten to 15 pounds attached to the cord pulling on the stirrup usually suffices.

7. Foot strap to support the foot at a right angle.

8. The foot of the bed is elevated for counter traction.

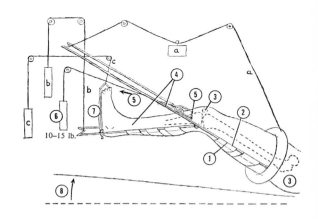

Management

Several times daily check the entire apparatus and note and adjust:
  a. Tension of the canvas slings.
  b. The line of pull and position of the pulleys; keep the limb and apparatus always properly balanced and suspended.
  c. Alignment of fragments; place pressure pads between the limb and side bars to maintain desired alignment.
  d. The ring of the splint; too much pressure may cause ulceration in the groin.
  e. Position and angle of the Pearson attachment; too much flexion or hyperextension of the knee is undesirable.
  f. Sagging of the limb at the site of fracture, producing a posterior bow; tighten the canvas slings.
  g. Forward bowing; lessen the tension of the slings.

Check the position of the fragments by x-ray at first every two days, then every few weeks, and make necessary adjustments.

Once length is restored, normal alignment achieved, and the fragments are in apposition, reduce the weight to 10 pounds, or in muscular individuals to 15 pounds; just enough weight to counteract muscle retraction is all that is necessary.

Avoid distraction of fragments by too much weight; distraction is the prime cause for delayed union and nonunion.

Beginning immediately and continuing throughout the period of immobilization, encourage the patient to exercise the lower leg, foot and toes on a regular regimen.

After a week or two institute quadriceps exercises; about the fourth week add flexion exercises of the knee. These exercises are most beneficial if performed under direct supervision of a physiotherapist.

In adults union is rarely achieved under 12 to 14 weeks; check for union clinically and by x-ray.

If there is doubt as to the adequacy of the union continue immobilization with reduced traction four to six more weeks, or eight weeks if necessary.

When union is sound remove the traction apparatus and permit the patient to exercise the limb at all joints freely in bed for several days.

Then allow the patient up on crutches, walking with protected weight bearing on the affected limb.

Crutches are discarded when sound union is a certainty.

A caliper is not needed; if union is not sound a caliper may predispose to angulation or even refracture and stiffness of the knee joint; never use one.

Institute an intense regimen of physical therapy to restore soft tissues of the thigh and knee joint to normalcy.

Never employ forceful passive manipulative maneuvers to hasten recovery of motion at the knee joint.

Many months of intensive therapeutic exercises and hard work may be necessary to achieve the maximum level of recovery.

Not infrequently some restriction of motion at the knee is permanent.

INTERNAL FIXATION FOR FRACTURES OF THE SHAFT OF THE FEMUR (INTRAMEDULLARY NAILING)

REMARKS

Let it first be emphasized that this is a formidable procedure for the patient and a technically difficult operation even for the most skillful surgeon. Many serious complications may arise during the execution of the operation or may follow improper nailing or poor postoperative management.

On the other hand, it is the most effective method of treating selected fractures of the shaft of the femur when performed by experienced surgeons.

It should never be performed:

In children;

In adolescents;

In young women except as a last measure;

In severely comminuted fractures;

In potentially infected or infected fractures;

In open fractures as a primary treatment.

Never attempt the procedure unless all the essential instruments are on hand; always have a sterile hacksaw on the table.

Never take this operation lightly because you may encounter technical obstacles which will tax to the utmost your ability and skill.

Intramedullary nailing is indicated in:

Fractures of the shaft from 2 inches below the lesser trochanter to 7 inches proximal to the adductor tubercle.

Transverse and short oblique or short spiral fractures; these readily lend themselves to this procedure.

Fractures with a third fragment, providing the surgeon is an experienced one; these usually require supplemental fixation.

Multiple fractures at different levels of the shaft, again a procedure only for the experienced surgeon.

This is also a most valuable method in the management of pathologic fractures and in treatment of delayed union, nonunion, and malunion.

The advantages of the method are:

External fixation is not needed;

The hospitalization period is cut to the minimum;

Early ambulation is possible;

Early and effective mobilization of the knee and other joints of the limb can begin at once;

Convalescence is shortened;

In properly treated cases the incidence of delayed union, nonunion and malunion is definitely diminished;

General and local complications are less frequently encountered than with other methods.

Always insert the nail under vision.

Never do a bilateral nailing at one time.

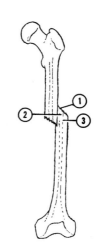

Prereduction X-Ray

1. Short oblique fracture of the upper third of the shaft.
2. Marked overriding of fragment.
3. Distal fragment is displaced laterally.

Operative Technique

1. The patient is in the complete lateral position lying on the unaffected side. The hip and knee on the affected side are flexed.

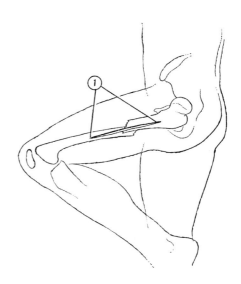

1. Make an incision on the posterolateral aspect of the thigh beginning 3 inches above the level of fracture and terminating 3 inches below.

Operative Technique (Continued)

1. Divide the fascia lata in the line of the skin incision exposing the posterior portion of the vastus lateralis.

2. Retract the vastus lateralis anteriorly.

3. This exposes the lateral intermuscular septum.

4. Make an incision along the anterior margin of the intermuscular septum down to the bone.

5. Expose the posterolateral aspect of the femur and fracture site by subperiosteal dissection.

Note: In the middle third the second perforating branches of the profunda artery and vein are encountered crossing the wound; these must be ligated.

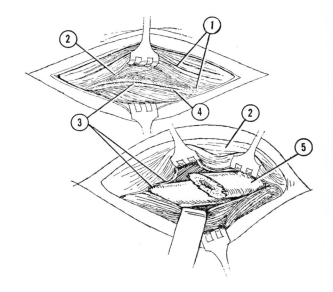

1. Elevate the distal fragment into the wound.

2. Determine the exact diameter of the medullary canal by passing long-handled drills, ranging in size from 8 to 12 mm., into the canal of the distal fragment until the one of correct diameter is found; it should fit snugly but not tightly.

3. Then pass the drill into the canal of the proximal fragment; if the canal is small ream it out to a diameter of at least 10 mm.

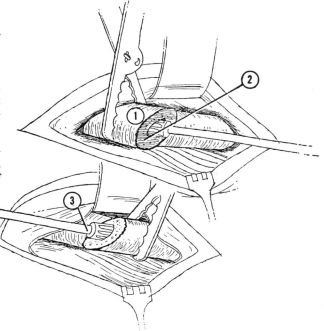

1. Now determine the correct length of the Küntscher nail to be used. Pass a guide wire of known length first in the canal of the distal fragment until it strikes the subchondral layer of bone; measure this distance.

2. Then pass a wire into the canal of the proximal fragments until it abuts against the cortex of the trochanter. Measure this length; the total of the two measurements a + b minus one inch will give the correct length of the nail.

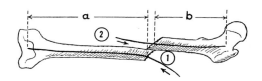

1. Place the nail in the canal of the proximal fragment with its eye directed posteromedially.

2. Acutely flex the fragment, and drive the nail through until it is felt protruding from the trochanter.

3. Make a small incision over the protruding nail and hammer the nail through until its distal end is level with the end of the proximal fragment.

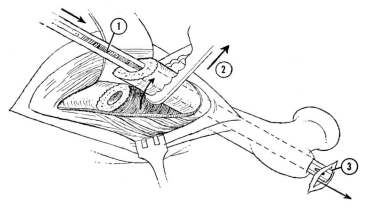

Operative Technique (Continued)

1. Align the fragments.

2. While the corrected position is held by the surgeon an assistant drives the nail into the distal fragment.

3. Two to 2.5 cm. of the nail is left protruding above the tip of the trochanter.

Note: During the insertion of the nail be sure that alignment is maintained at all times lest the nail be driven through the cortex of the distal fragment.

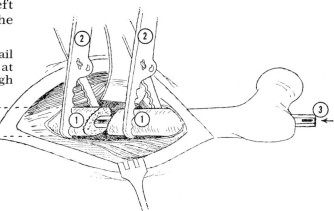

Postoperative Reduction X-Ray

1. The fragments are now in apposition and normal alignment.

2. The proximal end of the nail protrudes approximately 2 to 2.5 cm. above the tip of the trochanter.

3. The eye of the nail faces posteromedially.

4. The distal end of the nail is 1 to 1½ inches above the articular surface of the distal end of the femur.

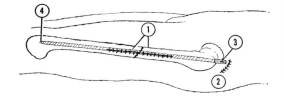

Postreduction X-Ray (Segmental Fractures)

1. Fracture in the upper third of the femur.

2. Fracture at the juncture of the middle and lower thirds of the femur.

3. Fragments adequately stabilized and aligned by intramedullary nail.

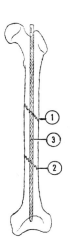

Postreduction X-Ray (Comminuted Fracture with Large Third Fragment)

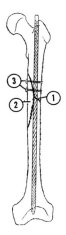

1. Comminuted fracture of the juncture of the upper and middle thirds of the femur.

2. Large third fragment.

3. Fragment secured to the proximal major fragment with two screws. (A circumferential loop of wire may be used instead of screws; don't tighten the wire too much.)

Postoperative Management

Place the extremity in balanced suspension for seven to ten days.

During this period encourage active flexion and extension of the knee just as soon as postoperative reaction permits. Take the leg out of the apparatus when the patient can actively raise the extended leg off the bed.

Warn the patient against the feeling of security provided by the nail.

Allow the patient out of bed on crutches without weight bearing on the leg at the end of the third week.

At the end of six weeks allow the patient weight bearing with crutches, keeping the knee stiff.

The crutches are not discarded until there is x-ray evidence of consolidation of the callus in the vicinity of the fracture—12 to 16 weeks.

Caution: Do not be fooled by the presence of exuberant callus which does not enter into the union of the fragments and is eventually absorbed.

Healing may be slow and it may take months before consolidation is complete and union firm enough to permit unprotected weight bearing.

Extract the nail only when x-rays show complete obliteration of the fracture site. This rarely occurs in less than one year.

Progressive intensive exercises of the thigh, leg and foot muscles and graduated exercises at the knee joint must continue during the entire convalescent period.

Never manipulate the joint forcefully to increase its range of motion.

What Might Happen During the Operation — Guard Against These Mishaps — Be Prepared to Deal with Them

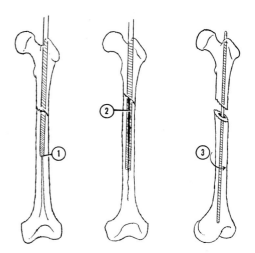

1. The nail jams in the medullary canal.

2. The diameter of the nail is too large and the shaft splits.

3. The diameter of the nail is too small; the fragments do not impact and the limb distal to the fracture usually rotates outward.

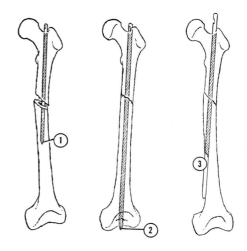

1. The nail is too short.
2. The nail is too long.
3. The nail perforates the cortex.

Some Late Complications of Fractures of the Shaft of the Femur

DELAYED UNION

REMARKS

If after a period of four or five months union is not sufficient to permit unprotected weight bearing, the healing process must be designated as delayed union.

The patient will be saved much time and the residual disability lessened if definitive measures are taken.

This complication is encountered in fractures treated by the conservative method and by internal fixation; however, it is more frequent in the former.

In cases treated by conservative methods, stabilize the fragments with an intramedullary nail and place slabs of cancellous bone around the fracture site.

In cases treated by internal fixation, add cancellous bone around the fracture site.

These cases can also be treated by two long compression plates and supplemental cancellous grafts.

A. X-Ray Appearance of Delayed Union

1. Fracture line is plainly visible.
2. Callus fails to bridge the fracture site and is inadequate in amount.

B. Postoperative X-Ray

3. Fragments fixed by intramedullary nail.
4. Slabs of cancellous bone surround the fracture site; more bone is applied to the inner than the outer aspects of the fracture.

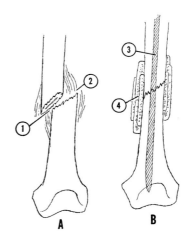

A   B

NONUNION

REMARKS

When the ends of the fragments become sclerotic and rounded, nonunion is definitely established.

The most effective treatment is fixation by intramedullary nailing and reinforcement of the fracture with slabs of cancellous bone.

In some instances treated by primary intramedullary nailing the nail breaks at the level of the fracture site; the nail should be removed and replaced.

These cases can also be treated by two long compression plates and supplemental cancellous grafts.

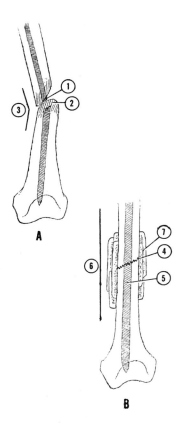

A. X-Ray of Nonunion

1. The nail is broken.
2. The ends of the fragments are rounded and sclerotic.
3. There is angular deformity at the fracture site.

B. Postoperative X-Ray

4. Bone ends are freshened.
5. The broken nail is replaced.
6. Alignment is restored.
7. Cancellous bone slabs surround the fracture site.

MALUNION

REMARKS

Minimal angular deformities are acceptable.

Moderate and severe deformities should be corrected.

Do an osteotomy at the apex of the deformity, fix the fragments with an intramedullary nail, and reinforce the osteotomy site with cancellous bone slabs — or fix the fragments with two compression plates and reinforce the osteotomy site with cancellous bone slabs.

A. X-Ray Appearance of Malunion

1. Union with severe angular deformity.

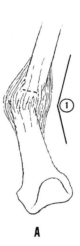

B. Postoperative X-Ray

2. The deformity is corrected and normal alignment restored by osteotomy.

3. An intramedullary nail stabilizes the fragments.

4. Cancellous bone slabs surround the osteotomy site.

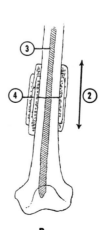

Page 1339

STIFFNESS OF KNEE

REMARKS

Stiffness of the knee is the result of one of several factors:
    Periarticular and intramuscular adhesions.
    Adhesions between the anterior surface of the femur at the site of
        fracture and the overlying quadriceps muscle mass.
    Fixation of the patella to the anterior surface of the femur.
This complication can be eliminated or its intensity minimized by:
    Early institution of exercises of leg, foot and toes.
    Active contraction of the quadriceps.
    Later (three or four weeks after placing the leg in traction), active
        flexion of the knee joint.
    Daily passive manipulation of the patella to prevent intra-articular
        adhesions.
    Continuance of this program on a graduated scale throughout the
        entire convalescent period.
    Avoidance of forceful manipulation of the knee joint to increase
        the range of motion. In the event that permanent stiffness
        results, lengthening of the quadriceps apparatus must be con-
        sidered.

FRACTURES OF THE SHAFT OF THE FEMUR IN CHILDREN

REMARKS

All fresh fractures in children can be treated adequately by skin traction.

Skeletal traction is indicated only in neglected cases with marked overriding.

Open reduction and internal fixation is never indicated and when performed is frequently followed by serious complications.

Overriding not exceeding 1 cm. and minimal angulation are acceptable. With growth the angulation disappears and the shortening is corrected.

In the event that skeletal traction is desirable, use a threaded wire inserted through the tibial crest distal to the proximal tibial epiphysis. In displaced fractures end to end apposition is undesirable because the subsequent acceleration of growth will result in a longer leg than on the opposite side.

Skin traction has its hazards; observe the following precautions:

Make traction on legs with strips of foam rubber secured by an elastic cotton bandage.

Don't apply the bandages too tightly because circulatory embarrassment may result.

Check the circulatory status of the limbs several times daily.

Cyanosis or pallor of the toes, swelling and pain indicate circulatory trouble; take the bandage off immediately and inspect the limb.

Failure to observe these warnings may result in sloughs or ischemic necrosis, a tragic complication.

Undisplaced incomplete fractures and spiral or oblique fractures with only minimal displacement can be treated by a plaster cast. Immobilize these fractures six to eight weeks.

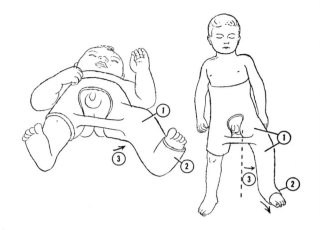

Plaster Spica for Undisplaced Incomplete Fractures and for Spiral and Oblique Fractures with Minimal Displacement

1. Hip and knee are slightly flexed.
2. Foot is at a slight angle.
3. Leg is in slight abduction.

Displaced Femur Shaft Fractures in Young Children (Under Five Years)

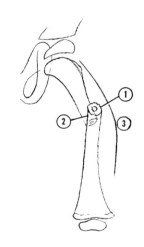

Prereduction X-Ray

1. Fracture at the juncture of the upper and middle thirds of the shaft.
2. Moderate overriding.
3. Lateral bowing.

Reduction and Immobilization (Bryant Traction)

1. Apply overhead traction to both legs; use strips of foam rubber secured by elastic cotton bandage.
2. Use pulleys and weights, not fixed traction.
3. The weight should just lift the buttocks off the mattress.
4. Use a restraint.

Note: In high femoral shaft fractures the legs should be widely abducted.

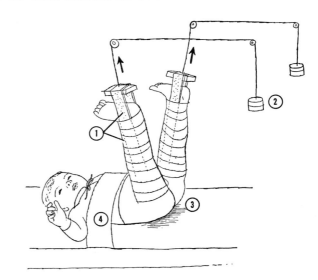

Postreduction X-Ray

1. Alignment is restored.
2. Slight overriding; this is acceptable.
3. Much callus about the fracture site.

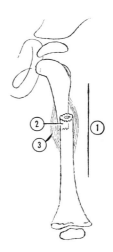

Management

Make frequent inspections of the limbs. Check for evidence of circulatory embarrassment.

If the circular bandages slip, rewrap the legs.

Maintain traction until the callus is no longer tender (four to six weeks).

Then remove the traction and keep the child in bed for another seven to ten days.

Now allow the child up on crutches (if of walking age), permitting partial weight bearing.

Crutches will be discarded voluntarily just as soon as the child is able to bear full weight on the affected limb with confidence.

No physical therapy is necessary.

Displaced Femoral Shaft Fractures in Older Children (Over Five or Six)

Reduction and Immobilization (Russell Traction)

1. Make skin traction on the lower leg. (Use foam rubber strips instead of adhesive plaster.)
2. The knee is supported in a canvas sling lined with a sheet of foam rubber and supported from an overhead beam.
3. Pulley systems *A* and *B* maintain the limb in the desired position.
4. The leg rests on one or two pillows with the knee flexed slightly.
5. Three to 6 pounds usually suffices to restore alignment and reduce excessive overriding.
6. Abduct the leg 45 to 60 degrees.
7. Elevated foot of bed for counter traction.
8. Foot plate to prevent rotation.

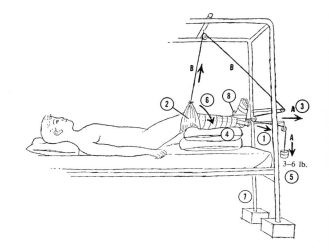

A. In the event that angulation is not corrected by single leg traction, apply skin traction to the opposite leg.

B. 1. Reduce weight on the affected limb.

   2. Increase weight on the unaffected limb; this tilts the pelvis downward on the unaffected side, correcting adduction of the distal fragment on the affected side.

Note: This is especially applicable to fractures of the upper and middle thirds with adduction of the proximal fragment.

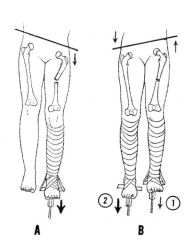

A   B

Prereduction X-Ray

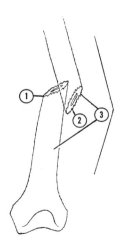

1. Fracture of the middle third of the shaft.

2. Marked overriding.

3. Adduction of the upper fragment and abduction of the lower fragment.

Postreduction X-Ray

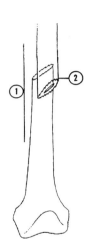

1. Alignment is almost restored to normal.

2. Overriding of fragments in the anteroposterior plane; this amount is acceptable (should not be over 1 cm.).

Management

Observe the same precautions relative to skin traction recorded on page 1341.

Check traction apparatus several times daily and make necessary adjustments.

Check constantly for evidence of circulatory embarrassment.

Maintain the limb in traction until the callus is no longer tender – six to eight weeks.

Now take the traction apparatus off and keep the child in bed one more week.

Allow the child up on crutches permitting partial weight bearing.

The crutches will be discarded voluntarily just as soon as full weight can be borne on the limb with confidence.

No physical therapy is necessary.

FRACTURES OF THE LOWER END OF THE FEMUR

Supracondylar Fractures of the Femur

REMARKS

These are rare lesions and always the result of severe violence.

There is always severe soft tissue damage, accompanied by massive hemarthrosis. The posteriorly displaced distal fragment may lacerate the popliteal vessels at the time of the initial injury or during manipulative reduction. Always check the circulatory status of the limb. A pulsating hematoma in the back of the knee indicates a rupture of the popliteal artery.

Always check for any neurologic deficit.

Reparative process following severe soft tissue injury may result in formation of numerous intra- and extra-articular adhesions; hence immobilize the knee in flexion no longer than is absolutely necessary—usually six weeks.

Closed methods of treatment are preferred to open methods unless closed methods have failed.

These fractures are reduced by traction and manipulation but flexion of the knee maintains the reduced position.

The obliquity of the fracture line may be such that engagement of fragments cannot be achieved by flexion alone; these may require continuous traction or internal fixation.

Prereduction X-Ray
(Supracondylar Fracture)

1. This distal fragment tilts backward into the popliteal space and is displaced upward.

2. The distal end of the proximal fragment is displaced downward (it may pierce the suprapatellar pouch and quadriceps apparatus).

3. The femur is shortened.

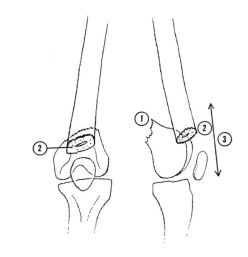

Reduction by Traction and
Manipulation (Under General
Anesthesia)

With aseptic technique, aspirate blood from the joint cavity, then,

1. Pass a threaded wire immediately below the tibial tubercle for traction.

2. Fix a wire tautener to threaded wire.

While traction is maintained by an assistant,

3. The patient fits snugly against the perineal post.

4. The foot on the opposite side is bound to a foot plate.

5. The affected leg is flexed 45 to 60 degrees at the hip.

6. The cord attached to the spreader is tied to an elevated foot plate.

7. The lower leg with the foot in plantar flexion remains free.

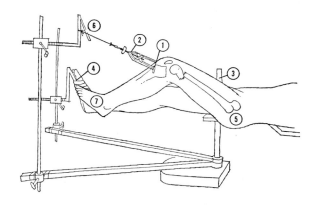

Reduction by Traction and Manipulation (Under General Anesthesia) (Continued)

1. Make strong mechanical traction in the line of the femur until length is restored.

2. The surgeon makes upward pressure on the distal fragment and downward pressure on the proximal fragment.

Correct any medial or lateral displacement.

3. After reduction is achieved, relax the traction slightly to engage the fragments.

Note: Now take check x-rays; if satisfactory, apply a plaster spica.

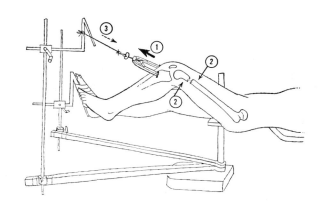

1. The plaster spica extends from the costal margin to the toes on the affected side.

2. The knee is flexed at the position required to maintain reduction.

3. The protruding ends of the wire are incorporated in the plaster.

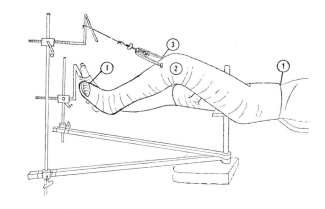

Postreduction X-Ray

1. Normal alignment is restored.
2. The flexed position of the knee maintains reduction.

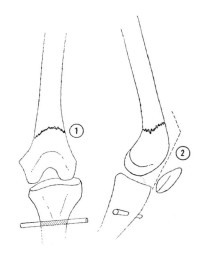

Postreduction Management

Encourage static contractions of the quadriceps and exercises for the toes.

Remove the plaster spica at the end of six weeks; also remove the threaded wire.

Now institute a program of physical therapy in the form of radiant heat and gentle massage, to be given daily.

Put the patient on a regulated regimen of progressive active exercise for the quadriceps, knee and foot; these are best performed under supervision if possible.

When the patient has achieved good quadriceps power, allow him out of bed on crutches without weight bearing.

After two weeks allow partial weight bearing on crutches.

Generally after two more weeks the crutches can be discarded.

ALTERNATE METHOD

REMARKS

Employ this method when, because of obliquity of the fracture site or severe comminution, reduction cannot be achieved and maintained by traction and manipulation as described on pages 1347 and 1348.

First aspirate the knee and insert a threaded wire just below the tibial tubercle for skeletal traction; then place the patient on a Böhler-Braun splint.

1. One assistant makes steady traction on the line of the femur.

2. A second assistant fixes the iliac crests.

3. After the length of the femur is restored, the surgeon grasps the distal fragment with both hands and elevates it forward.

4. The assistant relaxes the traction slightly to engage the fragments.

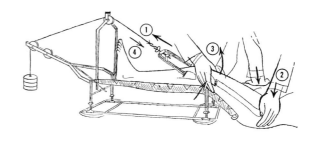

1. Place a felt pad behind the distal fragment.

2. The angle of the splint is behind the site of the fracture.

3. Determine the direction of traction which will hold the fragments in the desired position, then adjust the height of the pulley. (Use x-ray to check the position of the fragments at this point.)

4. Ten to 12 pounds usually suffices to maintain the desired position.

5. Elevate the foot of the bed for counter traction.

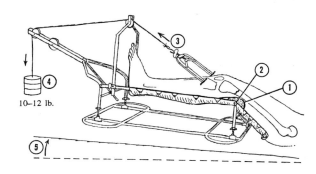

Postreduction Management

Check the traction apparatus and make the necessary adjustments several times daily.

Take check x-rays daily for the first few days, then every two or three days until maintenance of the position is assured.

Use lateral pressure pads to correct any lateral displacement.

Check constantly for evidence of pressure points.

Exercise the ankle, foot and toes, but not the knee, except for static quadriceps contraction.

After six weeks sufficient consolidation exists to take the leg out of traction and begin flexion and extension exercises at the knee joint.

Now insist on an intensive regimen of regulated exercises. After one or two weeks allow the patient up on crutches with no weight bearing on the affected limb. After two more weeks protected weight bearing is permitted, and after two more weeks the crutches can be discarded.

OPERATIVE REDUCTION AND INTERNAL FIXATION

REMARKS

This method is employed only if the methods previously described fail.

Generally, the added surgical trauma predisposes to more formation of soft tissue adhesions than the conservative methods and hence prolongs convalescence.

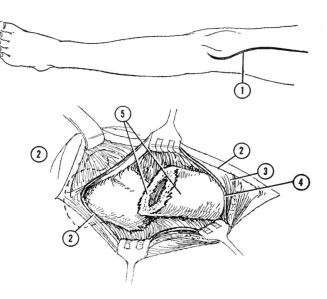

1. Make a 5 to 6 inch incision on the anterolateral aspect of the distal end of the thigh between the rectus femoris and the vastus lateralis. At the upper end of the patella the incision curves laterally to the level of the joint line, then gently anteriorly.

2. Divide the fascia lata and the lateral aponeurotic expansion and the joint capsule in the line of the skin incision; this exposes the intra-articular portion of the femur.

3. Develop the interval between the rectus femoris and the vastus lateralis, exposing the vastus intermedius.

4. Incise longitudinally the vastus intermedius and the periosteum.

5. By subperiosteal dissection expose the ends of the bone fragments.

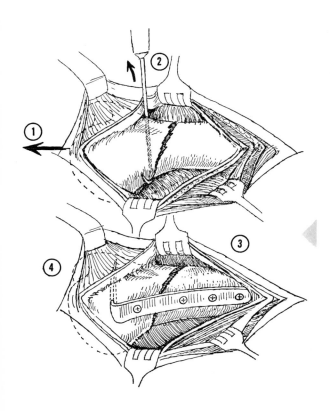

After washing all clots and loose fragments from the wound,

1. Make downward traction on the leg.

2. With a sharp curette or bone hook engage and elevate the distal fragment into its normal position.

3. Fix the fragments with a blade plate (Blount plate) or compression plate.

4. Place the plate subperiosteally and subsynovially.

Page 1351

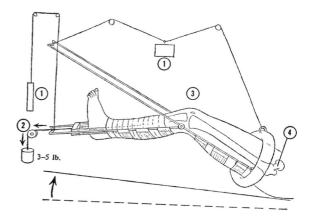

After closure of the wound,

1. The limb is placed in balanced traction and suspension.

2. Light skin traction is employed — 3 to 5 pounds.

3. The knee is flexed 30 degrees.

4. The hip is flexed 30 degrees.

Postoperative Management

Check the traction apparatus several times daily and make necessary adjustments.

Institute active foot and toe exercises immediately.

After seven to ten days institute active contraction of the quadriceps.

After the third week begin acitve flexion and extension exercises at the knee joint.

Remove the traction apparatus after six or eight weeks and allow the patient to exercise actively in bed for another week.

Then allow the patient up on crutches with protected weight bearing; after two more weeks the crutches should be discarded.

This timetable can be shortened considerably if the compression plate is used.

Intercondylar Fractures of the Femur

REMARKS

These fractures are always complicated by severe soft tissue damage and massive hemarthrosis; always aspirate the knee joint before and as many times as necessary after reduction.

Varying degrees of incongruity of the articular surface of the femur result by displacement of the fragment; this incongruity must be corrected.

These lesions are best treated by skeletal traction and manipulative reduction as depicted for supracondylar fractures of the femur (pp. 1347 and 1348); in addition the condyles are replaced in relation to each other by either manual compression or a screw clamp (Böhler or Forrester clamp).

Open reduction is indicated if this method fails.

OPEN REDUCTION AND INTERNAL FIXATION OF INTERCONDYLAR FRACTURES

REMARKS

This method is employed only if the method of reduction by manipulation and skeletal traction fails.

Prereduction X-Ray

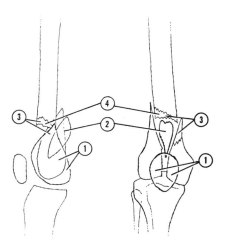

1. The distal fragment is split longitudinally into the joint.

2. The condylar fragments are held separated by a loose fragment drawn between them.

3. The ends of the fragments are comminuted.

4. The distal fragments are displaced backward and upward into the popliteal space.

Operative Reduction and Internal Fixation

1. Make a 5 to 6 inch incision on the anterolateral aspect of the distal end of the thigh between the rectus femoris and the vastus lateralis; at the level of the upper pole of the patella continue the incision first laterally and then gently anteriorly.

2. Divide the fascia lata and the lateral aponeurotic expansion and the joint capsule in the line of the incision; this exposes the intra-articular portion of the femur.

3. Incise longitudinally the vastus intermedius and the periosteum; by subperiosteal dissection expose the ends of both fragments.

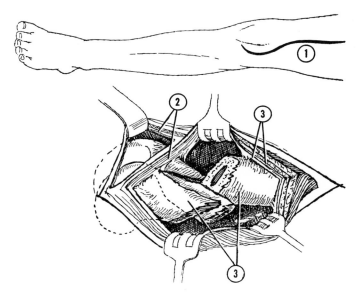

Operative Reduction and Internal Fixation (Continued)

Wash out all loose fragments and clots from the joint cavity and the fracture site, then:

1. While an assistant makes traction on the leg, lever the proximal ends of the condylar fragments into the wound.

2. Restore the condylar fragments into normal relation to each other.

3. Secure the fragments by inserting two threaded wires across the fracture site through stab wounds made in the skin slightly posterior to the incision. Cut the pin below the level of the skin. (Screws or bolts may be used instead of wires.)

4. Approximate the distal and proximal fragments into normal position.

5. Secure the fragments with a blade plate (Blount plate) placed subperiosteally and subsynovially; or use a compression plate.

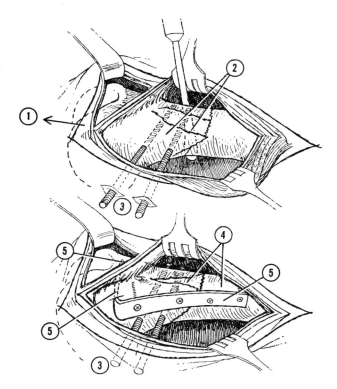

After closure of the wound:

1. The limb is placed in balanced traction and suspension.

2. Light skin traction is employed (3 to 5 pounds).

3. The knee is flexed 30 degrees.

4. The hip is flexed 30 degrees.

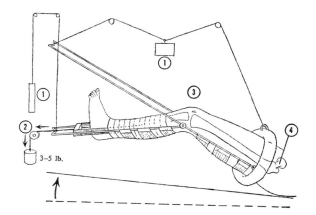

Postoperative Management

This is similar in every respect to that of supracondylar fractures treated by open reduction (p. 1352), except that threaded wires are removed at the end of the sixth week under local anesthesia.

Fractures of a Single Condyle of the Femur

REMARKS

These are usually the result of direct violence forcing the knee joint into varus or valgus.

Generally the fracture line is vertical and in the sagittal plane.

Rarely a fracture in the frontal plane occurs, when the force is applied with the knee moderately flexed.

The collateral ligament on the affected side usually remains intact while the contralateral collateral ligament is stretched or partially or completely torn.

In fractures in the frontal plane (usually involving the extreme posterior portion of the condyles) the fragment may not be controlled by ligamentous attachments; the fragment may be a free body.

CONDYLAR FRACTURES IN THE SAGITTAL PLANE

REMARKS

Always determine the integrity of the collateral ligament on the opposite side. If intact, proceed with the conservative method of treatment; if disrupted, first repair the ligament, then reduce and secure the fragment by the open method.

Some fractures comprise one or more cracks without displacement; these require nothing more than immobilization in a long leg plaster cast for four or five weeks.

Appearance on X-Ray

1. Fracture of the medial femoral condyle without displacement.

2. Here a long leg plaster cast suffices.

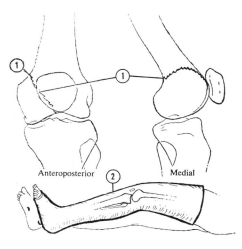

Anteroposterior   ②   Medial

Prereduction X-Ray

1. Fracture of the lateral femoral condyle.

2. The fragment is displaced upward.

3. The fragment is displaced slightly backward.

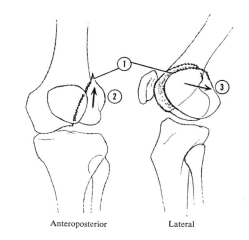

Anteroposterior   Lateral

Reduction by Manipulation and Traction

(The knee is first aspirated.)

1. The patient lies on a fracture table, snugly against the perineal post.

2. The feet are fastened to foot plates.

3. Make moderate downward mechanical traction on the affected side.

4. Manually correct any anteroposterior displacement.

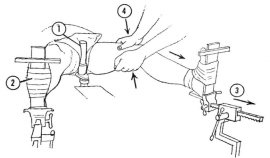

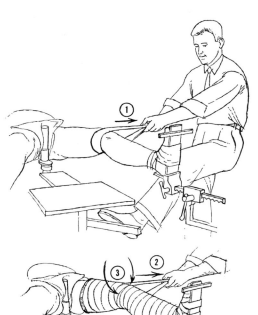

1. With a muslin bandage an assistant applies traction in the lateral direction. (For a fracture of the medial condyle apply traction in the medial direction.)

2. While traction is maintained apply a long leg plaster cast.

3. Mold and compress well the plaster around the condyles.

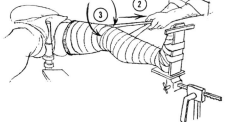

Postreduction X-Ray

1. The lateral condyle is restored to its anatomic position in both planes.
2. Regularity of the articular surface is restored.

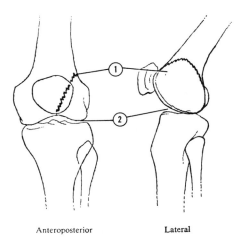

Anteroposterior   Lateral

Immobilization

1. Apply a plaster cast from the groin to the toes.
2. The knee is slightly flexed.
3. The foot is at a right angle.

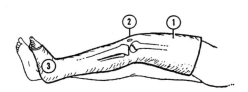

Postreduction Management

Encourage static contractions of the quadriceps and exercises for the toes.

Remove the plaster cast at the end of six weeks.

Now institute a program of physical therapy in the form of radiant heat and gentle massage, to be given daily.

Place the patient on a regulated regimen of progressive active exercises for the quadriceps, knee and foot. These are best performed under supervision if possible.

When the patient has achieved good quadriceps power allow him out of bed on crutches without weight bearing.

After two weeks begin partial weight bearing on crutches.

Generally after two more weeks the crutches can be discarded.

OPERATIVE REDUCTION AND INTERNAL FIXATION

REMARKS

This method is employed when reduction cannot be achieved by the closed method.

It is also employed when the lesion is complicated by a tear of the opposite collateral ligament of the knee joint.

The ligament is first repaired and then the fracture is reduced and fixed.

Prereduction X-Ray

1. Fracture of the medial femoral condyle.

2. The condylar fragment is displaced upward.

3. The condylar fragment is displaced and tilted backward.

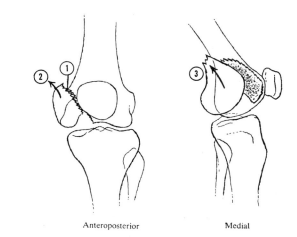

Anteroposterior   Medial

Operative Reduction and Internal Fixation

1. Make a 5 to 6 inch incision on the anteromedial aspect of the thigh in the interval between the rectus tendon and the vastus medialis muscle. Continue the incision downward around the patella.

Note: For lateral condylar fractures a similar approach is made on the lateral side of the joint between the rectus femoris and the vastus lateralis.

2. Divide the fascia lata, the medial aponeurotic expansion and joint capsule in the line of the incision.

3. Proximally develop the interval between the tendon of the rectus femoris and the vastus medialis.

4. Split the vastus intermedius longitudinally and expose the distal end of the femur and condyle by subperiosteal dissection.

5. Divide the synovial membrane exposing the knee joint.

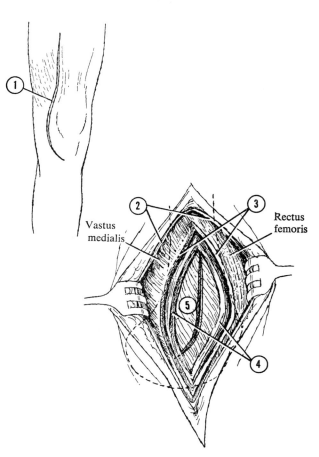

Vastus medialis

Rectus femoris

Page 1359

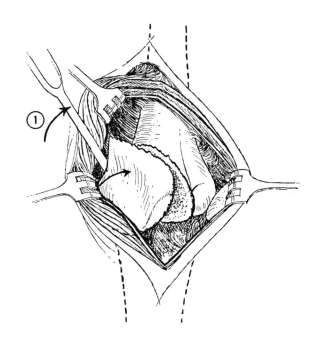

Operative Reduction and Internal Fixation (Continued)

1. Under direct vision lever the medial condyle into its normal position.

2. Secure the fragment with one or two screws.

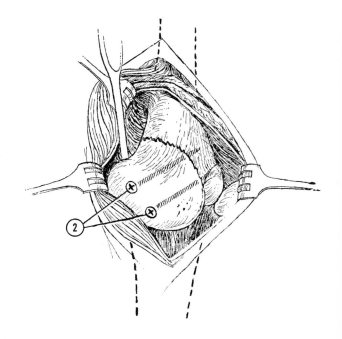

Postreduction X-Ray

The condylar fragment is in its normal position and secured with two screws.

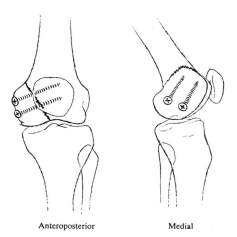

Anteroposterior   Medial

Immobilization

1. Apply a plaster cast from the groin to the toes.
2. The knee is slightly flexed.
3. The foot is at a right angle.

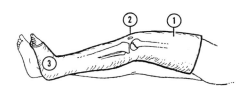

Postoperative Management

Encourage static contractions of the quadriceps and exercises for the toes.

Remove the plaster cast at the end of six weeks.

Now institute a program of physical therapy in the form of radiant heat and gentle massage, to be given daily.

Place the patient on a regulated regimen of progressive active exercises for the quadriceps, knee and foot. These are best performed under supervision if possible.

When the patient has achieved good quadriceps power allow him out of bed on crutches without weight bearing.

After two weeks begin partial weight bearing on crutches.

Generally after two more weeks the crutches can be discarded.

CONDYLAR FRACTURES IN THE FRONTAL PLANE

REMARKS

Large condylar fragments may be reduced by traction and manipulation as described for fractures in the sagittal plane.

Occasionally the fragment is displaced and rotated backward so that the manipulative methods fail; open reduction is now necessary.

Small, completely detached fragments of the posterior portion of the femoral condyles act as loose bodies; these should be excised.

Prereduction X-Ray

1. Fracture of the posterior portion of the medial femoral condyle.

2. The fragment is displaced backward.

3. It is rotated backward.

Operative Reduction and Internal Fixation

1. The incision begins just posterior to the biceps tendon; it extends downward to the level of the horizontal flexion crease; it continues horizontally across the popliteal space in the flexion crease and continues distally for 2 inches between the tendon of the semitendinosus and the medial head of the gastrocnemius.

2. Divide the deep fascia in the line of the incision.

3. Develop the interval between the tendon of the semitendinosus and the medial head of the gastrocnemius exposing the posterior joint capsule.

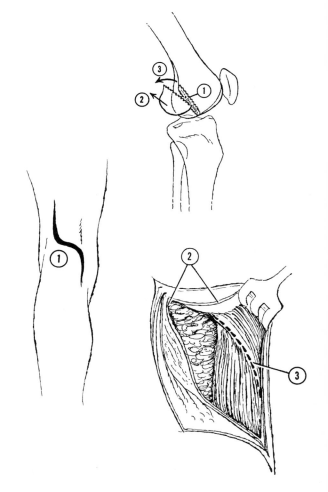

1. Divide the joint capsule longitudinally, exposing the posterior aspect of the medial femoral condyle.

2. Lever the condylar fragment into its normal position.

3. Secure the fragment with two screws.

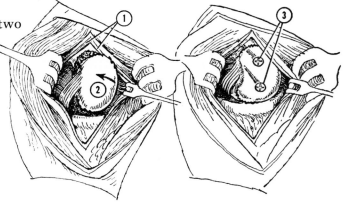

Postreduction X-Ray

The condylar fragment is in its normal position and fixed by two screws.

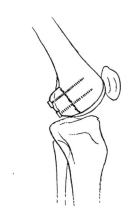

Immobilization

1. Apply a long leg plaster cast from the groin to the toes.
2. The knee is slightly flexed.
3. The foot is at a right angle.

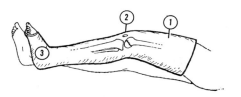

Postoperative Management

Encourage static contractions of the quadriceps and exercises for the toes.

Remove the plaster cast at the end of six weeks.

Now institute a program of physical therapy in the form of radiant heat and gentle massage, to be given daily.

Place the patient on a regulated regimen of progressive active exercise for the quadriceps, knee and foot. These are best performed under supervision if possible.

When the patient has achieved good quadriceps power allow him out of bed on crutches without weight bearing.

After two weeks begin partial weight bearing on crutches.

Generally after two more weeks the crutches can be discarded.

Separation of the Distal Femoral Epiphysis

REMARKS

This lesion is generally the result of severe violence

As a rule the epiphysis is displaced anteriorly; in rare instances it may be displaced backward or laterally. Lateral displacement may accompany an anterior or posterior displacement of the lower margin of the diaphysis. Displacement into the popliteal fossa may traumatize or compress the vessels and nerves; always check for circulatory embarrassment and neurologic deficits.

Always reduce the displacement without delay; procrastination for a few days may jeopardize the circulation of the limb and render the reduction difficult.

In young children minor displacements with good alignment are acceptable; with growth the deformity will disappear.

Lateral displacements producing valgus or varus deformities are not acceptable; even in young children these deformities diminish only slightly with growth.

Simple separations adequately reduced and treated rarely cause growth disturbances.

Crushed epiphyses may be complicated by premature closure or partial closure of the epiphysis, resulting in shortening or valgus or varus deformities or deformities in the sagittal plane.

Always warn the parents of these possibilities; take check x-rays for several years during the growth period to note the behavior of the epiphysis.

Open reduction is rarely indicated except in irreducible cases with gross displacement.

FORWARD DISPLACEMENT OF THE DISTAL FEMORAL EPIPHYSIS

Prereduction X-Ray

1. The femoral epiphysis is displaced forward.

2. The end of the diaphysis is displaced into the popliteal fossa.

Note: The degree of displacement may vary from minor amounts to complete separations.

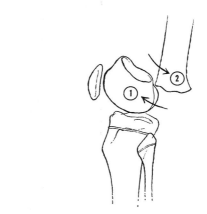

Manipulative Reduction

Note: If a massive hemarthrosis is present always aspirate the joint before reduction is executed.

1. Place the patient on a fracture table.

2. Fasten the unaffected foot to a foot plate.

3. With the knee flexed 30 to 45 degrees make strong manual traction in the long axis of the thigh.

4. Correct any displacement by making pressure on the epiphysis and the lower end of the shaft in opposite directions.

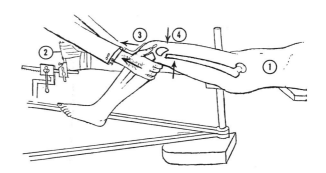

1. While an assistant makes upward pressure on the lower end of the thigh,

2. Reduce displacement by flexing the knee beyond a right angle.

(Now check position by x-ray.)

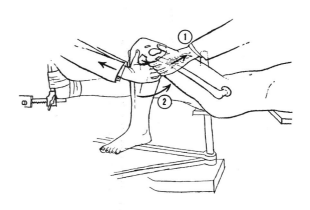

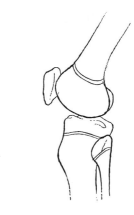

Postreduction X-Ray

The epiphysis is restored to its normal anatomic position.

Immobilization

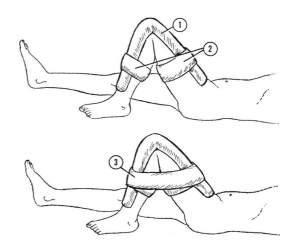

1. Apply an anterior plaster slab to the flexed leg.

2. Secure the slab to the thigh and calf with circular plaster bandages.

3. The degree of flexion is determined by the amount of swelling present and fixed by a circular bandage around the thigh and calf.

Postreduction Management

At the end of three to four weeks remove the plaster slab, decrease the flexion to 45 degrees and apply another similar plaster splint.

At the end of two to three more weeks remove the second splint.

Now institute graduated flexion and extension exercises to restore quadriceps power and joint motion.

When complete extension is achieved, allow the patient up on crutches and permit protected weight bearing.

Discard the crutches when the quadriceps is sufficiently strong to stabilize the knee adequately.

IRREDUCIBLE DISPLACEMENT OF THE DISTAL FEMORAL EPIPHYSIS

REMARKS

This method is used in late cases in which some healing has occurred between the epiphysis and the diaphysis.

These cases can be reduced if preliminary traction is applied for 24 to 48 hours before reduction is attempted.

Preliminary Traction

1. The patient lies in a fracture bed.
2. Insert a threaded wire through the upper end of the tibia; don't traumatize the proximal epiphyseal plate of the tibia.
3. Flex the hip 90 degrees.
4. Make vertical traction with 25 or 30 pounds of weight.

Note: At the end of 24 to 48 hours the fragments are usually disengaged to permit manipulative reduction as depicted for fresh separations (p. 1365); the subsequent management is the same as for fresh separations.

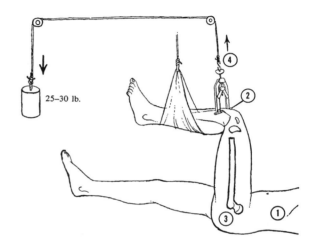

BACKWARD DISPLACEMENT OF THE DISTAL FEMORAL EPIPHYSIS

Prereduction X-Ray

1. The femoral epiphysis is displaced backward.
2. The distal end of the shaft of the femur is displaced forward.

(Varying degrees of lateral displacement of the epiphysis may be present.)

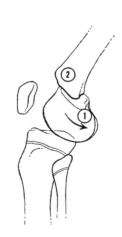

Manipulative Reduction

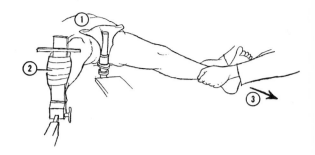

1. Place the patient on a fracture table.
2. Fasten the unaffected foot to a foot plate.
3. Make straight traction on the limb to restore length.

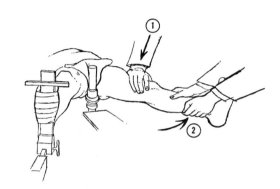

While traction is maintained,
1. An assistant makes downward pressure on the distal end of the shaft and
2. The operator hyperextends the knee, effecting the reduction.

Immobilization

1. Apply a plaster cast from the groin to the toes.
2. The knee is in full extension.
3. The foot is at a right angle.

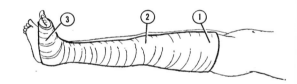

Note: Mold the plaster well around the condyles of the femur.

Postreduction Management

Remove the plaster cast after six weeks.

Institute graduated exercises to restore power to the quadriceps and motion at the knee joint.

Allow the patient up on crutches with protected weight bearing.

Discard the crutches when the quadriceps is powerful enough to stabilize the knee joint adequately.

INJURIES OF THE SOFT TISSUES AND BONY ELEMENTS OF THE KNEE JOINT

ANATOMIC FEATURES

The knee joint is the most massive articulation of the body. Its exposed position makes it vulnerable to many types of injuries involving both its bony and soft tissue components.

The knee joint is a compound articulation comprising the femorotibial and patellofemoral joints. From a functional point of view it is capable of both hinge and gliding motion; in fact the patellofemoral joint functions solely as a gliding joint.

The bony architecture of the joint provides little stability; only a small portion of the femoral condyles articulate with a corresponding small area on the tibial plateaus at any one time during motion.

Although the menisci deepen the articular surfaces of the tibial plateaus, this configuration adds little to the stability of the knee joint.

The stability of the knee joint is entirely dependent upon the ligamentous apparatus and the muscles that motorize the joint.

CAPSULE OF THE KNEE JOINT

The knee joint is enveloped by a fibrous capsule; the posterior and lateral portions of the capsule are intimately related with the posterior and lateral ligaments forming tight supports in these regions. The posterior structures protect the joint from hyperextension while the lateral structures prevent any abnormal lateral motion.

On the other hand, anteriorly, the capsule is loose and redundant and superiorly it bulges under the quadriceps apparatus to form the suprapatellar pouch. The loose arrangement of the capsule permits free flexion of the joint; anteriorly, the joint depends for stability on an efficient quadriceps apparatus.

The anterior capsule is taut only when the knee is completely flexed.

1. Capsule on lateral aspect of the joint is closely applied to the lateral ligaments.

2. Capsule on anterior aspect of joint bulges to form the suprapatellar pouch.

3. Quadriceps muscle.

4. Patella.

5. Patellar tendon.

6. Medial collateral ligament.

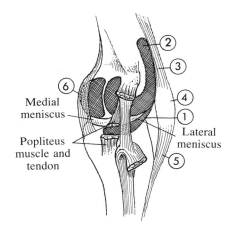

LIGAMENTS OF THE KNEE JOINT

The ligaments of the knee comprise a very intricate apparatus designed to stabilize the joint and to protect it from abnormal stresses in any direction. These ligaments surround the joint on all sides and function synergistically in such a manner that regardless of the position of the knee stability is maintained.

The most stable position of the knee is full extension. In this position all ligaments are taut. As flexion is performed some of the ligaments or parts of the ligaments begin to relax in order to permit flexion of the joint. This is especially true of the posterior ligament.

COLLATERAL LIGAMENTS

MEDIAL COLLATERAL LIGAMENT

This is a broad, strong, triangular ligament on the medial side of the joint. It is composed of two layers, a deep and a superficial layer.

The deep layer spans the interval from the femoral condyle to the upper margin of the tibia; it extends forward as far as the midlateral line; posteriorly it blends with the posterior ligament. The ligament is made up of short fibers closely applied to the capsule and at the joint line is firmly attached to the medial meniscus. The larger superficial layer runs from the medial femoral condyle to a point 5 to 7 centimeters below the joint line. Its anterior fibers blend with the fibers of the medial patellar retinaculum while its posterior fibers extend far backward to form a cup-like structure closely applied to the convex posterior surface of the medial femoral condyle. At the level of the joint line the superficial fibers blend with the deep fibers. Also some superficial fibers blend with the fascia of the thigh.

The arrangement of the fibers of the superficial ligament is such that regardless of the position of the knee some of its fibers remain taut, thereby providing the necessary stability.

Page 1371

Medial Collateral Ligament

1. Superficial layer of the ligament.
2. The posterior portion of the ligament is cupped around the medial
femoral condyle.
3. The ligament is firmly attached
to the medial meniscus.

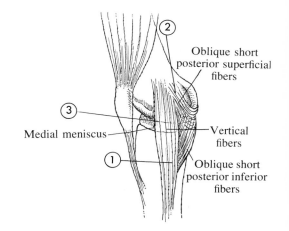

FIBULAR COLLATERAL LIGAMENT

On the lateral side of the joint the fibular collateral ligament guards
against lateral displacement of the joint.

It consists of a tough bundle of fibrous strands running from the
lateral femoral condyle to the head of the fibula. This ligament is reinforced by fibers from the iliotibial band which is also a stabilizer of the
knee on its lateral aspect. Some fibers of the iliotibial band run from
the femoral condyle to the upper margin of the tibia; these fibers are
often referred to as the lateral tibial collateral ligament.

This ligament is not attached to the lateral meniscus; between the
ligament and the meniscus lies the tendon of the popliteus muscle.

Fibular Collateral Ligament

1. Fibular collateral ligament.
2. Lateral meniscus.
3. Popliteus tendon and muscle.

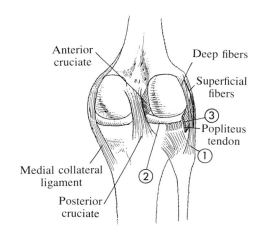

POSTERIOR LIGAMENT (OBLIQUE POPLITEAL LIGAMENT)

Essentially this structure is the posterior portion of the fibrous capsule reinforced by many fibrous strands converting it into a tough, strong ligament. It is attached above to the entire posterior aspect of the femur immediately above the condyles, and below to the entire posterior aspect of the tibia and also to the fibula. Medially this structure blends with the medial collateral ligament.

It functions primarily as a checkrein to hyperextension; in this position it is extremely tight and affords much stability to the knee joint. When the knee is in even the slightest amount of flexion, the ligament becomes lax and no longer is able to stabilize the joint in any direction.

Posterior Ligament

1. Note broad area covered by the ligament.
2. Insertion of the ligament into the tibia.

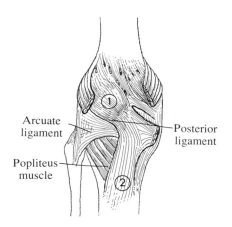

Arcuate ligament

Posterior ligament

Popliteus muscle

QUADRICEPS MECHANISM (ANTERIOR LIGAMENT)

From a functional point of view, the quadriceps apparatus, when in tone, serves as the anterior ligament of the knee joint.

The four quadriceps muscles of the thigh terminate distally in a complex but ingenious apparatus; they end in a common tendon, the quadriceps tendon, whose central portion inserts into the patella and whose lateral portions form the medial and lateral retinacula which in turn become continuous with the fascia of the leg. The central portion of the apparatus is continued distally from the patella to the tibial tubercle by the patellar tendon.

This mechanism is capable of powerful extension of the knee, and also reinforces the posterior and lateral ligaments. When this apparatus fails the remaining ligaments, especially the lateral ligaments, are not capable of providing total stability and are unable to cope with even normal stresses. Soon they become lax and marked instability of the joint ensues.

Quadriceps Mechanism

1. Quadriceps muscles of the thigh.
2. Quadriceps tendon.
3. Patella.
4. Medial and lateral retinacula.

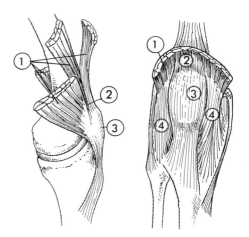

The efficiency of the quadriceps muscles is enhanced by the patella, which is strategically placed in the quadriceps tendon; it provides a fulcrum when extension of the knee is performed. The loss of the patella should not be taken lightly and whenever possible should be avoided. Don't ever remove the patella if there is another choice.

The patella is not a sesmoid bone; the patellofemoral joint is formed like any other synovial joint.

CRUCIATE LIGAMENTS

The cruciate ligaments are intra-articular but extrasynovial structures; they are fan-shaped and each is twisted on itself. The ingenious arrangement of their fibers serves as a guide, permitting specific movements and also providing much stability to the knee joint. In addition, these ligaments augment the strength of the lateral and posterior ligaments.

The anterior cruciate ligament runs from the anteromedial aspect of the tibial plateau, just anterior to the tibial spine, to the posterolateral aspect of the intercondylar notch of the femur.

It is primarily concerned with stabilizing the knee in the anteroposterior plane; it prevents forward displacement of the tibia on the femur.

The posterior cruciate ligament takes origin on the posterior aspect of the tibia just behind the articular surface. It extends forward, upward and inward and inserts into the medial aspect of the anterior margin of the intercondylar notch.

In addition to its other functions, this ligament's prime function is to prevent backward displacement of the tibia on the femur.

Cruciate Ligaments

1. Anterior cruciate ligament.
2. Posterior cruciate ligament.
3. Note fan-shaped configuration of the ligaments.
4. Anterior attachment of the anterior cruciate is in front of the tibial spine.
5. Posterior cruciate ligament—its posterior attachment is on the back of the tibia.
6. Anterior cruciate ligament—its posterior attachment is on the posterolateral side of the notch.
7. Menisci—note the relation of the posterior cruciate ligament to the menisci.

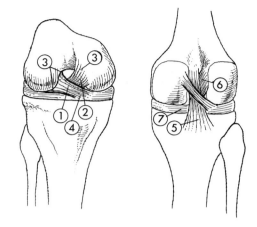

MUSCULAR APPARATUS OF THE KNEE JOINT

Even more than the ligamentous apparatus the muscles motorizing the knee joint play an important role in the stability of the knee joint. As previously noted the quadriceps muscle is the most important and, when in tone, is capable of powerful extension of the knee joint; it is the most important single structure contributing to the stability of the joint. The effectiveness of the lateral and posterior ligaments depends heavily on the efficiency of this muscle.

On the posterior aspect of the thigh are the hamstring muscles; these are powerful flexors of the knee joint; but in addition the mode of insertion of the medial hamstring muscles as they wind around the tibia to gain insertion into the anterior aspect of the tibia contributes much to the lateral and rotatory stability of the joint.

Flexors of the Knee Joint

1. Medial hamstring muscles.
2. Insertion of the medial hamstrings into the anteromedial aspect of the upper end of the tibia.

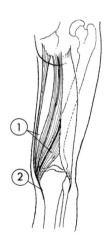

SPRAINS OF THE LIGAMENTS OF THE KNEE JOINT

REMARKS

Sprains of the ligaments of the knee are common injuries, especially in young males engaged in contact sports. These sprains are the result of abnormal motion. The severity of the lesion varies. A mild injury is one in which a few fibers are torn but the integrity of the ligament is not lost, nor has the ligament been elongated. In other words, the force producing the lesion is contained before serious damage to the ligament is done (Grade I). A moderate sprain (Grade II) is more serious; many fibers are torn and although there is no dissolution of the ligament it is elongated. An elongated ligament can no longer function as a stabilizer of the joint; its efficiency is markedly reduced. Complete disruption of the ligament (Grade III) results in total loss of function.

It becomes apparent that before treatment can be instituted the severity of the lesion must be adequately evaluated.

Mechanism of Sprains

The function of a ligament is to prevent abnormal motion of the joint in a particular direction. If the stress applied to a joint is of sufficient intensity to produce abnormal motion, the protecting ligament will be injured. The grade of the injury is governed by the intensity of the force.

In the knee joint, the forces producing ligamentous injuries are those forcing the knee into abnormal abduction, adduction, extension, internal rotation, external rotation, forward and backward displacement or a combination of any of these.

A common combination of forces is one in which the foot is forced in external rotation and an abduction force is applied at the outer aspect of the knee, forcing the thigh to rotate inward and the knee to flex.

In this mechanism the first structure to suffer is the medial collateral ligament, first the deep layer that is firmly attached to the medial meniscus and then the superficial layer.

If the force continues, stress is put on the anterior cruciate, which may not be able to contain it and gives way. With failure of the anterior cruciate, and if the force still continues, the posterior cruciate may be involved. It becomes apparent that the extent of implication of any one structure or of all structures in the path of abnormal stresses depends upon the intensity of the stresses acting.

Another mechanism is the reverse of the abduction and external rotation mechanism just described; it is the adduction–internal rotation injury which first involves the lateral ligaments, then the lateral meniscus and the anterior and the posterior cruciates.

Less common is the hyperextension type of injury; the first structure receiving the stress is the posterior ligament, followed by the posterior cruciate and finally the posterior portions of the lateral ligaments.

Abnormal stress forcing the tibia directly backward results in sprains of the posterior cruciate whereas stresses forcing the tibia forward produce sprains in the anterior cruciate.

Abduction–External Rotation Mechanism

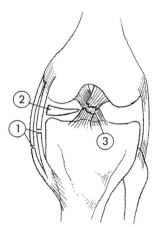

1. The foot is fixed; the leg rotates outward.
2. The knee is flexed.
3. Abducting stress is applied to the outer aspect of the knee.
4. Thigh rotates inward.

Pathology Resulting from Abduction–External Rotation Injuries

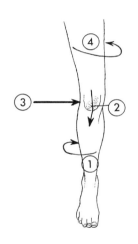

1. Tear of the superficial and deep layers of the medial collateral ligament (tear may extend into the posterior capsule).
2. Tear of the medial meniscus.
3. Complete tear of the anterior cruciate.

Adduction–Internal Rotation Mechanism

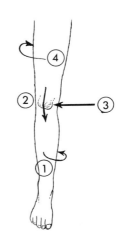

1. The foot is fixed and the leg is rotated inward.
2. The knee is flexed.
3. Adducting stress applied to inner side of the knee.
4. The thigh rotates outward.

Pathology Resulting from Adduction–Internal Rotation Injuries

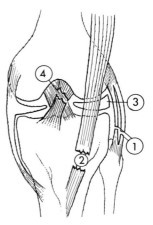

1. Tear of the fibular collateral ligament.
2. Tear of the lateral tibial collateral ligament (fibers from the iliotibial band).
3. Tear of the lateral meniscus.
4. Tear of the anterior cruciate.

Management of Sprains of the Ligaments of the Knee Joint

REMARKS

Before intelligent treatment can be instituted, correct assessment of the severity of the lesion is most essential.

This assessment can only be reached by a careful examination of the injured part and correct interpretation of the findings.

In general, in sprains of Grade I in which only a few fibers are damaged and in sprains of Grade II in which many fibers are disrupted but the continuity of the ligament is not lost, conservative treatment with emphasis on protection of the injured part until healing is complete is the treatment of choice.

On the other hand, ligaments suffering Grade III sprains, in which there is total disruption of the ligament, should be repaired surgically and the repair should be done as soon as conditions permit—today and not tomorrow.

TREATMENT OF GRADE I SPRAINS

REMARKS

These lseions are characterized by an absence of certain features. There is no abnormal mobility in any direction, no pain on normal motion, no locking of the joint, and no effusion or blood in the joint.

The positive findings are minimal local swelling, tenderness directly over the site of involvement of the ligament and pain when the affected ligament is stretched.

Maneuvers to Test Stability of the Joint

1. No abnormal rocking.
2. The anterior and posterior drawer signs are negative.
3. No demonstrable change in the width of the joint space when abduction or adduction forces are applied to the knee.

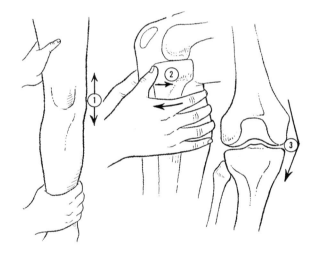

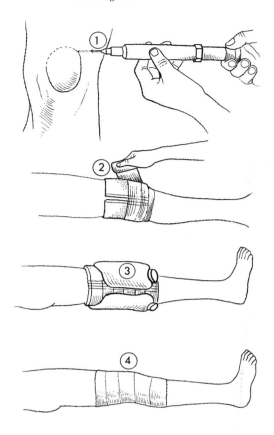

Local Treatment

1. Aspirate hematoma, if present.
2. Apply a compression bandage to the knee.
3. Apply ice packs.
4. After the local symptoms subside, protect the knee with an elastic wrapping.

Allow early resumption of normal activity.

Keep the patient under observation! You may have failed to recognize an injury to the meniscus. Institute a regimen of quadriceps exercises immediately.

TREATMENT OF GRADE II SPRAINS

REMARKS

The findings are similar to those in injuries of Grade I but they are of greater intensity.

There is no abnormal motion either in the lateral or anteroposterior direction.

There is pain on putting the ligament on the stretch, and tenderness over the entire ligament on pressure but more exquisite over the site of maximum injury. Any lateral or rotatory motion is painful; locking may be present or absent; local swelling is always present and later an effusion of the knee follows.

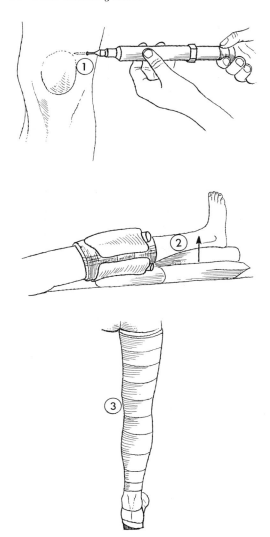

Local Treatment

1. Aspirate the knee joint and inject a steroid preparation; don't allow the capsule of the joint to be distended. Aspirate as frequently as necessary.

2. Apply a compression bandage, elevate the limb and apply ice packs; after 36 to 48 hours apply heat.

3. After seven to ten days apply a walking cast and institute a program of quadriceps exercises. Protect the joint until complete healing of the ligaments occurs; the time varies with the severity of the damage—usually the joint must be protected for four to six weeks.

Note: After removal of the cast apply a compression elastic bandage. Do not permit full activity as long as there are symptoms. If the patient is permitted to participate in strenuous athletics, protect the knee with adequate adhesive strapping.

TREATMENT OF GRADE III SPRAINS

REMARKS

These lesions are characterized by complete rupture of one or more ligaments.

There is immediate complete loss of function; pain is severe and the patient is aware of complete loss of stability of the joint.

The pertinent features are: demonstrable abnormal motion, the direction of which depends on the structures injured; evidence of local swelling at the site of injury followed by distention of the capsule by an effusion, blood or both; all movements produce pain, particularly those which separate the torn ends of the ligament. Locking of the joint may or may not be present.

The following tests will point to the ligaments involved.

Don't hesitate to use an anesthetic or to take stress x-rays if there is doubt about the diagnosis.

With the knee in extension, abnormal abduction indicates:

1. The medial tibial collateral ligament is torn.

2. The tear extends into the posterior ligament.

3. The anterior cruciate is disrupted.

4. The medial meniscus may or may not be torn.

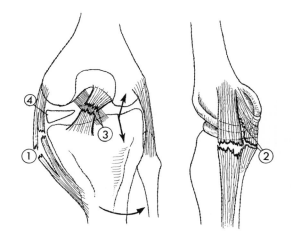

A knee stable in extension but unstable in 20 to 30 degrees of flexion indicates:

A. When there is abnormal abduction

    1. The medial tibial collateral ligament is torn and the posterior ligament is intact.

    2. The medial meniscus may or may not be damaged.

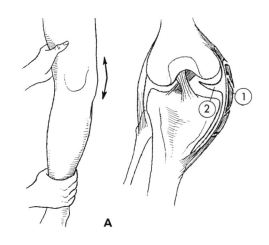

A

B. When there is abnormal adduction
1. The fibular collateral ligament is torn.

Note: The lateral collateral ligament is torn and the posterior ligament is intact.

2. The lateral meniscus may or may not be torn.

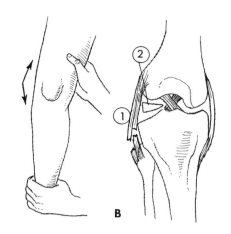

With the knee flexed at 90 degrees and the leg externally rotated 30 degrees:
1. Abnormal anterior displacement indicates
2. Tear of the deep tibial collateral ligament, of the superficial tibial collateral and possibly a tear of the anterior cruciate ligament.

Note: This combination causes rotatory instability.
Isolated tears of the anterior cruciate ligament are indeed rare.

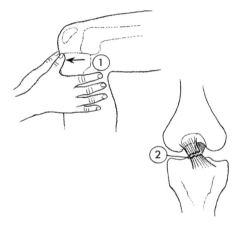

1. Abnormal posterior displacement indicates
2. Tear of the posterior cruciate ligament and attenuation or tear of the posterior capsule.

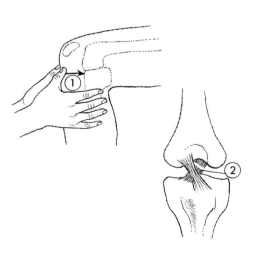

PRINCIPLES OF TREATMENT

As the result of the pioneer work of O'Donoghue, it is now generally accepted that ligaments disrupted by trauma should be repaired surgically.

The repair should be done immediately; early repair is almost invariably successful; late repair or reconstruction of the ligaments is not nearly as successful.

Prompt surgical repair presumes that a definitive diagnosis and assessment of the severity of the lesion be made early.

In combined lesions all ligaments must be repaired; it is wrong to repair a lateral ligament and not the anterior cruciate if severed. All ligaments play an important role in the stability of the knee joint; loss of one of the ligaments will definitely impair the stability and reduce the functional capacity of the joint; this applies to the cruciate ligaments.

The true nature and the severity of the lesions can only be adequately evaluated by visualization of the structure involved.

SURGICAL MANAGEMENT OF GRADE III SPRAINS

RECENT COMPLETE RUPTURE OF THE TIBIAL COLLATERAL LIGAMENT

REMARKS

The lesion is caused by momentary subluxation of the knee joint when the flexed knee with the tibia fixed is suddenly abducted and the femur is rotated internally.

The severity of the lesion depends upon the intensity of the subluxating force. Forces of great intensity may also produce a rupture of one or both cruciate ligaments or a tear of the internal semilunar cartilage, or both of these lesions.

Forces of lesser intensity may produce only sprains of the fibers of the ligament or partial tears without dissolution of the continuity of the ligament.

Surgical repair of all completely torn ligaments is the method of choice.

Mechanism of Injury

1. The subluxating force is applied to the outer aspect of the limb.
2. The foot is fixed.
3. The knee is flexed.
4. The tibia is abducted.
5. The femur is internally rotated.

Note: The severity of the lesion is governed by the intensity of the subluxating force.

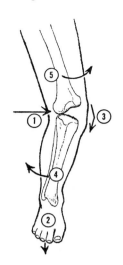

Position of the Patient for X-Ray Examination

1. The knees are bound together.
2. The knees are flexed 15 to 20 degrees.
3. The feet are wedged apart by sandbags.

Note: Widening of the medial joint space is significant only when it is demonstrable with the knees extended, indicating a tear of the posterior capsule in addition to a tear of the tibial collateral and possibly the anterior cruciate ligament.

With the knees flexed 15 to 20 degrees, mild or moderate widening is insignificant; severe widening indicates disruption of the tibial collateral and possibly the anterior cruciate ligament.

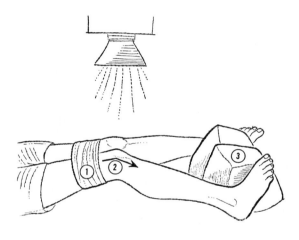

Preoperative X-Ray of Isolated Lesion

1. The medial joint space is widened.
2. The small bony fragment may be avulsed from the epicondyle of the femur.

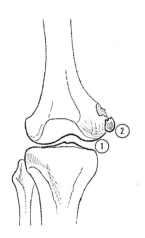

Page 1385

Preoperative X-Ray of Combined Lesions

1. Wide separation of the medial joint space.

2. Subluxation of the joint is reproduced.

Note: Such wide separation can only be produced when the anterior cruciate ligament and the tibial collateral ligament are torn; in this joint the medial meniscus was also torn.

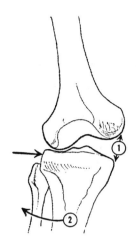

Maneuvers To Permit Diagnosis of Combined Lesions of the Tibial Collateral Ligament

A. 1. The knee is extended.
   2. An abduction force is applied to the extended knee.

Note: No abnormal abduction rocking is elicited if the anterior cruciate is intact; if present, it indicates a complete lesion of the tibial collateral ligament and also of the anterior cruciate ligament and posterior capsule.

B. Drawer Sign
   1. The knee is flexed 90 degrees.
   2. The femur is fixed.
   3. Severe anterior displacement indicates a tear of the anterior cruciate and the tibial collateral ligaments.
   4. Posterior displacement indicates a tear of the posterior cruciate ligament and the posterior capsule.

Note: A better method to demonstrate a tear of the posterior cruciate is by supporting the extended leg with the heel in the examiner's palm; the head of the tibia drops backward, producing a recurvation deformity.

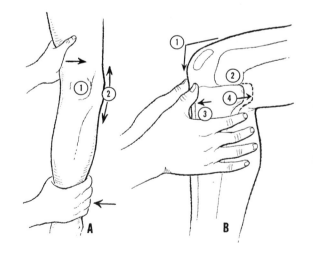

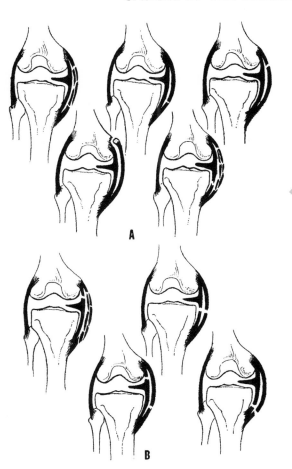

A and B. Types of Isolated Lesions

Note that both the superficial and deep portions of the ligament may be avulsed from the femoral or tibial insertions.

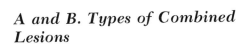

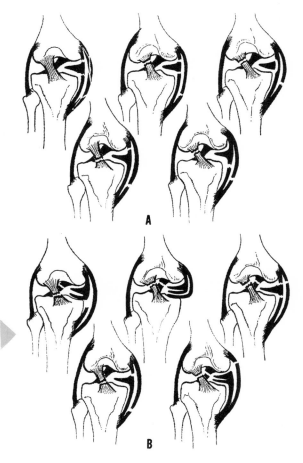

A and B. Types of Combined Lesions

Note that lesions of the tibial collateral ligament may be associated with lesions of one of the menisci or one or both cruciate ligaments.

Types of lesions of the anterior and posterior cruciate ligaments and various methods of repair are depicted on pages 1397 and 1398, 1401 and 1402.

Operative Repair of Isolated Lesions

1. Make an S-shaped incision on the anteromedial aspect of the knee; it begins 2 cm. above the medial femoral epicondyle and ends 8 cm. below the articular margin of the inner tibial condyle.

2. Divide the deep fascia by a vertical incision extending the full length of the skin incision.

3. Retract the edges of the fascia and expose and examine the entire ligament.

4. Abduct the tibia on the femur. This maneuver demonstrates the site and extent of the tear.

Note: Repair the deep and superficial layers of the ligament separately if possible. Repair the deep fibers first.

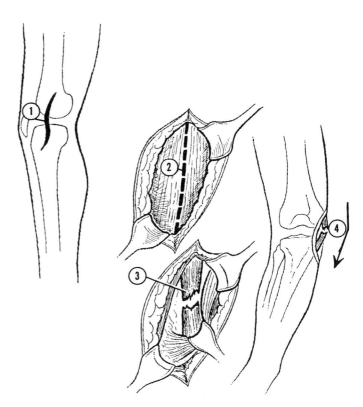

Methods of Repair of the Deep Fibers

1. Repair of the upper portion of the ligament.
2. Repair of the midportion of the ligament.
3. Repair of the lower portion of the ligament.

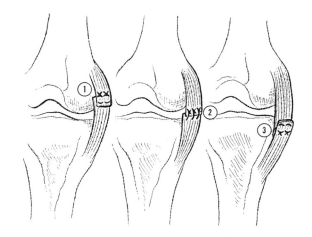

ALTERNATE METHODS

1. The femoral attachment is anchored in a slot in the femur.
2. The tibial attachment is anchored in a slot in the tibia.

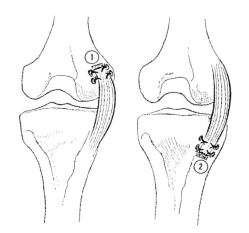

Methods of Repair of the Superficial Fibers

1. The ends of the ligament are approximated by interrupted sutures or
2 and 3. The end of the ligament is anchored in a slot in the tibia.

The femoral attachment of the superficial fibers is secured in the same manner as depicted for repairs of the femoral attachment of the deep fibers of the tibial ligament.

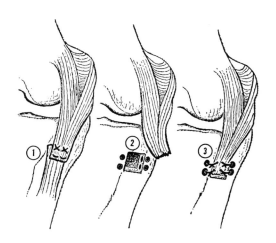

Operative Repair of Combined Lesions

1. Make an S-shaped incision in the anteromedial aspect of the knee; it begins 2 cm. above the femoral epicondyle and terminates 8 cm. below the articular margin of the medial tibial condyle.

2. Divide the deep fascia the entire length of the skin incision.

3. Retract the edges of the fascia and expose the entire tibial collateral ligament and estimate the extent of damage.

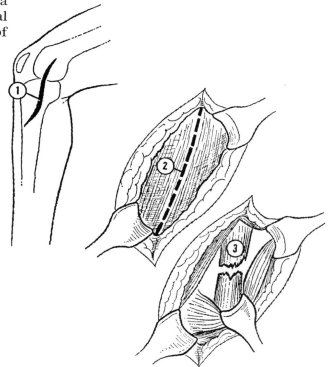

1. Retract the outer skin flap, exposing the parapatellar region, and make an incision in the capsule and synovialis.

2. Through the capsular incision inspect all intra-articular structures and note the extent of the damage to each.

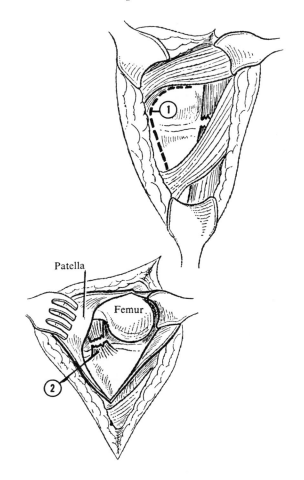

Patella

Femur

Order of Repair

First: Remove the medial meniscus, if torn. (See page 1424.)

Next: Repair the anterior cruciate (pages 1397 and 1398).

Then: Repair the deep layer of the tibial collateral ligament (page 1389).

Finally: Repair the superficial layer of the tibial collateral ligament.

Method of Repair of the Anterior Cruciate Ligament

When the ligament is avulsed from the tibia with or without a fragment of bone:

1. Reattach the end of the ligament by a mattress suture passing through two drill channels made in the medial tibial condyle.

2. If the bony fragment is large, anchor it to its tibial bed with a screw.

When the femoral attachment of the anterior cruciate is torn:

3. Reattach the end of the ligament by a mattress suture passing through two drill channels made obliquely through the lateral femoral condyle.

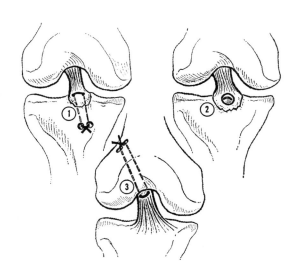

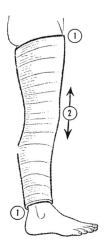

Immobilization

1. Apply a well padded plaster cylinder extending from the groin to just above the malleoli.
2. The knee is in full extension.

Postoperative Management

Begin graduated quadriceps exercises immediately.

Remove the plaster cylinder at the end of three weeks and apply another; this should fit snugly. Now permit weight bearing.

Step up the intensity of the quadriceps exercises.

Remove the second plaster cylinder six to eight weeks after operation; permit weight bearing with crutches.

Institute exercises to restore joint motion and increase the intensity of the quadriceps exercises.

Discard the crutches when the quadriceps is sufficiently strong to stabilize the knee adequately (usually two to three weeks).

RECENT COMPLETE RUPTURE OF THE FIBULAR COLLATERAL LIGAMENT

REMARKS

This lesion is rare and is usually produced by forceful adduction of the leg on the femur.

Stretching or rupture of the common peroneal nerve is a common associated lesion. Always check for this complication.

In severe lesions the lateral portion of the capsule is torn and the cruciate ligaments may be implicated.

A fragment of bone is often avulsed from the head of the fibula.

Following injury to the common peroneal nerve the prognosis is grave, even when immediate surgical repair is achieved.

Maneuvers to Permit Diagnosis of Lesions of the Fibular Ligaments

In isolated lesions:

1. Adduction rocking with the knee extended. (The drawer sign is negative in isolated lesions.)

In combined lesions:

2. Marked adduction rocking with the knee extended. (The drawer sign is positive, indicating a tear of the anterior cruciate ligament.)

Note: In the extended position any adduction rocking also indicates a tear of the posterolateral capsule.

Isolated lesions are indeed rare.

In severe lesions the fascia lata is always attenuated or torn, and occasionally the biceps tendon.

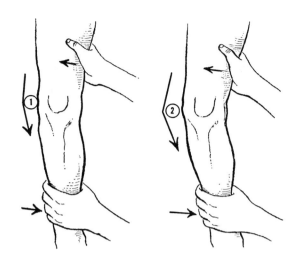

Types of Lesions

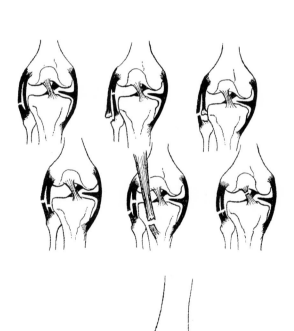

Preoperative X-Ray

X-ray taken while the tibia is forcefully adducted:

1. The lateral joint space is widened.

2. A small flake of bone may be avulsed from the head of the fibula.

Page 1393

Operative Repair

1. Make a vertical incision on the lateral aspect of the knee, beginning 1 inch above the lateral epicondyle and terminating 1 inch below the head of the fibula.

2. Divide the deep fascia on the line of the skin incision; reflect the skin edges and expose the fibular ligament to determine the extent of the damage. Always visualize the common peroneal nerve.

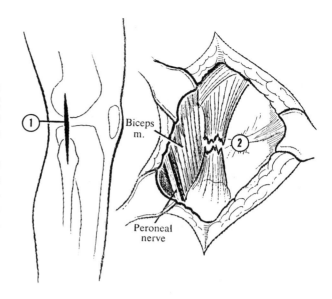

FOR ISOLATED LESIONS

1. Approximate the edges of the tear in the capsule and the deep capsular fibers of the ligament by interrupted sutures.

2. Approximate the edges of the tear in the superficial portion of the ligament.

3. Reinforce the ligament by taking a segment of the tendon of the biceps femoris muscle.

4. Anchor the proximal end of the tendon in a slot made in the lateral aspect of the lateral femoral condyle.

5. Fasten the tendon to the fibular collateral ligament with interrupted sutures.

Note: If the nerve is ruptured, approximate the ends by fine interrupted sutures.

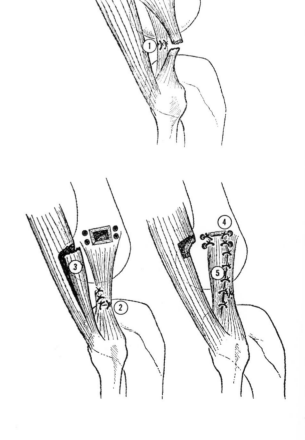

Operative Repair (Continued)

Methods of reattachment of the distal end of the fibular collateral ligament:

1. Reattachment of the ends of the ligament by interrupted sutures.

2. Anchorage of the end of the ligament in a slot made in the head of the fibula.

Note: If a fragment of bone is avulsed from the head of the fibula it may be excised or, if large, replaced in its original site.

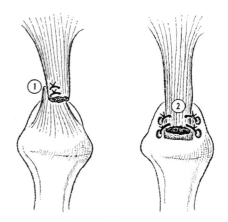

In combined lesions

When the anterior or the posterior cruciate ligaments are torn, repair is effected in the same manner as depicted on pages 1397 and 1398, 1401 and 1402.

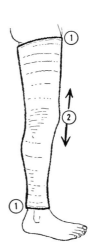

Immobilization

1. Apply a plaster cylinder from the groin to just above the malleoli.
2. The knee is in full extension.

Postoperative Management

Begin graduated quadriceps exercises immediately.

Remove the plaster cylinder at the end of three weeks and apply another cylinder; this should fit snugly. Now permit weight bearing.

Step up the intensity of the quadriceps exercises.

Remove the second plaster cylinder six to eight weeks after the operation; now permit weight bearing with crutches.

Institute exercises to restore joint motion and increase the intensity of the quadriceps exercises.

Discard the crutches when the quadriceps is sufficiently strong to stabilize the knee adequately (usually two to three weeks).

In the event that a repair of the external peroneal nerve has been performed, after removal of the cast fit the patient with a brace with a drop-foot stop.

Electrical stimulation of the paralyzed muscles is helpful to maintain volume and tone.

RECENT RUPTURES OF THE ANTERIOR CRUCIATE LIGAMENT

REMARKS

Isolated lesions are rare but they may result from severe hyperextension of the knee or from a force driving the femur backward on the fixed tibia while the knee is flexed.

The ligament may be avulsed from the lateral femoral condyle or avulsed from the tibial spine, or a portion of the tibial spine may be avulsed with the ligament attached. This last lesion is usually encountered in children, adolescents and young adults.

In most instances lesions of the anterior cruciate ligament are combined with lesions of the tibial collateral ligament and lesions of the medial meniscus resulting from severe abduction or rotatory forces. (These have been discussed previously.)

These lesions are always accompanied by hemorrhage and synovial effusion into the joint.

Adequate examination may not be possible in recent cases unless the joint is aspirated and the patient given a general anesthetic.

Always bear in mind the possibility of a concomitant meniscal lesion; it may not be possible to eliminate this complication at the time of the initial examination.

Always take x-rays in the anteroposterior, lateral and axial planes to visualize the tibial spine adequately.

Except for avulsions of the tibial spine which can be reduced by conservative measures, all lesions of the anterior cruciate ligament should be exposed and repaired surgically.

Early surgical repair produces far better results and more stable knees than conservative measures.

Diagnostic Maneuver (Anterior Drawer Sign)

Note: In fresh lesions swelling, spasm and pain may preclude execution of this maneuver; therefore always administer a general anesthetic and aspirate the knee before performing the test.

1. The knee is flexed to a right angle.
2. The femur is fixed.
3. Anterior displacement of the tibia may indicate a lesion of the anterior cruciate ligament.

Note: This is not a very reliable test.

Operative Repair for Detachments of the Distal and Proximal Ends of the Anterior Cruciate Ligament

(Perform the operation with a tourniquet applied around the upper third of the thigh.)

1. Expose the intercondylar region of the tibia with a medial parapatellar incision.
2. After flushing out of the joint cavity all blood clots, identify the lesion in the anterior cruciate ligament.

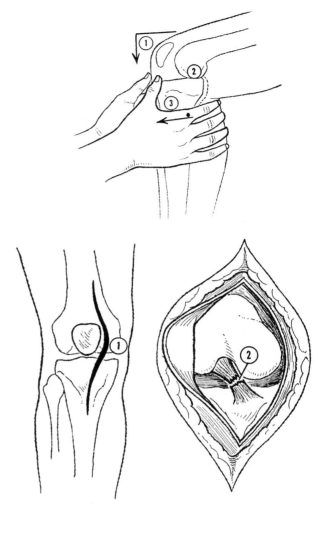

For detachment of the distal end of the anterior cruciate ligament:

1. Make two parallel drill channels in the medial condyle of the tibia. They begin on the anteromedial surface of the condyle 4 cm. below the tibial brim and are directed obliquely upward, backward and inward, and issue from the superior surface of the tibia through the original site of the attachment of the ligament. (These channels may also be made from within the joint—outward.)
2. Secure the ligament to its raw bed by a mattress suture tied on the anterior surface of the tibia.

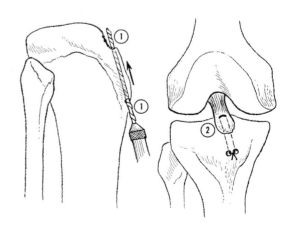

Operative Repair for Detachments of the Distal and Proximal Ends of the Anterior Cruciate Ligament *(Continued)*

For detachment of the proximal end of the anterior cruciate ligament:

Note: This is an exceedingly rare lesion and usually is encountered in combination with lesions of the tibial collateral ligament.

1. Pass a suture (stout silk) through the proximal end of the anterior cruciate ligament.

2. Make a 2 inch vertical incision on the lateral aspect of the thigh immediately above the lateral femoral epicondyle.

3. Make two drill channels 1 cm. apart in the lateral femoral condyle; they are directed downward and inward and issue through the area normally providing attachment for the proximal end of the ligament.

4. Pass the ends of the suture through the drill channels, pull the ligament taut, and tie the ends of the suture on the lateral aspect of the femur.

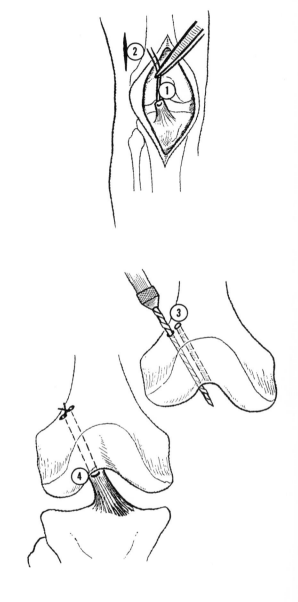

Operative Repair for Detachments of the Distal and Proximal Ends of the Anterior Cruciate Ligament (Continued)

1. Apply a well padded plaster cylinder extending from the groin to just above the malleoli.
2. The knee is in full extension.

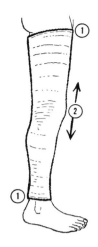

Postoperative Management

Begin graduated quadriceps exercises immediately.

Remove the plaster cylinder at the end of three weeks and apply another; this should fit snugly. Now permit weight bearing.

Step up the intensity of the quadriceps exercises.

Remove the second plaster cylinder six to eight weeks after the operation. Permit weight bearing with crutches.

Institute exercises to restore joint motion and increase the intensity of the quadriceps exercises.

Discard the crutches when the quadriceps is sufficiently strong to stabilize the knee adequately (usually two to three weeks).

RECENT RUPTURE OF THE POSTERIOR CRUCIATE LIGAMENT

REMARKS

This is a rare isolated lesion.

Usually it is the result of a direct force driving the tibia posteriorly while the foot and femur are fixed and the knee is flexed.

One of two lesions may be encountered: (1) rupture of the femoral attachment of the ligament or (2) avulsion of the tibial attachment with a fragment of bone.

Hemarthrosis and synovial effusion are always present immediately after the injury.

In fresh cases, give the patient a general anesthetic and aspirate the joint before examining the joint for tears of the ligaments.

Always take an x-ray in the anteroposterior, lateral and axial planes.

Surgical repair is the treatment of choice.

Diagnostic Maneuver (Posterior Drawer Sign)

1. The knee is flexed at a right angle.
2. The femur is fixed.
3. Backward displacement of the tibia indicates a lesion of the posterior cruciate.

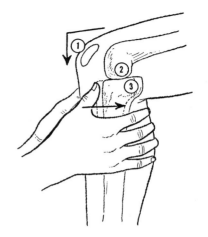

Preoperative X-Ray

1. Avulsion of a fragment of bone from the tibia at the site of the inferior attachment of the posterior cruciate ligament.

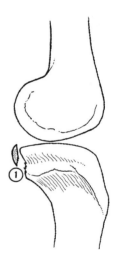

Operative Repair for Lesions of the Posterior Cruciate Ligament

1. Make a vertical S-shaped incision centered over the posterior joint line.

2. Divide the deep fascia and develop the interval between the inner head of the gastrocnemius and the tendon of the semitendinosus.

3. Cut the inner head of the gastrocnemius and displace the muscle together with the neurovascular bundle laterally, exposing the posterior capsule of the joint.

When a fragment of bone is avulsed with the ligament:

Identify the fragment of bone and the corresponding defect in the tibia.

Curette the defect free of blood clots and debris.

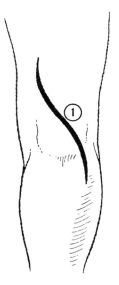

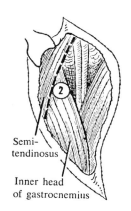

Semi-
tendinosus

Inner head
of gastrocnemius

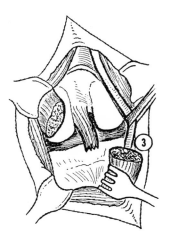

Operative Repair for Lesions of the Posterior Cruciate Ligament (Continued)

Secure the fragment in its normal position by one of the following methods:

1. Fasten the fragment in position by interrupted sutures passing through the surrounding capsular tissue.

2. If the fragment is large, anchor the fragment to the tibia with a screw.

3. If the fragment is very small, anchor it to its normal site in the tibia by a stout mattress suture passing through parallel drill channels 1 cm. apart in the medial tibial condyle. The ends of the suture are tied on the anterior surface of the tibia.

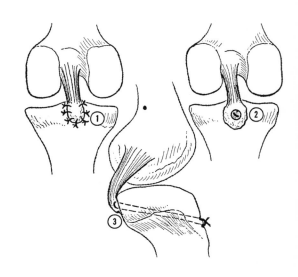

When the superior end of the ligament is detached from the femur:

1. Open the capsule and identify the posterior cruciate ligament.

2. Make two parallel drill channels in the medial femoral condyle from just above the epicondyle to the site of the attachment of the ligament. (These channels can also be made from within the joint—outward.)

3. Secure the end of the ligament to the medial femoral condyle by a mattress suture passing through the distal stump of the ligament and the drill channels in the medial femoral condyle; tie the ends of the suture over the medial epicondylar area.

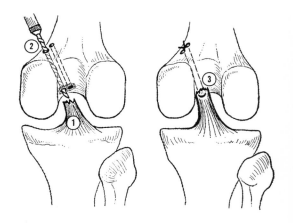

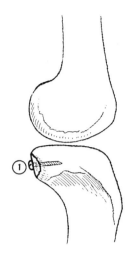

Postoperative X-Ray

1. Large bony fragment is anchored to the tibia with a screw.

Immobilization

1. Apply a plaster cylinder from the groin to just above the malleoli.
2. The knee is flexed 15 to 20 degrees.

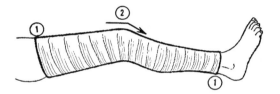

Postoperative Management

Begin quadriceps setting and drill immediately; increase the intensity of the exercise as the postoperative pain subsides.

After 10 or 14 days remove the plaster cylinder and apply a snug fitting plaster cylinder holding the leg in full extension.

Permit weight bearing three or four weeks after operation.

Six or eight weeks after the operation remove the plaster cylinder.

Now institute a program to restore normal quadriceps tone and volume and normal joint function.

AVULSION OF THE TIBIAL SPINE

REMARKS

This lesion is comparable to detachment of the anterior cruciate ligament, with a fragment of bone, from its tibial attachment.

It is most commonly encountered in adolescence and is usually the result of backward displacement of the femur with the tibia fixed and the knee flexed.

The degree of displacement of the bony fragment varies from no displacement to marked displacement.

Hemarthrosis is always present and the anterior drawer sign is positive when the bony fragment is completely detached.

Types of Fractures

A. PREREDUCTION X-RAY

1. Avulsion of the anterior tibial spine with minimal displacement.

B. PREREDUCTION X-RAY

1. Avulsion of the anterior tibial spine.
2. The fragment is moderately displaced.

C. PREREDUCTION X-RAY

1. Avulsion of the anterior tibial spine with marked displacement.
2. The fragment lies deep in the intercondylar notch of the femur.

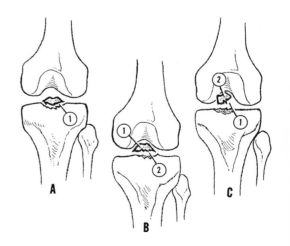

Page 1404

Conservative Management (Reduction by Hyperextension of the Knee)

Note: Before reduction is attempted the patient is given a general anesthetic and the knee is aspirated of blood and synovial fluid.

1. Force the knee gently and firmly into a position of hyperextension.

2. Then bring the knee back to the position of 180 degrees (full extension) and take check x-rays.

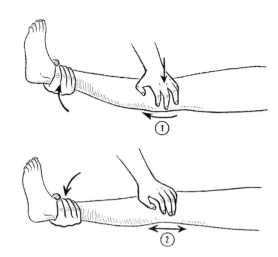

Postreduction X-Ray

1. The fragment is shown in its normal anatomic position.

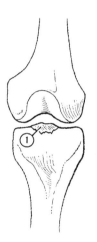

Immobilization

1. Apply a well padded plaster cylinder from the groin to just above the malleoli.

2. The knee is fully extended.

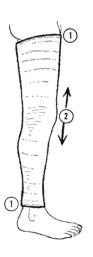

Postreduction Management

Begin graduated quadriceps exercises immediately.

Remove the plaster cylinder at the end of three weeks and apply another; this should fit snugly. Now permit weight bearing.

Step up the intensity of the quadriceps exercises.

Remove the second plaster cylinder six to eight weeks after the operation; permit weight bearing with crutches.

Institute exercises to restore joint motion and increase the intensity of the quadriceps exercises.

Discard the crutches when the quadriceps is sufficiently strong to stabilize the knee (usually two to three weeks).

Operative Reduction

Note: This method is employed if closed methods fail to return the fragment to its normal anatomic position.

1. Expose the intercondylar region of the tibia with a medial parapatellar incision

2. After flushing out of the joint cavity all blood clots, identify the fragment and the defect in the superior aspect of the tibia.

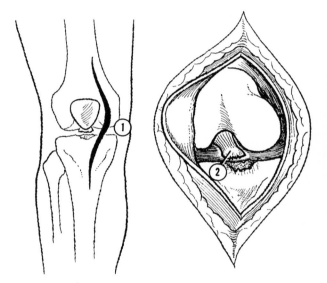

1. Make two parallel drill channels in the medial condyle of the tibia. They begin on the anteromedial surface of the condyle 4 cm. below the tibial brim and are directed obliquely upward, backward and inward, and issue from the base of the defect in the intercondylar region of the tibia.

2. If the fragment is large, perforate it with two small drill holes and pass through them a stout silk suture.

3. If the fragment is small, pass the suture through the inferior end of the cruciate ligament.

4. Pass the ends of the suture through the drill holes in the tibial condyle, pull the fragment snugly in place, and tie the ends of the suture on the anterior surface of the tibia.

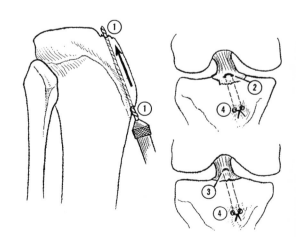

Immobilization

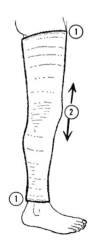

1. Apply a well padded plaster cylinder from the groin to just above the malleoli.

2. The knee is in full extension.

Postoperative Management

Begin graduated quadriceps exercises immediately.

Remove the plaster cylinder at the end of three weeks and apply another; this should fit snugly. Now permit weight bearing.

Step up the intensity of the quadriceps exercises.

Remove the second plaster cylinder six to eight weeks after the operation; permit weight bearing with crutches.

Institute exercises to restore the joint motion and increase the intensity of the quadriceps exercises.

Discard the crutches when the quadriceps is sufficiently strong to stabilize the knee adequately (usually two to three weeks).

COMPLETE AVULSION OF THE EPIPHYSIS OF THE TIBIAL TUBERCLE

REMARKS

This lesion is the result of violent contracture of the quadriceps with the knee flexed.

The tibial epiphysis may be one of two types (depicted below); the character of the avulsion is governed by the type of epiphysis present.

Complete extension is not lost because the lateral expansions of the quadriceps apparatus are not completely torn from the tibia.

The lesion is most common before the age of 18 when the epiphysis is not as yet fused to the head of the tibia.

Operative repair is the treatment of choice.

Types of Epiphyses of the Tibia

Type I: The tibial tubercle is continuous with the superior portion of the epiphysis.

Type II: The tibial tubercle arises from a separate center of ossification.

Types of Fractures

A. PREREDUCTION X-RAY

1. The entire anterior prolongation of the tibial epiphysis is pulled away from the anterior surface of the tibia; the base of prolongation is intact.

B. PREREDUCTION X-RAY

1. The anterior prolongation is pulled away from the anterior surface of the tibia.
2. The base of the epiphyseal prolongation is fractured.

C. PREREDUCTION X-RAY

1. A small separate epiphysis of the tubercle is avulsed and pulled upward.

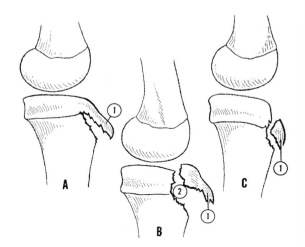

Operative Reduction

1. Make a hockey stick incision on the medial aspect of the knee; the lower limb crosses the anterior crest of the tibia just below the tibial tubercle.
2. Reflect the skin and the deep fascia outward, exposing the patellar tendon and the avulsed epiphysis.

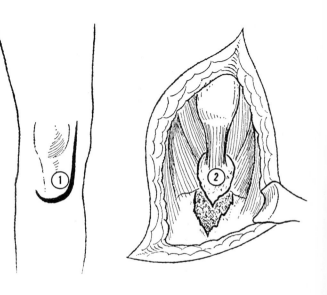

Operative Reduction
(Continued)

1. Grasp the epiphysis with a towel clip and place it in its anatomic position on the anterior surface of the tibia.

2. Anchor the epiphysis in its position by interrupted sutures passing through surrounding soft tissues. (Internal fixation is rarely justified.)

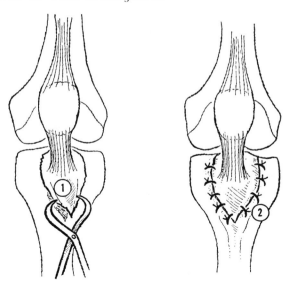

Postoperative Management

1. Apply a compression bandage around the knee.

2. Place the limb on a posterior plaster splint extending from the upper third of the thigh to the toes.

3. The knee is extended fully and the foot is at a right angle.

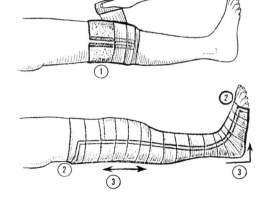

After ten days remove the splint and

1. Apply a plaster cylinder from the groin to just above the malleoli.

2. The knee is extended.

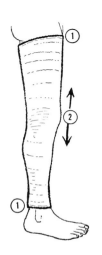

Now institute a regulated program of progressive quadriceps exercises.

Remove the cast at the end of five to six weeks and permit protected weight bearing with crutches. Now increase the intensity of the quadriceps and flexion exercises.

After eight or nine weeks permit unprotected weight bearing; continue the exercises until maximum restoration of quadriceps power and extension and flexion of the knee are achieved.

PELLEGRINI-STREDA DISEASE (COMPLICATION OF SPRAIN OF THE MEDIAL COLLATERAL LIGAMENT)

REMARKS

This disorder results from minor direct or indirect trauma to the inner aspect of the knee; often it is a complication of lesions of the medial collateral ligament.

This lesion can be aborted if all strains about the knee joint are adequately managed by a period (four weeks) of complete immobilization in a plaster cylinder.

Never forcefully manipulate a knee with this complication; overzealous activity enhances formation of more heterotopic bone.

X-Ray of Early Lesion

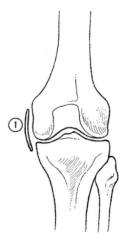

1. Elongated amorphous calcareous deposit in the substance of the tibial collateral ligament.

Note: This usually appears two to three weeks after the injury.

X-Ray of Late Lesion

1. Formation of discrete heterotopic bone in the region of the medial epicondyle.

2. Ossified ligament is attached to the epicondyle.

Note: These conditions are usually present in neglected cases ten to twelve weeks later, when the proliferative stage is completed.

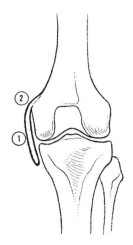

Management (Early)

Always anticipate and try to abort this complication in ligamentous injuries, especially of the tibial collateral ligament.

1. Apply a nonpadded plaster cylinder to the limb from the groin to just above the malleoli.

2. The knee is extended.

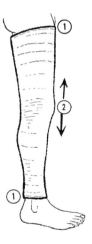

Permit weight bearing and quadriceps drill immediately.

Never institute overzealous treatment in the form of massage and forced activity; these enhance the development of the lesion.

In early established cases recognized within three or four weeks, again apply a nonpadded cast for four to six weeks; at the end of this time the calcareous deposit is usually absorbed. Now institute gentle exercises to develop joint motion.

Injection of 1 cc. of Hydrocortone into the ligament will enhance absorption of calcareous deposit or prevent its occurrence.

Never operate on early cases.

Never forcefully manipulate the knee or institute strenuous exercises.

Late Management

If the mature bony mass is tender and interferes with normal motion of the knee, it must be excised by sharp dissection.

X-Ray of Early Case before Treatment

1. Crescent plaque of amorphous calcareous deposit in the medial ligament.

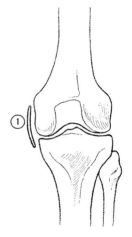

X-Ray of Early Case after Five Weeks of Plaster Immobilization

Calcareous deposit is completely absorbed.

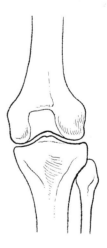

X-Ray of Late Neglected Case

Large mass of heterotopic bone is attached to the femoral epicondyle.

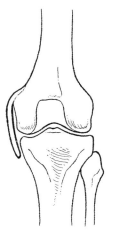

X-Ray of Same Case after Excision of Bony Mass

1. Heterotopic bone is excised; only a small spicule remains in the region of the femoral epicondyle.

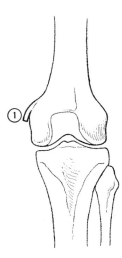

DISLOCATIONS OF THE KNEE JOINT

REMARKS

These lesions are always accompanied by severe damage to the capsule and the ligamentous and muscular apparatuses of the knee joint.

Menisci may be displaced.

Always check for palsy of the external popliteal nerve; this is a common complication in lateral dislocations. Permanent paralysis is a common sequel.

Check for injury to the popliteal artery. This may be evident at the time of the initial examination if the artery is completely torn, or not until the third or fourth day if the artery is only stretched or contused.

Fracture of the tibia may complicate the dislocation.

These lesions should always be treated surgically and all disrupted ligaments repaired. Conservative treatment is justified only if conditions exist which contraindicate surgical repair.

Types of Dislocation

1. Anterior dislocation.
2. Posterior dislocation.
3. Lateral dislocation.

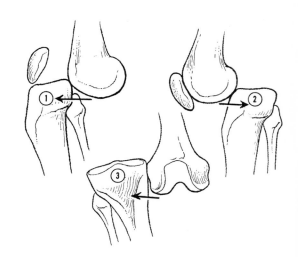

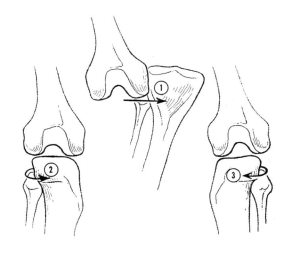

Types of Dislocation
(Continued)

1. Medial dislocation.

2 and 3. Rotatory dislocations; these are extremely rare.

Prereduction X-Ray

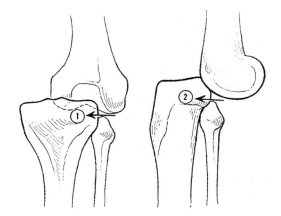

1. The tibia is dislocated medially.
2. The tibia is dislocated anteriorly.

Manipulative Reduction

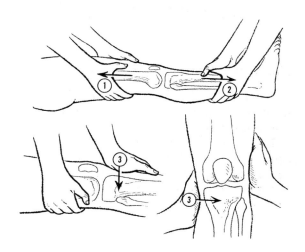

(Should be performed under general anesthesia as soon as possible after the accident.)

1. An assistant fixes and makes counter traction on the thigh.

2. Another assistant makes straight traction on the leg (this usually reduces the dislocation).

3. The surgeon makes direct pressure over the displaced bones.

Postreduction X-Ray

1. The tibia and
2. The femur are in normal relation to one another.

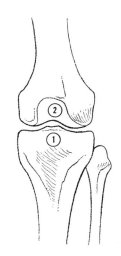

Immediate Postreduction Management

1. Aspirate the joint of blood and synovial fluid.
2. Apply a compression bandage extending from the groin to midcalf.
3. Apply a posterior plaster splint from the groin to the toes.
4. The foot is dorsiflexed 90 degrees.
5. The knee is flexed 20 degrees.

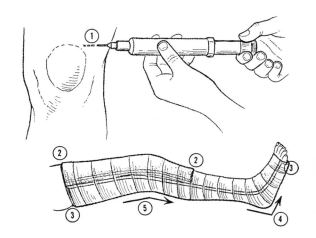

WHEN CONSERVATIVE MANAGEMENT IS DEEMED BEST FOR THE PATIENT

Postreduction Management

1. Elevate the limb, surround the knee with bags of ice and keep it at complete rest.
2. At the end of seven to ten days apply a nonpadded plaster cylinder from the groin to just above the malleoli; the knee is flexed 10 to 15 degrees.

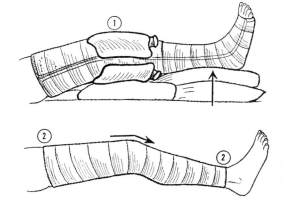

Now institute progressive quadriceps exercises.

After three or four weeks apply another plaster cylinder and permit weight bearing with crutches.

Remove the plaster fixation after 12 to 14 weeks. Institute more intensive exercises to develop quadriceps and restore joint motion.

Permit use of crutches until the quadriceps is sufficiently strong to stabilize the knee joint.

Note: Some restriction of motion is the usual sequel.

SURGICAL REPAIR OF THE DISRUPTED LIGAMENTS OF THE KNEE JOINT

REMARKS

When surgical treatment is deemed best for the patient (and there are few exceptions), the treatment should be instituted as soon as conditions permit—within a few hours after the injury if possible. All disrupted ligaments must be repaired.

Operative technique varies with the type of pathologic condition present; in general most of the procedures to be performed can be executed through a medial parapatellar incision.

Always inspect the inside of the joint and the surfaces of the patella and femoral condyle for loose osteochondral fragments.

If the posterior cruciate and the posterior ligaments are torn, a posterior incision may have to be made.

If there is a peroneal nerve deficit which requires surgical attention, a second operation should be performed two or three weeks after the first.

The technique of repairing specific structures—the cruciate ligaments, collateral ligament, posterior ligament and the removal of the menisci if torn—is the same as that previously described in this book for isolated or combined lesions of these structures.

Irreducible Dislocation of the Knee Joint

REMARKS

Interposition of soft tissue between the articular surfaces precludes closed reduction.

These lesions require operative intervention.

Appearance on X-Ray

After manipulation and traction,

1. The articular surfaces are widely separated.

2. The tibia is displaced anteriorly.

3. The tibia is displaced medially.

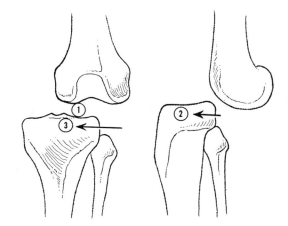

X-Ray after Open Reduction

1. The articular surfaces of the femur and tibia are in normal relation to one another.

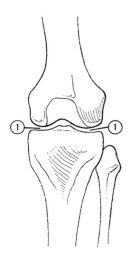

TEARS OF THE SEMILUNAR CARTILAGES

REMARKS

Tears of both semilunar cartilages are sustained by the same mechanism; namely, the menisci are swept into the interior of the joint when the femur is forcefully internally rotated while the knee is flexed and the tibia fixed. If at this time the knee is extended the menisci are crushed between the femoral condyles and the tibial plateaus, or the menisci are torn from their peripheral attachments.

The medial cartilage is more frequently implicated than the lateral, the ratio being seven to one.

The posterior horn is the segment most frequently involved.

One injury will predispose the knee to repeated trappings of the affected meniscus.

With each redisplacement of the meniscus the original tear may be extended or new tears sustained.

Locking of the knee joint (inability to extend the knee fully) occurs in approximately 25 per cent of initial lesions and in approximately 50 per cent of recurrent lesions.

Synovial effusion invariably accompanies every original tear; it becomes manifest within a few hours after the injury. In subsequent trappings of the meniscus varying amounts of synovial effusion occur.

Buckling or giving way of the knee joint is the most common symptom of tears of the menisci.

Always test for lesions of the collateral ligaments and cruciate ligaments. These are not infrequent complications.

Meniscal tears are rare in women; always eliminate a subluxating patella in these cases.

In recent injuries of the knee followed by synovial effusion, the diagnosis of internal derangement may be very difficult or impossible. When in doubt treat the case as for traumatic synovitis until the diagnosis is established.

Once the diagnosis of a meniscal tear is made, excise the involved cartilage.

In initial lesions wait two or three weeks before excising the cartilage; allow the tissues to return to normal and treat the lesion as for a traumatic synovitis.

Remember that both menisci are occasionally involved; always check clinically and at the time of operation for dual lesions.

Between attacks there may be no clinical manifestations except slight atrophy of the quadriceps; the diagnosis can only be established upon the history.

Most Common Varieties of Meniscal Tears

1. Bucket-handle tear: this is the most common lesion encountered (medial meniscus).

2. Multiple longitudinal and bucket-handle tears: significant of numerous trappings of the meniscus (medial meniscus).

3. Longitudinal tear traversing the posterior horn: relatively common lesion (medial meniscus).

4. Longitudinal tear traversing the anterior horn: relatively rare lesion (medial meniscus).

5. Multiple scoring of the inferior surface and one small complete longitudinal tear: indicative of numerous trappings of the meniscus (medial meniscus).

6. Incomplete tear of the peripheral attachments of the posterior segment (medial meniscus).

7. Incomplete transverse tear (lateral meniscus): a rare lesion but more frequently encountered in the lateral menisci.

Diagnostic Tests

AREAS OF MAXIMUM TENDERNESS

Direct pressure over areas 1-2-3 invariably elicits marked tenderness. Pressure over area 4 rarely elicits tenderness except in tears complicating the anterior horn.

Note: The same is true on the lateral side of the joint in lateral meniscal tears.

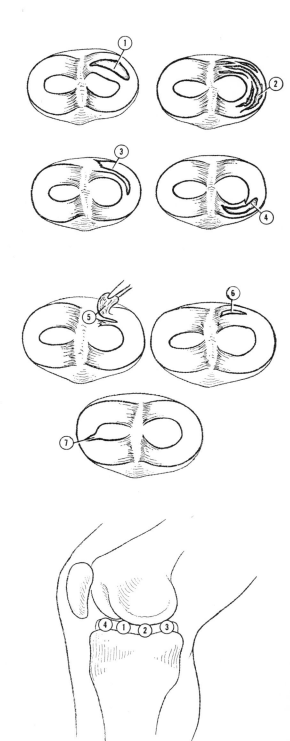

Diagnostic Tests (Continued)

McMurray's test

A test for lesions of the posterior horn, which is the segment most commonly involved.

1. The knee is fully flexed with the leg close to the buttock.

2. One hand fixes the knee.

3. The other hand grasps the foot.

4. For medial meniscal tears rotate the leg externally. (For lateral meniscal lesions rotate the leg internally.)

5. With rotation maintained extend the joint to a right angle; a click is felt or even heard as the femoral condyle passes over the meniscus.

Note: The more extended the knee at the moment the click is noted, the more anterior is the lesion.

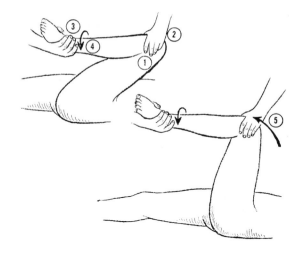

Compression test

1. The knee is in a position of full extension.

2. For lesions of the medial meniscus, the leg is adducted. (For the lateral meniscus the leg is abducted.)

Note: This maneuver compresses the meniscus and localizes the pain on the affected side.

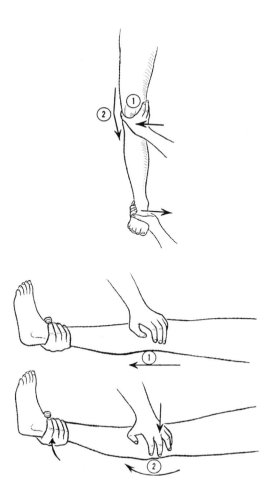

Extension test

1. The knee is in full extension.

2. Hypertension will elicit pain over the joint line on the side of the involved meniscus.

The Locked Knee Joint

REMARKS

Attempt to reduce a displaced meniscus causing locking as soon as possible.

A locked joint causes serious damage to the intra-articular structures and tends to stretch and fray the anterior cruciate ligament.

Remember that manipulation to unlock a locked knee is only a preliminary form of treatment; in all instances the implicated meniscus must be excised.

The best time of excision is two to three weeks after manipulation.

Don't execute repeated manipulations if the first or second attempts fail to reduce the displaced cartilage. Repeated manipulations will only extend the tear more anteriorly and stretch the anterior cruciate ligament. Here immediate surgical intervention is indicated.

Technique of Reduction for Locked Medial Meniscus

(General anesthetic is optional.)

1. With the hip and knee flexed, first abduct the leg.

2. While abduction is maintained, rotate the leg internally and externally.

3. When maximum amount of internal rotation is attained, extend the leg suddenly. Complete extension and a painless range of motion are the best indications of a successful reduction.

Note: For locking due to a lateral meniscus the above procedure is reversed; the leg is adducted and when the maximum amount of external rotation is attained, the leg is suddenly extended.

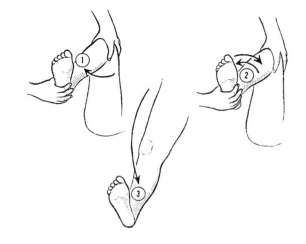

Postreduction Management

1. Aspirate the joint if the knee is distended.

2. Apply a compression bandage.

Institute a regulated program of quadriceps exercises immediately.

Allow weight bearing only when the effusion is gone and the quadriceps is strong.

Excise the meniscus when the tissues have approached a normal state, usually two or three weeks later.

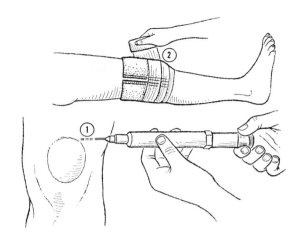

Excision of the Semilunar Cartilages

REMARKS

Once the diagnosis of a tear of a meniscus is established the only treatment is excision of the meniscus.

Be sure of the diagnosis. In cases involving women, always think of a subluxating patella in the differential diagnosis; in acute initial lesions, remember that traumatic synovitis may give a clinical picture identical to that of a torn meniscus.

If in doubt, wait a few weeks or months until the diagnosis is established.

In an initial lesion treat the patient as for a traumatic synovitis; after two or three weeks excise the meniscus. This procedure is also valid for locked knee joints requiring manipulation.

Failure to unlock a locked knee joint is an indication for surgical intervention.

Always check the status of the entire ligamentous apparatus before excision of a meniscus; combined lesions are common.

Always institute a program of quadriceps exercises for as long as possible before operation.

The method of excision of a meniscus depicted here has been developed and is taught by the author; however, there are many other methods. Employ that technique in which you excel, provided that you attain your goal, namely, to remove the cartilage in toto without damage to other structures.

Page 1423

Operative Technique of Excision of the Medial Semilunar Cartilage

1. Apply a tourniquet around the upper third of the thigh.

2. The knee is flexed 90 degrees over the end of the table.

3. Make a gently curved incision, beginning above the joint line just anterior to the tibial collateral ligament and terminating 0.5 cm. below the superior border of the tibial condyle, at the medial margin of the patellar tendon.

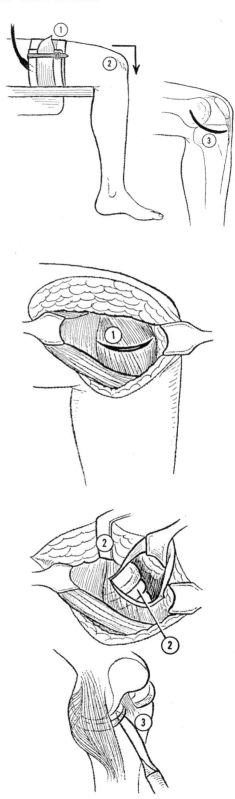

1. Incise the aponeurosis and capsule in the line of the skin incision.

2. Displace the infrapatellar fat pad laterally with a right angle, thin-bladed retractor. Now inspect the interior of the joint and estimate the extent of damage to the meniscus; also inspect the other intra-articular structures.

3. With a scalpel sever the anterior segment of the medial meniscus from the capsule and synovium, and from its anterior tibial attachment.

Operative Technique of Excision of the Medial Semilunar Cartilage (Continued)

1. Grasp the free end of the meniscus with a Kocher clamp.

2. Displace the tibial collateral ligament inward and backward with a thin-bladed retractor.

3. While traction is made on the meniscus toward the center of the joint, place a thin-bladed meniscectomy knife between the meniscus and the tibia, and from below upward divide the meniscal attachments to the inner surface of the tibial collateral ligament.

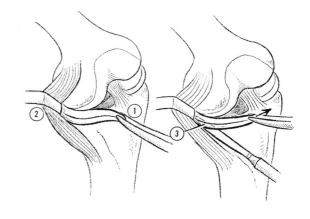

1. Now, an assistant firmly abducts and rotates the leg externally, opening the medial joint space.

2. Pass the blade of the meniscectomy knife in a horizontal plane along the posterior periphery of the tibial plateau, dividing the remaining peripheral tibial attachments of the meniscus.

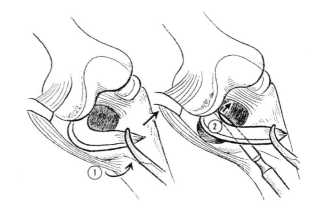

1. Rotate the tibia internally and displace the meniscus toward the center of the joint.

2. Divide the posterior attachment under direct vision.

Note: In order to facilitate closure of the wound, raise the end of the table so that the leg assumes a position of complete extension.

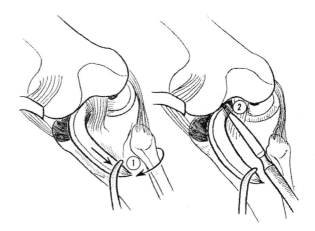

INDICATIONS FOR INCISIONS IN BOTH ANTERIOR AND POSTERIOR COMPARTMENTS

When the joint is unusually tight so that removal of the posterior segment is difficult.

When the posterior segment has been left behind in partial meniscectomy.

In the event that during removal of the meniscus through the anterior route the meniscus ruptures transversely.

When large cysts of the meniscus are encountered, rendering delivery of the meniscus through the anterior incision impossible.

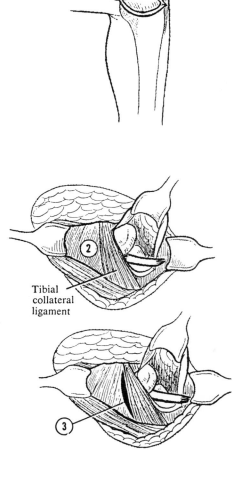

1. Extend the skin incision upward and posteriorly to a point 1 cm. behind the medial epicondyle.

2. Retract the skin edges and expose the aponeurosis behind the tibial collateral ligament.

3. Make an oblique curved incision in the aponeurosis, capsule and synovialis posterior to the tibial collateral ligament.

Tibial collateral ligament

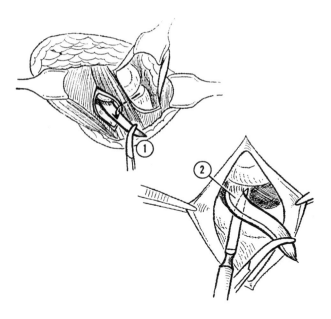

1. Pass the freed anterior half of the meniscus through the posterior incision.

2. With a meniscectomy knife divide the posterior peripheral and posterior central attachments of the meniscus.

Note: Remove the meniscus by sharp dissection; avoid tugging, tearing and laceration of tissues.

Operative Technique of Excision of the Lateral Semilunar Cartilage

1. Apply a tourniquet around the upper third of the thigh.

2. The knee is flexed 90 degrees over the end of the table.

3. Make a gently curved skin incision beginning in front of the fibular collateral ligament immediately above the joint line and terminating just lateral to the patellar tendon, 0.5 cm. below the head of the tibia.

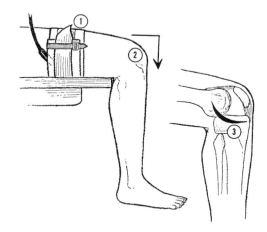

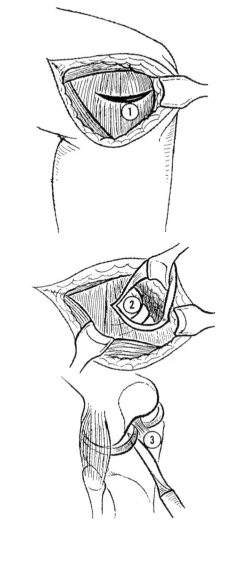

Operative Technique of Excision of the Lateral Semilunar Cartilage (Continued)

1. Incise the aponeurosis and capsule in the line of the skin incision.

2. Displace the infrapatellar fat pad toward the inner side of the joint with a thin-bladed retractor.

3. With a scalpel sever the anterior segment of the lateral meniscus from the capsule and synovialis and from its anterior tibial attachment.

1. Grasp the free end of the meniscus with a Kocher clamp.

2. Displace the fibular collateral ligament outward and backward with a thin-bladed, right angle retractor.

3. While traction is made on the meniscus toward the center of the joint, place the blade of the knife between the meniscus and the tibia and from below upward divide the capsular attachment of the meniscus.

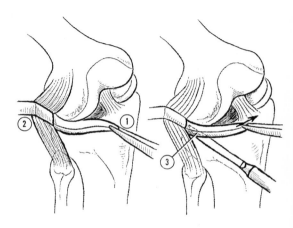

Operative Technique of Excision of the Lateral Semilunar Cartilage *(Continued)*

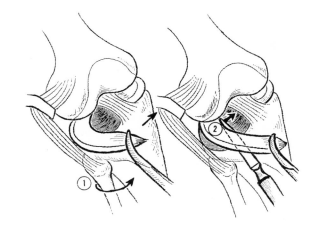

1. Now an assistant adducts and rotates the leg internally, opening the lateral joint space.

2. Pass the blade of the knife in a horizontal plane along the posterior periphery of the tibial plateau, dividing the remaining peripheral tibial attachment.

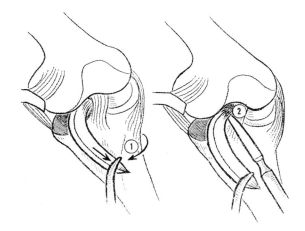

1. Rotate the leg externally and displace the meniscus toward the center of the joint.

2. Divide its posterior attachment under direct vision.

Note: Closure of the wound is facilitated by raising the end of the table and allowing the leg to assume the position of full extension.

INDICATIONS FOR INCISIONS IN BOTH ANTERIOR AND POSTERIOR COMPARTMENTS

When the joint is unusually tight so that excision of the posterior segment is difficult.

When the posterior segment has been left behind in partial meniscectomy.

In the event that during removal of the meniscus through the anterior incision the meniscus ruptures transversely.

When large cysts of the meniscus render delivery of the meniscus through the anterior incision impossible.

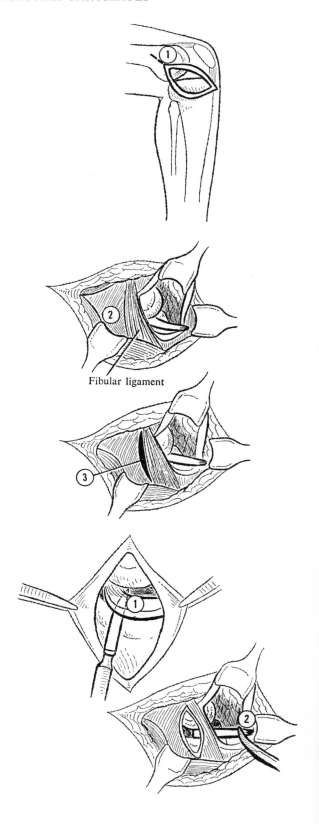

1. Extend the skin incision upward and posteriorly to a point 1 cm. behind and on the level of the lateral femoral epicondyle.

2. Retract the skin edges and expose the aponeurosis behind the fibular ligament.

3. Make an incision in the aponeurosis, capsule and synovialis, behind and parallel with the fibers of the fibular ligament.

Fibular ligament

1. With a meniscectomy knife divide the peripheral and central attachments of the meniscus.

2. Deliver the detached meniscus through the anterior incision.

Note: The anterior segment may first be passed through the posterior incision; the posterior segment is mobilized and the meniscus is then delivered through the posterior incision.

Postoperative Management

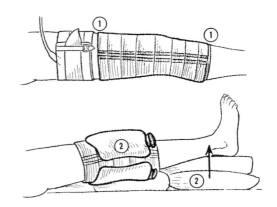

1. Before removal of the tourniquet apply a compression bandage around the knee extending from the mid-thigh to 6 inches below the knee.

2. Elevate the limb on hard pillows in full extension and surround the knee with bags of ice.

Maintain compression for seven or eight days.

Remove the sutures on the ninth or tenth postoperative day.

Begin quadriceps setting exercises on the second day. These should be done under supervision two or three times daily for 15 or 20 minutes.

As soon as the quadriceps drill is mastered, add straight leg exercises without resistance (usually on the third or fourth day).

Now add straight leg exercises against resistance of a rubber tubing (five minutes every hour).

Allow flexion exercises within the confines of the compression bandage.

After the tenth day, if no effusion is present, allow weight bearing with crutches; now increase the intensity of the quadriceps and flexion exercises.

After the third week the crutches can be discarded and quadriceps exercises against increasing loads (using a Delorne boot) are started.

Normal restoration of function is achieved in 10 to 12 weeks.

CAUTION

Don't permit weight bearing and strenuous exercises in the face of a massive effusion.

If a large effusion is present, aspirate the joint, apply a compression bandage and permit no weight bearing until the effusion has subsided and the quadriceps is sufficiently strong to stabilize the knee joint.

Don't permit exercises beyond the capacity of the quadriceps muscle; this leads to fatigue, which predisposes the ligamentous structure to harmful strains.

Don't permit unrestricted weight bearing until the quadriceps is strong enough to protect the joint against strains incident to weight bearing.

FRACTURES OF THE PATELLA

Remember that the patella plays an important role in the functional mechanics of the knee joint and it should not be indiscriminately removed.

By improving leverage the patella increases the strength of the quadriceps muscle; it protects the anterior aspect of the joint.

Its loss produces a permanent deformity of the joint which is often not acceptable to women.

Fractures resulting from indirect force are usually associated with rupture of the medial and lateral retinacula and separation of the fragments.

Fractures resulting from direct violence usually exhibit only minimal displacement of fragments and the patellar retinaculum remains intact.

X-ray study should always include anteroposterior, lateral and axial views. Axial views may reveal longitudinal and marginal fractures not seen in routine anteroposterior and lateral views.

Fissure and Comminuted Fractures of the Patella without Displacement

REMARKS

These may be the result of direct or indirect force.

No displacement of the fragments or incongruity of the articular cartilage exists.

The continuity of the quadriceps apparatus is intact.

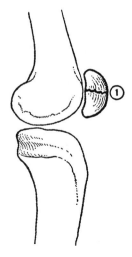

Appearance on X-Ray

1. Fissure fracture without separation of the fragments (caused by indirect force).

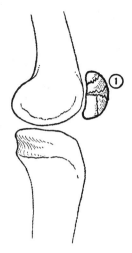

Appearance on X-Ray

1. Comminuted fracture with no displacement (caused by direct force).

Management

Aspirate the blood from the joint cavity under aseptic conditions.

Apply a posterior molded plaster splint from above the malleoli to the upper region of the thigh and place bags full of ice about the knee joint.

After two or three days, when swelling of the joint has decreased, apply a circular plaster cylinder from the groin to above the malleoli.

After 24 hours permit partial weight bearing with crutches.

Institute a regulated regimen of graduated exercises to maintain the quadriceps muscle at a high level of tone and power.

Remove the cast after four to six weeks, depending on the severity of the lesion.

Now institute an intensive program to restore normal joint motion and quadriceps power.

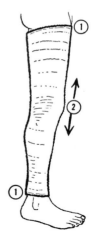

Immobilization

1. A plaster cylinder extends from the groin to just above the malleoli.
2. The knee is fully extended.

Transverse Fracture of the Patella with Minimal Displacement and No Comminution of Fragments

REMARKS

This fracture is rare.

The following method of treatment is justifiable only if perfect apposition of the articular surfaces can be achieved.

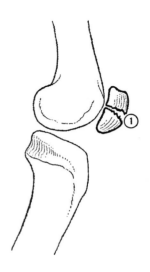

Prereduction X-Ray

1. Transverse fracture of the patella. Separation of fragments is minimal. The break is clean; no comminution exists.

Page 1434

Operative Reduction and Internal Fixation

1. Make a U-shaped incision with its apex over the inferior segment.
2. Reflect the skin upward and downward, exposing the apex and the base of the patella.
3. Identify the fracture and bring the fragments into accurate and firm contact with two towel clips

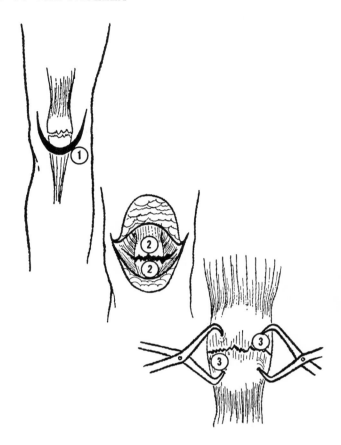

1. Flex the knee 15 or 20 degrees and make a drill channel through both fragments in the long axis of the patella; the drill hole passes through the center of the anteroposterior plane of both fragments.
2. Secure both fragments with a long screw.
3. The end of the screw should barely penetrate the upper pole of the patella.
4. Repair the rent in the medial and the lateral retinacula with mattress sutures.

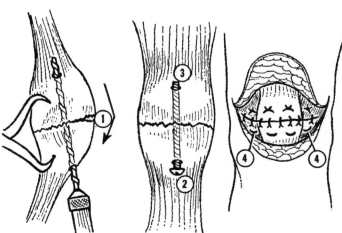

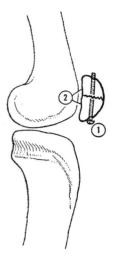

Postreduction X-Ray

1. A screw fixes both fragments firmly in perfect apposition.

2. No incongruity of the articular surface exists.

Immobilization

1. Apply a plaster cylinder from the groin to just above the malleoli.

2. The knee is fully extended.

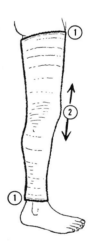

Postoperative Management

Institute rhythmic contractions of the quadriceps the day following the operation.

At the end of two weeks permit straight leg raising and protected weight bearing on crutches.

Remove the cast at the end of six weeks.

Institute a program of progressive exercises to develop maximum quadriceps power and joint motion.

Transverse Fracture of the Patella with Separation of Fragments

REMARKS

Retention of one large fragment and excision of all other fragments is the procedure of choice in:

1. Transverse fractures with fragments of approximately equal size and with wide separation—excise the lower fragment.

2. Transverse fractures with fragments of unequal size—excise the smaller fragment.

3. Comminuted fractures in which there is one large fragment—excise all the other fragments.

4. Polar fracture with comminution or separation—excise the smaller fragments.

Preoperative X-Ray

1. Transverse fracture in which fragments are approximately of equal size.

2. Fragments are widely separated.

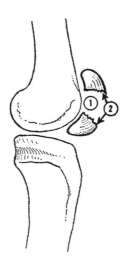

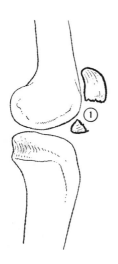

Preoperative X-Ray

1. Transverse fracture in which the fragments are of unequal size with wide separation.

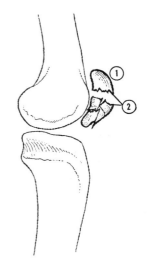

Preoperative X-Ray

Comminuted fracture with:
1. One large fragment and
2. Separation of fragments.

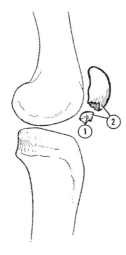

Preoperative X-Ray

Polar fracture with:
1. Comminution of smaller fragment and
2. Separation of fragments.

Operative Procedure

1. Make a U-shaped skin incision
with its base over the distal portion of
the patellar tendon.

2. Reflect the skin flaps upward
and downward, exposing the patella
and the parapatellar regions.

3. After washing out blood clots
and loose bony spicules, identify the
type of fracture present.

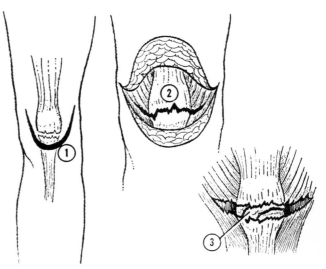

Operative Procedure (Continued)

By sharp dissection excise:

1. In transverse fractures with fragments of equal size, the lower fragment.

2. In transverse fractures of unequal size, the smaller fragment.

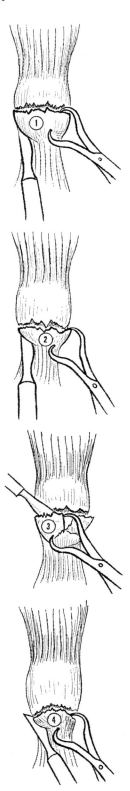

3. In comminuted fractures with one large fragment, all other fragments.

4. In polar fractures, the polar fragment or fragments.

Operative Procedure (Continued)

1. With a bone biter trim the margin of the remaining fragment to create a flat surface at right angles to the long axis of the patella.

2. Make two parallel drill channels in the fragment; they are directed downward and slightly posteriorly, opening on the fractured surface just anterior to the articular cartilage.

3. After trimming all devitalized tissue from the end of the tendon, pass a mattress suture of stout chromic catgut through the tendon and pass the ends of the suture through the drill holes in the large fragment.

4. Draw the ends of the suture taut and tie the ends on the anterior surface of the fragment.

5. Approximate the edges of the rents in the retinacula with interrupted sutures.

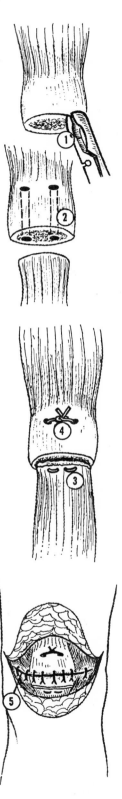

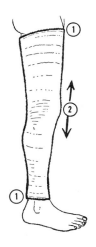

Immobilization

1. Apply a plaster cylinder from the groin to just above the malleoli.
2. The knee is fully extended.

Postoperative Management

Institute rhythmical contractions of the quadriceps the day following the operation.

At the end of two weeks permit straight leg raising and protected weight bearing on crutches.

Remove the cast at the end of six weeks.

Institute a program of progressive exercises to develop maximum quadriceps power and joint motion.

Severely Comminuted Fractures of the Patella

REMARKS

Total patellectomy is justifiable in extensively comminuted fractures which do not possess a fragment sufficiently large to provide a bony anchorage for the opposing tendon.

Preoperative X-Ray

1. Severely comminuted fracture of the patella.

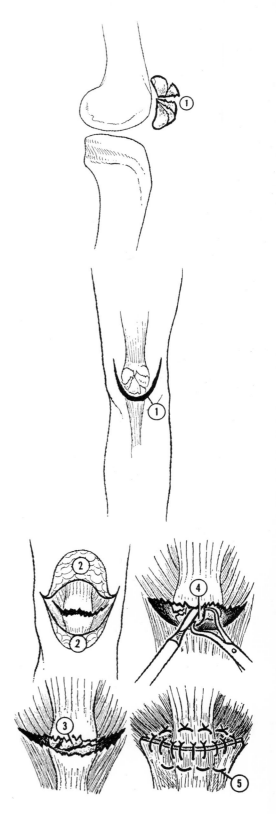

Excision of All Patellar Fragments

1. Make a U-shaped incision with its base over the distal end of the patellar tendon.

2. Reflect the skin flaps upward and downward.

3. Identify the fracture and the rents in the medial and lateral retinacula.

4. Grasp each fragment with a towel clip and enucleate it with sharp dissection.

5. After trimming away loose shredded fragments of the tendons and flushing the wound clear of loose fragments of bone and blood clots, overlap and plicate the edges of the tendon and the edges of the torn retinacula with mattress sutures (use No. 30 cotton).

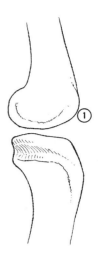

Postoperative X-Ray

1. The patella has been removed.

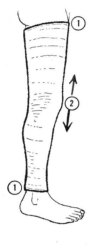

Immobilization

1. Apply a plaster cylinder from the groin to just above the malleoli.
2. The knee is fully extended.

Postoperative Management

Institute rhythmic contractions of the quadriceps the day following the operation.

At the end of two weeks permit straight leg raising and protected weight bearing on crutches.

Remove the cast at the end of six weeks.

Institute a program of progressive exercises to develop maximum quadriceps power and joint motion.

ALTERNATE METHOD: USING A PATELLAR PROSTHESIS

REMARKS

There is much to be said for this method. It:
1. Preserves the efficiency of the quadriceps apparatus.
2. Protects the anterior aspects of the knee joint.
3. Maintains a normal configuration of the knee joint.

4. Provides the anterior articular surface of the femur with an apposing smooth gliding surface.

This method should be employed only by those well versed in surgery of the knee joint.

The method, as described by D. S. McKeever, requires trimming and fitting the fragments into a vitallium prosthesis.

I believe this method is far superior to patellectomy; I employ it routinely if there are no contraindications.

X-Ray

Fragments of a comminuted fracture of the patella have been fitted into a vitallium prosthesis.

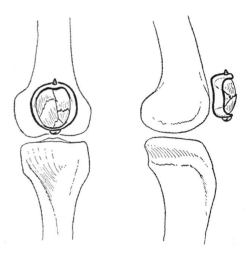

Marginal Fractures of the Patella

REMARKS

This lesion results from direct violence to the margins of the patella, shearing away a fragment of its periphery.

Displacement is minimal.

The retinacula of the quadriceps are intact.

Excision of the fragment is essential; if it is not excised, in most instances, late degenerative changes occur in the patellofemoral joint.

Always take x-rays in the axial view, which usually shows the lesion best.

In old cases this lesion must be differentiated from congenital anomalies of the patella.

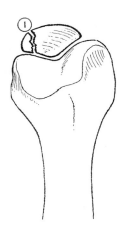

Preoperative X-Ray

1. Marginal fracture of the patella. Displacement is minimal.

Excision of Fragments

1. Make a small vertical incision directly over the fragment.

2. By sharp dissection enucleate the fragment from the fascial periosteal tissues of the patella and capsule.

3. Trim the edges of the main fragment and make them smooth.

4. Close the remaining defect with interrupted sutures.

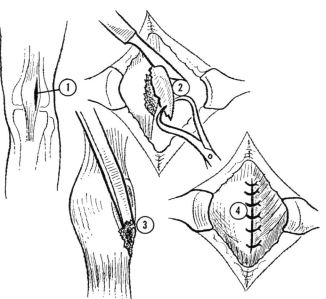

Postoperative Management

Apply a snug compression bandage around the knee.

Begin immediately quadriceps exercises and joint exercises on a regulated regimen.

After seven days allow partial weight bearing with crutches.

After one more week allow nonprotected weight bearing.

Osteochondral Fractures of the Patella

REMARKS

This lesion may be one source of loose bodies in the knee joint.

It results from forceful contraction of the quadriceps, following subluxation or dislocation of the patella with engagement of the medial border of the patella under the edge of the lateral femoral condyle; the trapped portion of the articular surface is sheared off the main body of the patella.

The lesion is usually encountered in children and adolescents, and occasionally in young adults.

Clinical manifestations are those of a loose body in the knee joint.

Always take axial x-ray views because routine anteroposterior and lateral views may fail to disclose the defect in the articular surface of the patella.

If the fragment is entirely cartilaginous, x-ray examinations will fail to reveal its presence.

The body may be depicted as a thin flake of bone. This appearance is not indicative of the true size of the body.

Preoperative X-Ray

1. Loose body in the infrapatellar region of the knee joint.

2. Corresponding defect in the inframedial aspect of the articular surface of the patella.

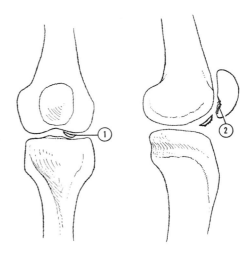

Removal of Loose Fragment (Median Parapatellar Incision)

1. Make a skin incision on the medial aspect of the knee, beginning 3½ inches proximal to the upper margin of the patella at the medial margin of the quadriceps tendon. The incision follows the medial border of the quadriceps tendon, the medial margin of the patella and the patellar ligament, and ends just distal to the lower border of the tibial tubercle.

2. Divide the deep fascia in the line of the incision.

3. Make a vertical incision in the quadriceps tendon 1 cm. lateral to its medial border and continue it distally around the medial margin of the patella and along the medial border of the patellar tendon.

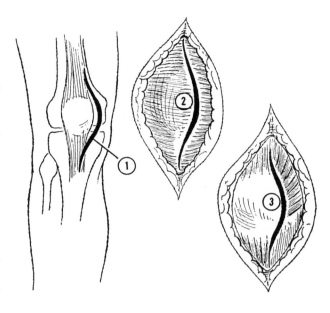

1. Divide the synovialis 1 cm. from the medial border of the patella and the patellar ligament.

2. Dislocate the patella laterally and rotate it in its vertical axis so that its articular surface faces anteriorly.

3. Locate the loose body and remove it.

4. Identify the defect in the articular surface of the patella and with a scalpel make smooth the irregular edges of the defect in the cartilaginous surface.

Note: Before closure flush the wound with a solution of normal saline in order to remove all blood clots and flakes of cartilage.

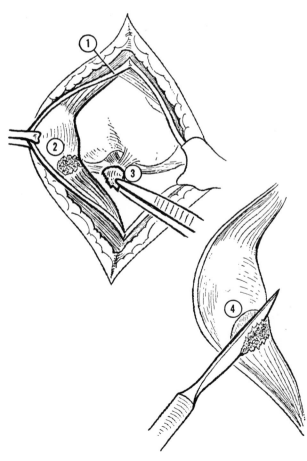

Postoperative Management

Immediately after operation apply a compression bandage around the knee joint.

Elevate the leg in bed and surround the knee with bags containing ice.

The following day institute quadriceps setting exercises and in four or five days allow the patient to raise the extended leg from the bed.

Begin flexion exercises on the seventh or tenth day.

Permit partial weight bearing on crutches after two weeks provided that the joint is not distended; if it is, aspirate the joint and apply a compression bandage.

Unprotected weight bearing is permitted after the third week.

Continue an intensive program of graduated exercises against resistance for the quadriceps and flexion exercises until normal function and power is restored.

RUPTURE OF THE EXTENSOR APPARATUS OF THE KNEE JOINT

REMARKS

Rupture of the extensor mechanism of the knee joint is caused by forceful contraction of the quadriceps muscle against a force acting in the opposite direction, such as is produced when the knee is suddenly flexed by the body weight.

Rupture of the quadriceps apparatus may occur at one of four levels; the site is generally governed by the age of the patient.

Rupture may occur:
1. At the level of the upper pole of the patella.
2. Through the patella.
3. At the level of the lower pole of the patella.
4. At the level of the tibial tubercle. (The tubercle may be avulsed from the tibia.)

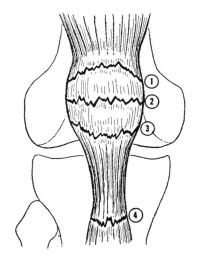

Immediate recognition of the lesion is imperative because repair of the apparatus in fresh cases gives excellent results whereas late repairs are difficult to achieve and frequently give poor results.

Don't sacrifice the patella in these lesions except as a last resort.

Avulsion of the Quadriceps Muscle from the Patella

REMARKS

This lesion occurs most frequently in individuals after the fourth decade.

Patients exhibit complete loss of the power of extension of the knee joint.

Generally the tear traverses the entire quadriceps tendon and extends laterally and medially through the lateral and medial retinacula.

Only rarely is the tear limited to the tendons of the rectus femoris and vastus intermedius muscles; in these cases the patient can actively extend the knee joint.

Immediate operative repair is imperative in all instances.

In late cases the repair should be reinforced by a flap of fascia lata as depicted below.

Old neglected cases exhibit a typical deformity of the knee joint as depicted below.

Typical Deformity in Neglected Cases

1. Retracted distal end of the quadriceps muscle.

2. Sulcus between the end of the quadriceps and the upper margin of the patella.

3. With contraction of the quadriceps the sulcus becomes more pronounced.

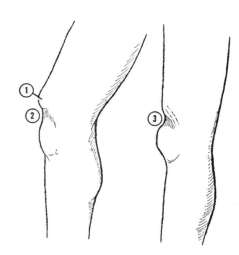

Operative Repair

TENDON TO TENDON REPAIR

This method is employed when sufficient tissue remains on the upper margin of the patella to permit a tendon to tendon repair.

1. Make a U-shaped skin incision with its convexity downward; it begins over the medial femoral condyle, crosses the leg just distal to the insertion of the patellar tendon, and ends over the lateral femoral condyle.

2. Reflect the skin flap and deep fascia upward, exposing the quadriceps tendon, the patella and the patellar tendon.

3. Identify the extent of the tear in the extensor mechanism and flush out all blood clots with a solution of normal saline.

4. Trim all loose strands of tissue and devitalized tissue at the edges of the tendon.

5. Grasp the proximal end of the tendon with a towel clip and pull it down until it approximates the distal end.

6. Join both ends of the tendons with mattress sutures (use No. 2 chromic catgut sutures).

7. Close the tears in the medial and lateral expansions of the tendon with interrupted sutures (use No. 1 chromic catgut sutures).

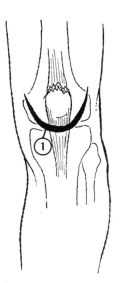

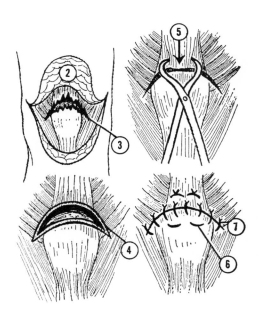

Operative Repair (Continued)

TENDON TO BONE REPAIR

This method is utilized when no tendon tissue suitable for tendon to tendon repair remains on the upper margin of the patella.

1. Make two drill channels through the patella in its longitudinal axis.

2. Approximate the end of the tendon to the bone by a mattress suture passing through the drill channels and tied on the anterior surface of the tendon.

3. Repair the tears in the lateral expansions of the quadriceps apparatus by interrupted sutures.

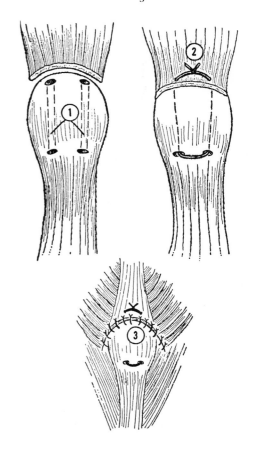

In old cases:

1. Extend the lateral limit of the skin incision upward on the lateral aspect of the thigh 5 or 6 inches.

2. Remove a wide rectangular strip of fascia lata, leaving its base attached.

3. Reflect the strip of fascia lata over the anterior aspect of the quadriceps apparatus and secure it to the underlying tissues by interrupted sutures.

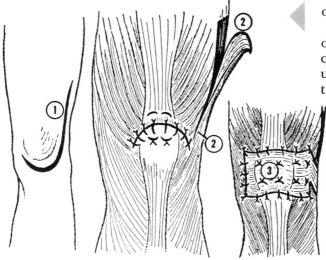

Postoperative Management

1. Apply a compression bandage around the knee.

2. Place the limb in a posterior plaster splint extending from the upper third of the thigh to the toes.

3. The knee is extended fully and the foot is at a right angle.

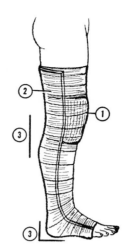

After ten days remove the splint and apply a plaster cylinder from the groin to just above the malleoli.

Now institute a regulated program of progressive quadriceps exercises.

Remove the cast at the end of five to six weeks and permit protected weight bearing with crutches.

Now increase the intensity of the quadriceps and flexion exercises.

After eight to nine weeks permit unprotected weight bearing. Continue the exercises until maximum restoration of quadriceps power and extension and flexion of the knee are achieved.

Avulsion of the Patellar Tendon from the Patella

REMARKS

This lesion usually occurs in the early decades of life.

Generally there is complete avulsion of the tendon from the inferior margin of the patella and a tear in the lateral patellar retinaculum.

Occasionally a piece of bone is avulsed from the lower pole of the patella.

Occasionally old cases are encountered in which there is marked shortening of the quadriceps muscle and formation of heterotopic bone in the interval between the patella and the tibial tubercle.

In most instances the patella is pulled upward.

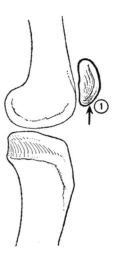

Preoperative X-Ray (Fresh Case)

1. The patella is pulled upward by the quadriceps muscle.

Preoperative X-Ray (Old Cases)

1. Upward displacement of the patella.

2. Heterotopic bone formation in the interval between the patella and the tibial tubercle.

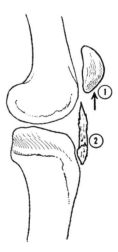

Operative Repair

1. Make a U-shaped skin incision with its convexity downward; it begins over the medial femoral condyle, crosses the leg just distal to the insertion of the patellar tendon and ends over the lateral femoral condyle.

2. Reflect the skin flap and deep fascia upward, exposing the quadriceps tendon, the patella and the patellar tendon.

3. Identify the defect in the patellar tendon.

4. Remove all loose fragments of bone and trim off all devitalized strands of tissue.

5. Grasp the patella with a towel clip and pull it down until the proximal end of the tendon apposes the distal end.

6. Join both ends of the tendon with mattress sutures passing close to the bone (use No. 2 chromic catgut sutures).

7. Close the tears in the lateral patellar retinaculum with interrupted sutures.

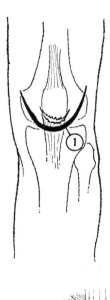

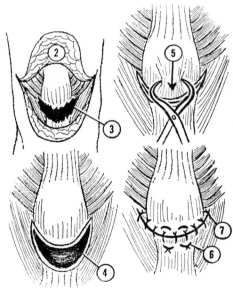

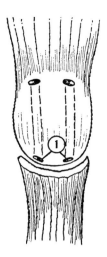

Operative Repair (Continued)

If the remaining tendon on the patella is insufficient to effect a repair, do a bone to tendon repair.

1. Make two drill channels through the patella in its longitudinal axis and opening on the inferior surface of the patella.

2. Approximate the patella to the tendon by a mattress suture passing through the drill channels and tied on the anterior surface of the patella.

3. Repair tears in the lateral patellar retinaculum with interrupted sutures.

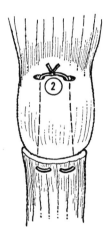

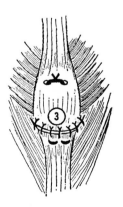

Operative Repair (Continued)

In old cases the patellar tendon may be completely disintegrated with the formation of heterotopic bone in the interval between the tibial tubercle and the tendon.

Here excise the heterotopic bone and reconstruct the patellar tendon.

1. Make a hockey stick skin incision in the median parapatellar region, beginning 2 inches above the base of the patella, and extending to just below the tibial tubercle; then it curves laterally to the lateral margin of the tibial crest.

2. Reflect the skin and deep fascia laterally, exposing the extensor apparatus and the defect in the patellar tendon.

3. Excise all scar tissue and heterotopic bone.

4. From the opposite thigh obtain a piece of fascia lata 2½ by 5 inches and place one end over the anterior surface of the patella.

5. Anchor the proximal end of the fascia lata strip to the periphery of the patella and the adjacent retinaculum with interrupted sutures placed deeply.

6. Divide the distal end of the strip into two halves.

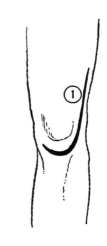

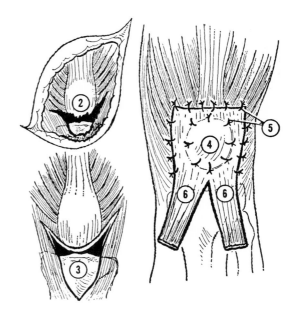

Operative Repair (Continued)

1. Cut out a bony ledge ½ inch deep from the tibial tubercle.

2. Make two drill channels in the longitudinal axis of the tubercle; the exits are in the raw surface of the ledge.

3. While downward traction is made on the patella with a towel clip, pass each fascial strip through a drill channel and secure it to itself with interrupted sutures.

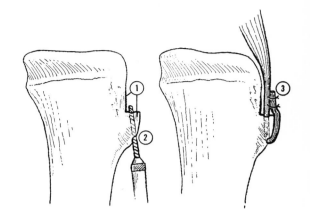

Postoperative Management

1. Apply a compression bandage around the knee.

2. Place the limb in a posterior plaster splint extending from the upper third of the thigh to the toes.

3. The knee is extended fully and the foot is at a right angle.

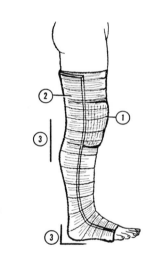

After ten days remove the splint and apply a plaster cylinder from the groin to just above the malleoli.

Now institute a regulated program of progressive quadriceps exercises.

Remove the cast at the end of five to six weeks and permit protected weight bearing with crutches.

Now increase the intensity of the quadriceps and flexion exercises.

After eight to nine weeks permit unprotected weight bearing. Continue the exercises until maximum restoration of quadriceps power and extension and flexion of the knee are achieved.

Avulsion of the Patellar Tendon from the Tibial Tubercle

REMARKS

This lesion is usually encountered in persons past middle life.

Occasionally the proximal portion of the tibial tubercle is fragmented or avulsed.

Immediate surgical intervention is imperative in order to prevent shortening of the quadriceps muscle.

Typical Deformity

1. The patella rides high.
2. Sulcus immediately over the tibial tubercle. (This sulcus may be obliterated by swelling but it is always palpable.)

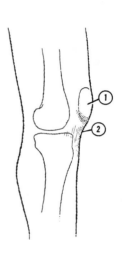

Preoperative X-Ray

1. The patella rides high.
2. Fragmentation of the proximal end of the tibial tubercle.

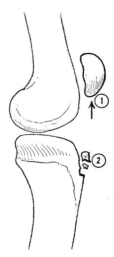

Operative Repair

1. Make a hockey stick incision on the medial aspect of the knee; the lower limb of the incision crosses the anterior tibial crest just distal to the tibial tubercle.

2. Reflect the skin and deep fascia outward, exposing the patella, the patellar ligament and the tibial tubercle.

3. Identify the lesion and trim away the shredded strands of tissue and periosteum from the end of the tendon and the upper end of the tubercle.

4. Identify the extent of the tear in the medial and lateral retinacula.

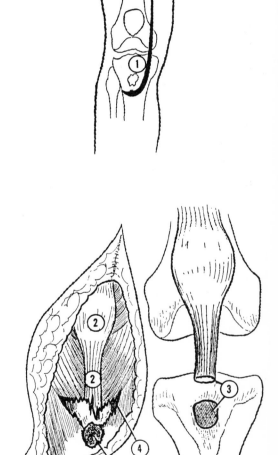

Operative Repair (Continued)

Reattach the tendon to the tibia as depicted below if the tendon is torn cleanly from the tubercle, or if the tendon is avulsed with a small fragment of bone after excision of the bony fragment.

1. With a sharp osteotome cut out a ledge from the tibial tubercle ½ inch deep and at right angles to the longitudinal axis of the tibia.

2. Make two drill channels through the tubercle which are directed upward and inward so that the exits are on the raw surface of the ledge.

3. Grasp the patella with a towel clip and make downward traction.

4. Secure the end of the tendon to the raw surface of the ledge with a mattress suture passing through the drill channels and tied on the anterior surface of the tubercle. (Use No. 2 chromic catgut suture.)

5. Repair the tears in the medial and lateral retinacula with interrupted sutures. (Use No. 1 chromic catgut sutures.)

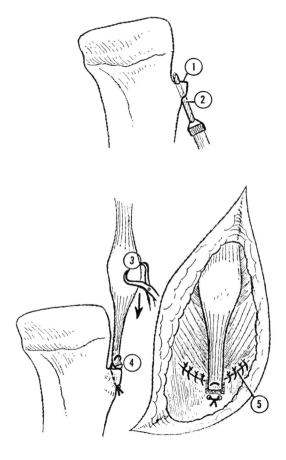

Operative Repair *(Continued)*

If a large piece of bone is avulsed with the tendon use one of the two following methods.

Replace the bone in its anatomic position and secure it with:

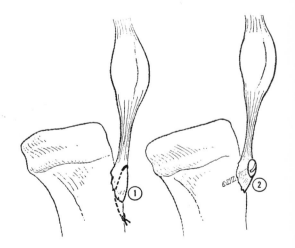

1. A mattress suture passing through two drill channels made in the tubercle and the bony fragment.

or

2. A screw fixing the bony fragment and tendon to the tibial tubercle.

Postoperative Management

1. Apply a compression bandage around the knee.

2. Place the leg in a posterior plaster splint extending from the upper third of the thigh to the toes; the knee is extended fully and the foot is at a right angle.

After ten days remove the splint and apply a plaster cylinder from the groin to just above the malleoli.

Now institute a regulated program of progressive quadriceps exercises.

Remove the cast at the end of five to six weeks and permit protected weight bearing with crutches.

Now increase the intensity of the quadriceps and flexion exercises.

After eight to nine weeks permit unprotected weight bearing. Continue the exercises until maximum restoration of quadriceps power and extension and flexion of the knee are achieved.

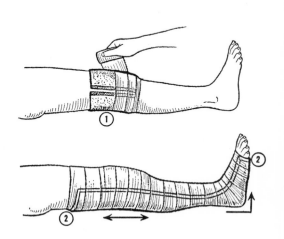

Page 1462

DISLOCATIONS OF THE PATELLA

Acute Lateral Dislocation of the Patella

REMARKS

In most instances, primary dislocation of the patella is possible because of some existing congenital alteration in the quadriceps apparatus or of the bony components of the knee joint.

Primary dislocation may occur in normal knee joints as the result of a direct force applied to the inner aspect of the patella, driving it laterally. This lesion is most common in young people engaged in strenuous activities.

Dislocations may be incomplete or complete. In all instances there is serious damage to the medial patellar retinaculum, vastus intermedius and medialis, and to the fibrous capsule, which may be lacerated.

Osteochondral fractures of the patella are not uncommon; always look for this complication.

Incomplete dislocations usually reduce spontaneously when the knee is extended; this may also occur in complete dislocations.

After spontaneous reduction the clinical findings are altered and may make the diagnosis difficult; however, severe tenderness along the medial border of the patella is a constant finding. Also, if seen before the swelling is marked, a definite defect can be palpated in the medial retinaculum. Negative findings rule out ligamentous injuries; there is no tenderness along the course of the lateral collateral ligament, and there is no pain when the tibia is forced in abduction or adduction, either with the knee extended or flexed.

Occasionally the findings mimic those of a torn semilunar cartilage. Don't make this error.

Acute lateral dislocations should be treated surgically; the retinaculum must be repaired. Failure to do this results in healing of the medial retinaculum with considerable laxity, a situation which predisposes to future dislocations.

The surgery should be performed as soon as possible—never later than 24 hours.

If there are no congenital predisposing factors, simple repair of the medial retinaculum suffices; if these factors exist, the patellar tendon should be transferred medially on the tibia.

Typical Deformity of Acute Traumatic Dislocation of the Patella

1. The knee is semiflexed.
2. The patella is displaced laterally over the lateral femoral condyle.
3. The quadriceps and patellar tendons are taut.

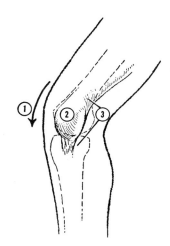

Prereduction X-Ray

1. The patella lies on the lateral aspect of the lateral femoral condyle.
2. The patella is displaced slightly downward.

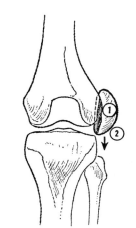

Manipulative Reduction (Under General Anesthesia)

1. Extend the knee gradually while
2. Medialward pressure is made upon the patella pushing it over the lateral femoral condyle.

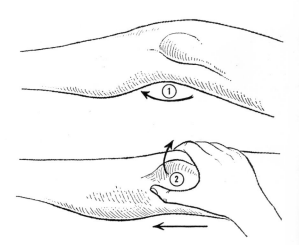

Manipulative Reduction (Under General Anesthesia) (Continued)

1. The patella is in its normal position.

2. Marked swelling is usually present. Always aspirate the joint if intra-articular tension is marked.

3. Aspirate blood and synovial fluid from the joint cavity.

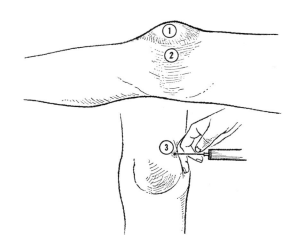

Operative Repair

(Perform the operation with a tourniquet applied around the upper third of the thigh.)

1. Expose the area by a medial parapatellar incision beginning at the upper pole of the patella and ½ inch medial to it. Continue the incision around the patella and then distally medial to the patellar tendon, terminating slightly below the tibial tubercle.

2. Retract the skin edges and divide the deep fascia to visualize the damage to the muscles, medial retinaculum and capsule. Flush out all debris and clots with normal saline solution and carefully inspect the inside of the joint for osteochondral fragments.

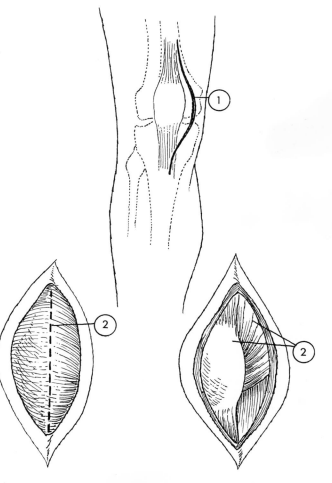

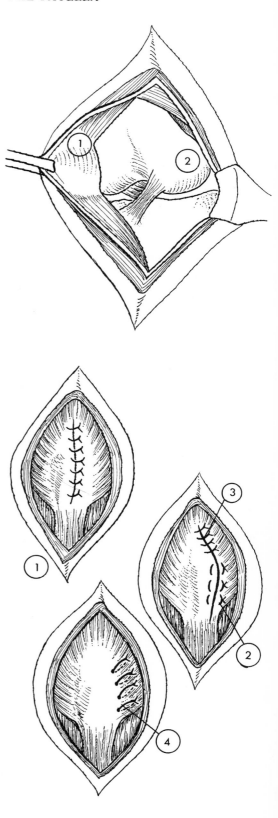

Operative Repair (Continued)

1. Bring the articular surface of the patella into view and examine it for evidence of damage to the cartilage.

2. Also inspect the articular cartilage of the lateral femoral condyle.

If there are no congenital alterations of the knee joint predisposing to dislocation:

1. Repair the capsule by bringing the edges together with interrupted sutures.

2. Overlap the edges of the tear in the medial retinaculum with mattress sutures.

3. Reattach the vastus medialis to the patella in case it has been torn from its attachment.

In case the tear is so close to the edges of the patella that closure is impossible:

4. Drill holes along the edge of the patella (don't damage the articular surface) and attach the retinaculum to bone.

Operative Repair (Continued)

If there exist congenital alterations predisposing to dislocation:

5. In addition to the above repair, transfer the tibial tubercle with the tendon attached to the inner side of the tibia.

The surgical technique is described on page 1473.

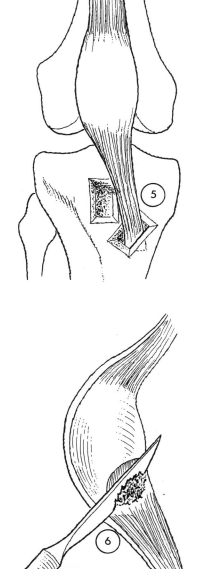

6. In case there is damage to the cartilage of the patella or of the lateral femoral condyle, shave off all loose fragments, leaving a clean, smooth surface.

Postoperative Management

Apply a compression bandage with the knee flexed 10 to 15 degrees.

After ten days remove the sutures and apply a plaster cylinder.

Four weeks after operation remove the cylinder and

Institute an intensive program of exercises to restore normal quadriceps power and full motion at all joints.

Recurrent Lateral Dislocation of the Patella

REMARKS

This lesion, in most instances, is secondary to some abnormality of the components of the knee joint.

The abnormality may be a congenital relaxation of the quadriceps mechanisms usually associated with a high riding patella; it may be a relaxation of the medial patellar retinaculum following faulty repair of these tissues or loss of tone of the vastus medialis following an acute traumatic dislocation.

There may be a congenitally flat, underdeveloped lateral femoral condyle and a flattening of the corresponding articular surface of the patella which permits lateral displacement of the patella.

There may be a congenital or acquired genu valgum. The congenital variety is invariably associated with a shortened iliotibial band and intermuscular septum; this contributes to the valgus deformity of the knee.

The lesion is encountered most commonly in girls; the first dislocation usually occurs during adolescence.

In late cases degenerative changes in the articular surface of the lateral femoral condyle and the patella are inevitable sequelae.

The dislocation occurs when the knee is extended from a flexed or semiflexed position; frequently it reduces when the knee is extended.

The treatment in all instances is surgical; the type of procedure performed depends on the age of the patient, the type of abnormality of the knee present, and the severity of the degenerative changes in the articular cartilage of the lateral femoral condyle and that of the patella.

Subluxation of the patella is frequently encountered in athletes. Special axial views (Hughston view) reveal the patella to be poorly seated in the patellar groove on the anterior surface of the femur. Also, with the knee flexed 90 degrees the patella points either directly upward or to the outer side instead of directly forward.

Normal Knee Joint

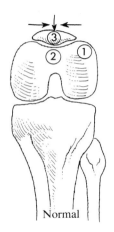

1. The lateral condyle is well developed.

2. The patellar groove is adequate.

3. The patella is deeply seated in the groove and its lateral articular surface is contained by the articular surface of the lateral condyle.

Congenital Abnormality of the Knee Joint

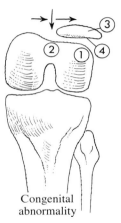

1. The lateral condyle is underdeveloped.

2. The patellar groove is inadequate; it is too shallow.

3. The lateral condyle does not contain the patella, predisposing the patella to lateral displacement.

4. The lateral articular surface of the patella is flat.

Preoperative X-Ray (When the Lateral Femoral Condyle is Underdeveloped)

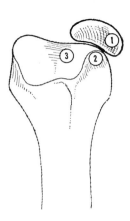

1. The patella lies on the lateral aspect of the femoral condyle.

2. The lateral femoral condyle is underdeveloped and flat.

3. The intercondylar groove is shallow.

Page 1469

Operative Stabilization of the Patella

INCISION

1. Make a hockey stick incision on the medial aspect of the knee beginning approximately 2 inches above the superior pole of the patella. The lower limb of the incision curves laterally just below the tibial tubercle and terminates lateral to the tibial crest.

2. Reflect the skin laterally, exposing the lower fibers of the vastus medialis, the patella, the patellar tendon and the tibial tubercle.

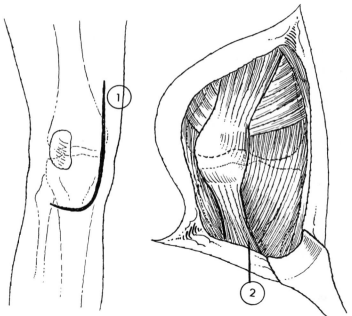

For Children and Adolescents in Whom the Quadriceps Apparatus is in Valgus

1. By sharp dissection free the patellar tendon.

2. With a sharp osteotome remove the insertion of the patellar tendon with a thin layer of bone from the tibial tubercle. (Don't injure the epiphyseal plate.)

3. Mobilize the tendon by splitting the lateral patellar retinaculum from below upward, and continue proximally as far as the fascia lateral to the vastus lateralis.

4. Pull the patellar tendon slightly downward and medially until the patella lies in a normal position between the condyles. Now select the new site of insertion on the medial side of the tibia that will maintain this position.

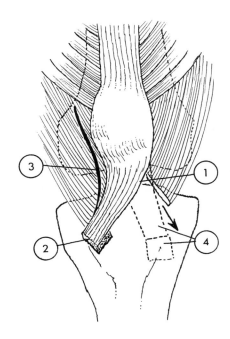

5. Raise an osteoperiosteal flap from above downward (from the new site of insertion on the tibia).

6. Pass drill holes through the elevated flap; secure with sutures the distal end of the patellar tendon and its bony insertion to the posterior surface of the osteoperiosteal flap.

7. Secure the patellar tendon to the adjacent periosteum with interrupted sutures.

8. Free the insertion of the vastus medialis to form a V-shaped mass.

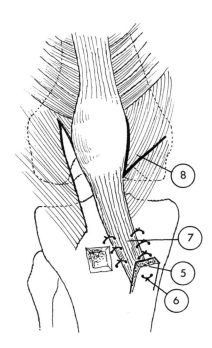

1. Pull the end of the vastus medialis downward and laterally and anchor it to the soft tissues on the posterior surface of the patella.

2. Leave the gap in the lateral retinaculum open.

3. Reflect the skin flap further laterally and expose the iliotibial band.

4. Divide the band transversely; also divide the intermuscular septum. (These are tight, contracted structures contributing to the valgus deformity.)

Note: Before the final sutures are placed always test the path of motion of the patella by flexing and extending the knee. The patella should ride in the groove without any interference.

Don't transfer the patellar tendon too far medially; this may cause a medial subluxation of the patella.

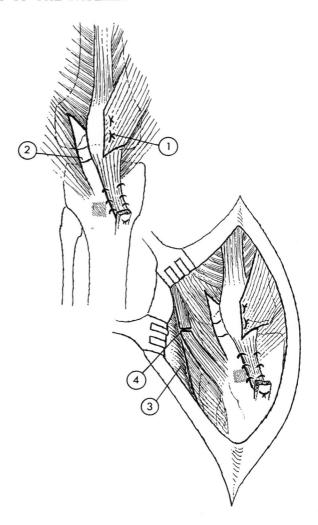

Postoperative Management

1. Immediately after the completion of the operation apply a posterior plaster splint extending from the toes to the upper thigh.

2. After two weeks remove the skin sutures and apply a plaster cylinder from just above the malleoli to the groin.

Now institute quadriceps exercises and permit partial weight bearing with crutches.

Six weeks postoperatively remove the plaster cylinder and institute an intensive program of graduated exercises to restore normal joint motion and normal quadriceps tone and volume.

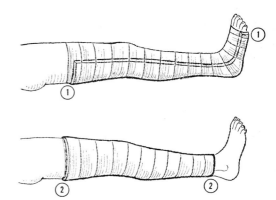

FOR ADULTS IN WHOM THE QUADRICEPS APPARATUS IS IN VALGUS AND THERE IS MINIMAL DEGENERATION OF THE ARTICULAR CARTILAGE OF THE PATELLA AND FEMUR

1. By sharp dissection free the patellar tendon.

2. With a sharp osteotome remove a rectangle of cortical bone 1¼ inches by ½ inch with the tendon attached.

3. Mobilize the tendon by splitting the lateral retinaculum from below upward as far as the fascia lateral to the vastus lateralis.

4. Make a corresponding defect on the anteromedial aspect of the tibia slightly below the original site of attachment of the patellar tendon (its bony axis is inclined 45 degrees with the vertical axis of the tibia) and remove the cancellous bone from the superior and inferior ends of the defect.

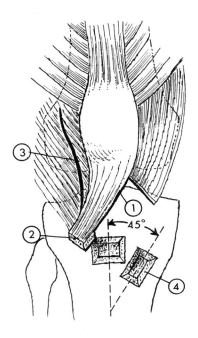

5. Place the tibial tubercle in the defect and then rotate it so that its vertical axis parallels that of the quadriceps.

6. Free the insertion of the vastus medialis to form a V-shaped mass.

7. Pull the end of the vastus medialis downward and laterally and anchor it to the posterior surface of the patella by interrupted sutures.

8. Leave the gap in the lateral patellar retinaculum open.

Note: Before inserting the last sutures always test the path of excursion of the patella by flexing and extending the knee. The patella should ride freely. Don't transfer the patellar tendon too far medially; this may cause a medial subluxation of the patella.

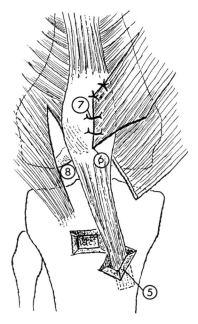

Postoperative Management

1. Immediately after completion of the operation apply a posterior plaster splint extending from the upper thigh to the toes.

2. After two weeks remove the skin sutures and apply a plaster cylinder extending from the upper thigh to just above the malleoli.

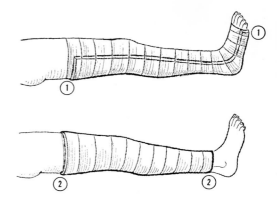

Now institute graduated quadriceps exercises and permit weight bearing.

Five weeks postoperatively remove the plaster cylinder and institute an intensive program of graduated exercises to restore normal joint motion and normal quadriceps power and volume.

For Adults in Whom the Quadriceps Apparatus is in Normal Alignment and the Changes in the Articular Cartilage of the Patella and Femur are Minimal

1. The incision begins 3 inches above the patella at the medial border of the quadriceps tendon; it swings around the patella and continues distally on the medial border of the patellar tendon; it terminates at the distal end of the tibial tubercle.

2. Deepen the incision between the vastus medialis and the medial border of the quadriceps tendon and along the medial border of the patella and patellar tendon. Inspect the inside of the joint for loose bodies.

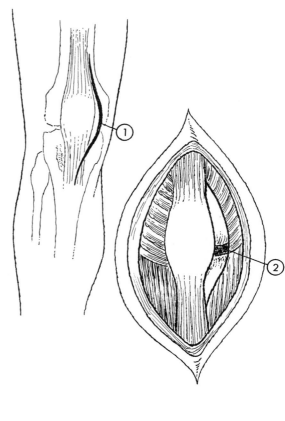

1. Free the patellar tendon.

2. Mobilize the tendon by splitting the lateral patellar retinaculum from below upward and continue proximally as far as the fascia lateral to the vastus lateralis.

3. By the use of mattress sutures overlap the vastus medialis and the medial retinaculum onto the quadriceps tendon, the patella and patellar tendon as far as the midline of the quadriceps tendon, the patella and its tendon.

4. Leave the gap in the lateral patellar retinaculum open.

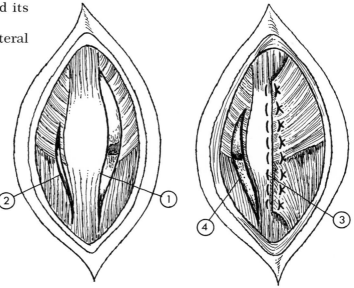

Immobilization

1. Apply a compression bandage.
2. Apply a posterior plaster splint from the toes to the upper thigh.

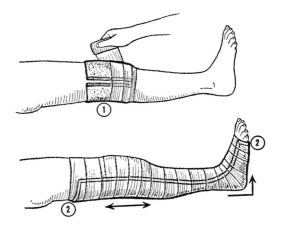

Postoperative Management

Institute quadriceps exercises within 48 hours.

Allow walking with crutches at seven to ten days.

At the end of three weeks remove the splint and institute a regulated program of quadriceps exercises and guarded movements at the knee. The splint is worn between exercise periods.

At the end of five weeks intensify the exercise program and start exercises against resistance.

Full flexion and extension should be achieved in three to four months.

FOR ADULTS IN WHOM THERE IS A VALGUS DEFORMITY OF THE QUADRICEPS MECHANISM AND ADVANCED DEGENERATION OF THE CARTILAGE OF THE FEMUR AND PATELLA

REMARKS

These are difficult lesions to treat; removal of the patella may be indicated; however, in my opinion the patella should be spared if at all possible. I prefer to cap the patella with a vitallium prosthesis and transfer the patellar tendon insertion medially. This procedure in my hands has given many satisfactory results.

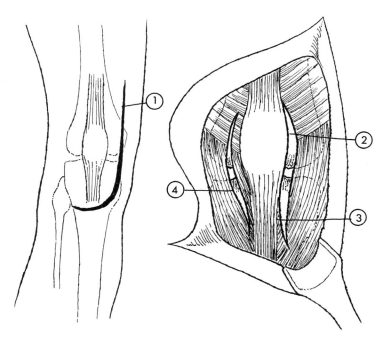

1. Make a hockey stick incision beginning 3 inches above the patella at the medial border of the quadriceps tendon; it extends distally as far as the distal end of the tibial tubercle, then swings laterally as far as the crest of the tibia.

2. Deepen the incision between the vastus medialis and the medial border of the quadriceps tendon and along the medial border of the patella and patellar tendon. Inspect the inside of the joint for loose bodies.

3. Free the patellar tendon.

4. Mobilize the tendon by splitting the lateral retinaculum from below upward as far as the fascia lateral to the vastus lateralis.

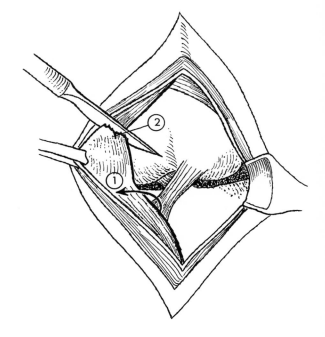

1. Rotate the patella on its vertical axis so that its articular surface faces anteriorly.

2. Remove the articular cartilage.

3. Trim the side of the patella down so that it fits into the prosthesis.

4. Cap the patella and fix the prosthesis with a screw.

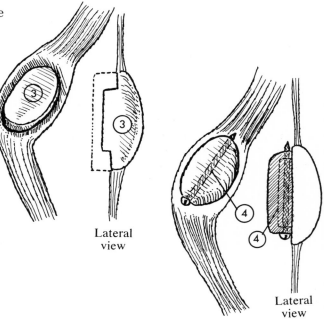

Lateral
view

Lateral
view

1. With a sharp osteotome remove a rectangle of bone 1¼ inches by ½ inch with the tendon attached.

2. Make a corresponding defect on the anteromedial aspect of the tibia slightly below the original site of attachment of the patellar tendon (its long axis inclines 45 degrees with the vertical axis of the tibia).

3. Remove the cancellous bone from the superior and inferior ends of the defect.

4. Place the tibial tubercle in the defect and rotate it so that its vertical axis parallels that of the quadriceps.

Note: Before placing the final sutures always test the path of excursion of the patella in the patellar groove; it should ride freely.

Don't transfer the tendon too far medially; this may cause a medial subluxation.

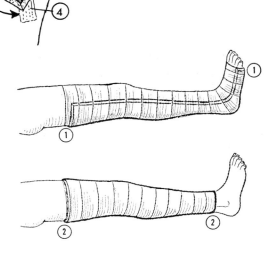

Postoperative Management

1. Immediately after completion of the operation apply a posterior splint extending from the upper thigh to the toes.

2. After two weeks remove the skin sutures and apply a plaster cylinder extending from the upper thigh to just above the malleoli.

Now institute graduated quadriceps exercises and permit weight bearing.

Five weeks postoperatively remove the plaster cylinder and institute an intensive program of graduated exercises to restore normal joint motion and normal quadriceps power and volume.

Patellectomy

REMARKS

In the face of severe degenerative changes of both the patella and femur, patellectomy may be indicated but it should be done only if there is no alternative. In addition, a quadriplasty should be done to improve the tone and direction of the quadriceps mechanism.

1. Over the anterior surface of the knee make a transverse U-shaped incision just distal to the patella.

2. Reflect the skin edges above and below and make a similar incision through the quadriceps expansion at the level of the distal one-third of the patella.

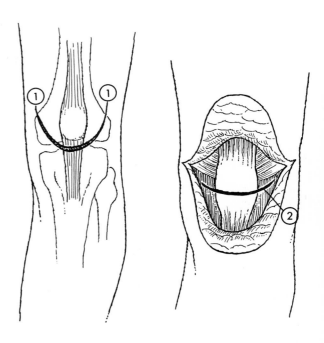

3. By sharp dissection excise the patella from the quadriceps tendon, the capsule and the quadriceps expansion and patellar tendon. Inspect the inside of the joint for any loose bodies and shave off any degenerated loose cartilage from the femoral condyles.

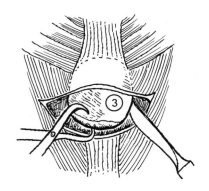

4. Pull the proximal portion of the capsule and quadriceps tendon downward and medially for ½ to ¾ inch so that they overlap the distal portion of the capsule by at least ½ inch. With mattress sutures secure the edges in this position.

5. Free the insertion of the vastus medialis from the quadriceps tendon in the form of a V.

6. Pull the end of the vastus medialis downward and laterally and secure it in this position with interrupted sutures.

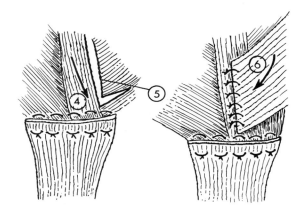

Immobilization

1. Apply a compression bandage.
2. Apply a posterior plaster splint from the toes to the upper thigh.

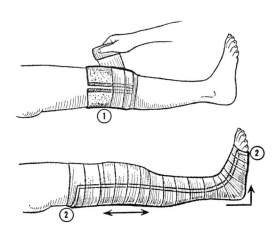

Postoperative Management

Institute quadriceps exercises within 48 hours.

After seven to ten days permit walking with crutches.

At the end of three weeks remove the splint and institute a regulated program of exercises and guarded movements at the knee. The splint is worn between exercise periods.

At the end of five weeks discard the splint and intensify the exercise program and add exercises against resistance.

Full flexion and extension should be achieved in four to six months.

Irreducible Dislocation of the Patella

REMARKS

These lesions are rare; the patella rotates about its long axis and its medial edge locks under the lateral border of the femoral condyle.

Reduction in most instances can be achieved by manipulation and extension of the knee joint.

Some cases defy manipulative reduction and require surgical intervention.

Tearing of the patellar retinaculum and of the attachment of the vastus medialis to the patella may occur in this lesion.

Prereduction X-Ray

1. The patella is dislocated laterally and inferiorly.

2. The articular surface faces outward and downward.

3. The medial edge of the patella is locked under the lateral border of the lateral femoral condyle.

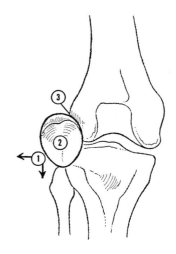

Operative Reduction

1. Make a midline skin incision over the anterior aspect of the knee joint.

2. Reflect the skin flaps and visualize the position of the patella and other soft tissue damage.

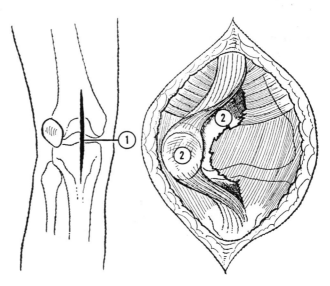

1. Grasp the patella with a towel clip; disengage its medial edge and derotate the quadriceps and patellar tendons.

2. Repair the tears in the patellar retinaculum.

3. Reattach the vastus medialis to the patella in case it has been torn from its attachment.

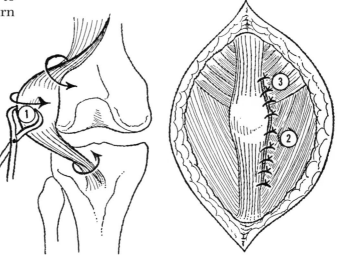

Postoperative Management

1. Immediately after completion of the operation apply a posterior plaster splint extending from the upper thigh to the toes.

2. After two weeks remove the skin sutures and apply a plaster cylinder extending from the upper thigh to just above the malleoli.

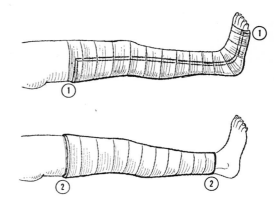

Now institute graduated quadriceps exercises and permit weight bearing.

Five weeks postoperatively remove the plaster cylinder and institute an intensive program of graduated exercises to restore normal joint motion and normal quadriceps power and volume.

ACUTE TRAUMATIC SYNOVITIS AND TRAUMATIC HEMARTHROSIS

REMARKS

Acute traumatic synovitis is a sequel of all types of knee injuries, especially internal derangements.

Occasionally the causative factor defies all diagnostic aids.

It is essential to recognize and correct the responsible agent in order to prevent recurrence of traumatic synovitis.

Traumatic synovitis differs clinically from traumatic hemarthrosis in that the fluid accumulates slowly over a period of 12 to 24 hours, the joint seldom becomes tense, and pain is never severe.

Traumatic hemarthrosis is the usual sequel to all types of intra-articular fractures. It may also accompany such lesions as maceration of the infrapatellar fat pad, rupture of one of the cruciate ligaments, tears of the synovialis, or tears in the vascular peripheral attachment of the menisci.

In traumatic hemarthrosis marked swelling is demonstrated one to two hours after the injury and pain is an outstanding feature.

MANAGEMENT OF ACUTE TRAUMATIC SYNOVITIS

In cases of small effusions with minimal distention apply a snug elastic compression bandage, prohibit full weight bearing for several days, and institute graduated quadriceps exercises.

In cases of massive effusion:

Aspirate the joint.

Apply an elastic compression bandage.

Immobilize the joint on a posterior plaster splint.

Institute graduated quadriceps exercises immediately on a regulated regimen.

If effusion reaccumulates repeat the aspiration of the joint.

After several days permit partial weight bearing on crutches.

Discard the posterior splint after seven to ten days and allow full weight bearing.

Always remember to look for and remedy the primary etiologic factor responsible for the effusion.

MANAGEMENT OF TRAUMATIC HEMARTHROSIS

Aspirate the joint.

Apply an elastic compression bandage.

Immobilize the leg on a posterior plaster splint; elevate the leg and surround the knee with bags containing ice.

Repeat the aspiration after one or two days if necessary.

After seven to ten days of complete rest institute graduated quadriceps exercises.

Now allow partial weight bearing with crutches.

After ten to 14 days discard the posterior plaster splint, permit full weight bearing, and step up the quadriceps and joint exercises.

Always search for and rectify the primary cause for the hemarthrosis.

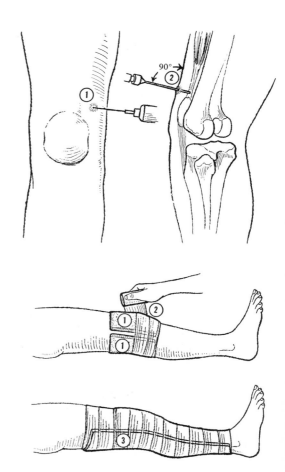

Aspiration of the Knee Joint

Perform the procedure with strict aseptic precautions.

1. Raise an intradermal wheal, using 1 per cent procaine and a fine hypodermic needle, on the outer aspect of the knee just above the superior pole of the patella.

2. After two to five minutes, pass into the joint cavity a large bore needle at a right angle to the skin.

Immobilization

1. Apply a sheet of foam rubber over the anterior and posterior aspects of the knee joint.

2. Make firm, even compression with a circular cotton elastic bandage.

3. Rest the limb on a posterior plaster splint extending from the upper thigh to just above the malleoli; secure the splint with a 3 inch cotton elastic bandage.

FRACTURES OF THE CONDYLES OF THE TIBIA

REMARKS

Most fractures of the condyles of the tibia are the result of severe abduction or adduction forces applied to the outer or inner aspect of the knee (the former is by far the most common) *or* of forces acting in the vertical direction on the tibial plateau; occasionally both forces are acting in some degree.

All these lesions are accompanied by damage to the ligamentous apparatus in varying degrees, from strain to complete rupture.

Fractures of the lateral condyle which result from abduction forces are frequently complicated by damage to the tibial collateral ligament, the anterior cruciate ligament and the lateral semilunar cartilage; in fractures of the medial condyle the opposite corresponding soft tissue structures are implicated.

Lesions of the medial condyle are exceedingly rare.

Only rarely is the continuity of the tibial collateral ligament disrupted completely; however, it is often severely strained and attenuated. The acting force is usually expended in producing a fracture of the lateral condyle.

Lesions of the ligaments are usually amenable to conservative treatment but may require surgical repair.

In the management of these lesions try to achieve the following:
1. Restore anatomic alignment of the tibial plateaus to as near normal as possible.
2. Repair all disrupted ligaments.
3. Fix the limb sufficiently long to allow adequate soft tissue healing.
4. Begin quadriceps exercises and continue them until the muscle approaches or, better, exceeds the quadriceps of the unaffected limb in power and volume. (This is the salvation of many severely disrupted knee joints.)

Remember that many severely damaged knee joints are capable of satisfactory function provided that the quadriceps is strong and powerful.

Fractures of the medial condyle are rare and are treated in a similar manner to fractures of the lateral condyle except that the forces necessary to achieve reduction are applied in the opposite direction.

Fracture of the Lateral Tibial Condyle without Fragmentation or Depression

REMARKS

In this lesion injury to the ligamentous apparatus is minimal.
All instances are amenable to conservative management.
The prognosis is excellent provided that postfracture care is adequate.

Prereduction X-Ray

Fracture of the lateral condyle without displacement.

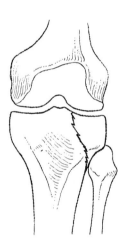

Management

1. Aspirate the knee joint.
2. Apply a circular cast from the groin to just behind the metatarsal heads.

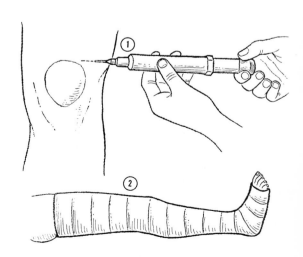

Postreduction Management

Allow crutch walking without bearing weight on the affected limb. Institute quadriceps exercises immediately.

Remove the cast after four weeks and apply a circular cotton elastic bandage around the knee joint.

Start flexion and extension exercises and increase the intensity of the quadriceps exercises.

After eight weeks, provided the quadriceps is strong, permit weight bearing on the affected limb with crutches.

Depressed Fractures of the Lateral Tibial Condyle without Fragmentation

Prereduction X-Ray

1. The lateral tuberosity is depressed.

2. The articular surface of the tuberosity is not fragmented.

3. There is a fracture of the head and the neck of the fibula. (This may or may not occur.)

Note: This type of fracture may have a complete tear of the tibial collateral ligament. Always check for this possibility.

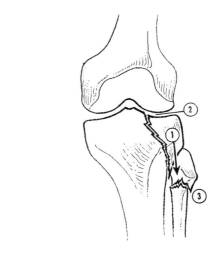

Reduction by Traction and Manipulation

Note: If the joint is distended, always aspirate the blood before proceeding with the reduction.

1. Fasten the patient's feet to the foot pieces of the fracture table.

2. The knees are extended.

3. Make moderate mechanical traction on the affected limb.

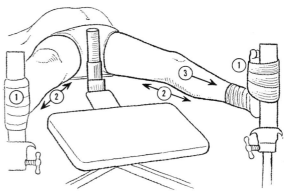

Reduction by Traction and Manipulation (Continued)

1. While traction is maintained an assistant makes manual lateral traction on the knee, using a muslin sling.

2. Traction is strong enough to force the extended knee into the varus position.

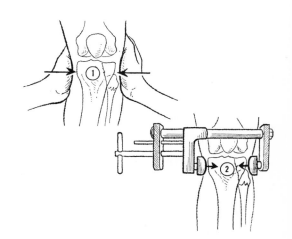

1. Now firmly compress the tibial tuberosity with the heels of the hands or

2. Squeeze the tuberosities together with a compression clamp.

Note: The clamp should be applied and released quickly.

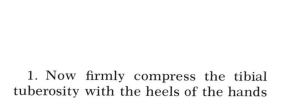

Immobilization

While lateral traction is maintained:

1. Apply a padded plaster cast from the groin to the toes.

2. Mold the plaster well around the tibial tuberosities.

3. The knee is extended.

4. The foot is at 90 degrees dorsiflexion.

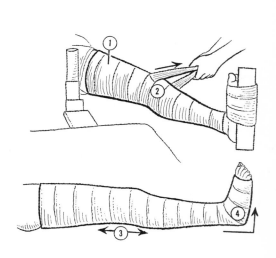

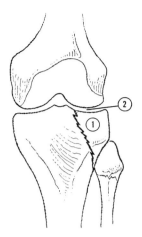

Postreduction X-Ray

1. The fragment is elevated to its normal anatomic position.

2. The congruity of the articular surfaces is restored.

Postreduction Management

Begin quadriceps drill immediately on a regulated schedule, first aided, and then unaided, five minutes every hour.

Follow this with straight leg-raising exercises against elastic resistance, then exercises against increasing loads.

After three weeks apply a new plaster cast, maintaining the same position; now permit ambulation on crutches without weight bearing on the affected extremity.

Remove the second cast four to six weeks after the reduction and institute exercises to restore joint motion. Apply a circular cotton elastic bandage around the knee joint.

Permit weight bearing at the end of 10 or 12 weeks.

Note: Don't discard the crutches until the quadriceps is sufficiently strong to stabilize the knee and protect the ligamentous apparatus during normal function; braces and knee cages should not be worn.

ALTERNATE METHOD

REMARKS

To be employed in those rare cases in which reduction cannot be achieved by traction and manipulation.

Operative Reduction

Apply a tourniquet around the upper third of the thigh.

1. The skin incision begins just anterior to the tibial collateral ligament immediately above the joint line. It curves gently downward and forward to the medial margin of the patellar tendon, then continues downward parallel to the margin of the tendon and terminates at the level of the distal end of the tibial tubercle.

2. Divide the aponeurosis along the line of the skin incision.

3. Open the capsule in the line of the upper arm of the skin incision.

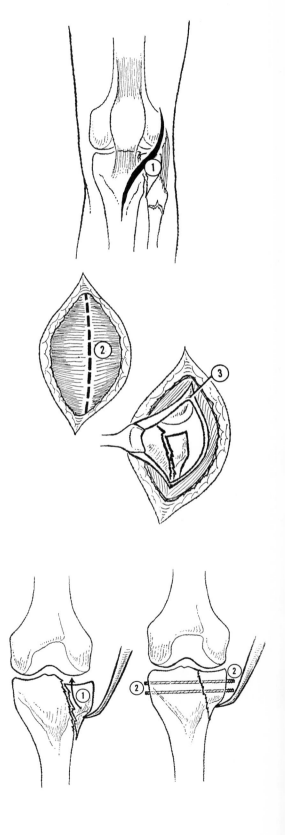

1. After flushing the wound with normal saline, elevate the tibial tuberosity into its anatomic position, using a stout curette.

2. While the corrected position is maintained (a compression clamp may be used), transfix the fragment with two pins which pierce the cortex of the opposite tibial condyle. Use Knowles or Haggie pins.

Immobilization

1. Apply a plaster cast from the groin to the toes.
2. The knee is extended.
3. The foot is dorsiflexed 90 degrees.

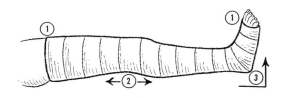

Postoperative Management

This phase is the same as that described for fractures treated by the conservative method except that the pins are withdrawn after eight weeks.

Fracture of the Lateral Condyle with Depression of the Central Portion of the Tibial Plateau

REMARKS

This lesion is relatively uncommon.

A large segment of the tibial plateau without fragmentation is depressed into the substance of the tibial condyle.

It is impossible to elevate this fragment by closed method; surgical intervention is essential.

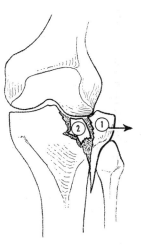

Prereduction X-Ray

1. The tuberosity is split and displaced laterally.
2. A large unfragmented portion of the tibial plateau is depressed into the tibial condyle.

Page 1493

Operative Reduction

Apply a tourniquet around the upper end of the thigh.

1. The skin incision begins just anterior to the tibial collateral ligament immediately above the joint line. It curves gently downward and forward to the outer margin of the patellar tendon 1 cm. below the articular surface of the condyle, then it continues downward parallel to the tendon and terminates at the level of the distal end of the tibial tubercle.

2. Divide the aponeurosis along the line of the skin incision.

3. Open the capsule in the line of the upper arm of the skin incision.

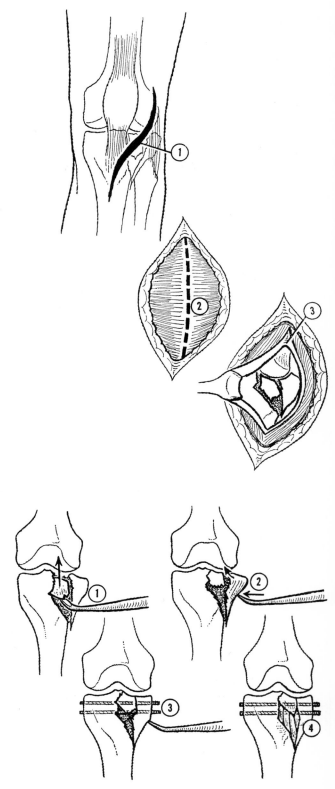

1. After flushing out the joint cavity with normal saline solution, elevate the depressed fragment into place, using a curette.

2. Elevate and compress the displaced outer fragment into its normal position.

3. While the corrected position is maintained (a compression clamp may be used), traverse the marginal fragment and the opposite tibial tuberosity with two threaded pins which are parallel to the articular surface and pierce the cortex of the inner tuberosity. Use Knowles or Haggie pins.

4. Pack the remaining defect with cortical bone struts long enough to support the central fragment.

Immobilization

1. Apply a plaster cast from the groin to the toes.
2. The knee is extended.
3. The foot is dorsiflexed 90 degrees.

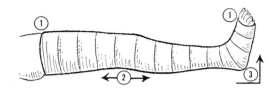

Postreduction X-Ray

1. The central fragment is elevated.
2. The congruity of the articular surface is restored.
3. Pins traverse both tuberosities.

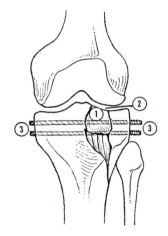

Postoperative Management

Begin quadriceps drill immediately on a regulated schedule, first aided and then unaided, for five minutes every hour.

Follow this with straight leg-raising exercises against elastic resistance, then exercises against increasing loads.

After three weeks apply a nonplaster cast, maintaining the same position; now permit ambulation on crutches without weight bearing on the affected extremity.

Remove the second cast eight weeks after the reduction and institute exercises to restore joint motion.

Permit weight bearing at the end of 10 or 12 weeks.

Note: Don't discard the crutches until the quadriceps is sufficiently strong to stabilize the knee and protect the ligamentous apparatus during normal function; braces and knee cages should not be worn.

The wires are removed at the end of eight weeks.

Fractures of the Lateral Condyle with Severe Fragmentation and Depression of the Tibial Plateau

REMARKS

This lesion is often associated with severe ligamentous damage; the lateral semilunar cartilage may be crushed and displaced into the lateral tuberosity. This type is by far the most common fracture encountered.

Comminution is usually severe and many small central fragments may be driven into the head of the tibia; these are devoid of blood supply.

These displaced fragments may preclude reduction by closed methods because it is impossible to elevate them into their position by traction and manipulation.

If the marginal fragment is relatively large, reduction by traction, manipulation and compression is indicated; the small central fragments are ignored and are crushed into the head of the tibia. Operative reduction is indicated when closed methods fail and in those cases with severe comminution and a small marginal fragment.

The prognosis in these lesions should always be guarded.

In many instances a serviceable joint may be salvaged, provided the quadriceps is developed and maintained at its maximum level of efficiency.

If the tibial collateral ligament is torn, this structure should be repaired first by a separate incision on the medial side of the joint as previously described; then proceed to reduce the lateral plateau fracture as described on page 1497.

COMMINUTED FRACTURE OF THE LATERAL TIBIAL CONDYLE WITH A LARGE MARGINAL FRAGMENT

Prereduction X-Ray

1. Comminution of the central plateau of the lateral condyle.

2. The marginal fragment is large and displaced downward and outward.

Note: This fracture should be reduced, immobilized, and managed in the same manner as depressed fractures of the lateral tibial condyle without fragmentation, page 1489.

If this closed method fails, operative intervention as depicted for comminuted fractures of the lateral tibial condyle with a small marginal fragment is indicated (see following).

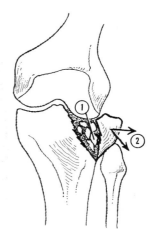

COMMINUTED FRACTURE OF THE LATERAL TIBIAL CONDYLE WITH A SMALL MARGINAL FRAGMENT

Prereduction X-Ray

1. Severe comminution and depression of the central portion of the tibial plateau.

2. The marginal fragment is small.

3. Fracture of the head and neck of the fibula. (This is a not infrequent associated lesion.)

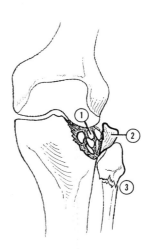

Operative Reduction

Apply a tourniquet around the upper end of the thigh.

1. The skin incision begins just anterior to the tibial collateral ligament immediately above the joint line. It curves gently downward and forward to the outer margin of the patellar tendon 1 cm. below the articular surface of the condyle, then it continues downward parallel to the tendon and terminates at the level of the distal end of the tibial tubercle.

2. Divide the aponeurosis along the line of the skin incision.

3. Open the capsule in the line of the upper arm of the incision.

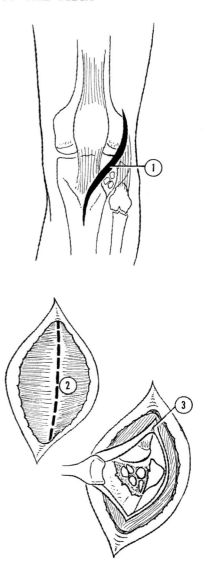

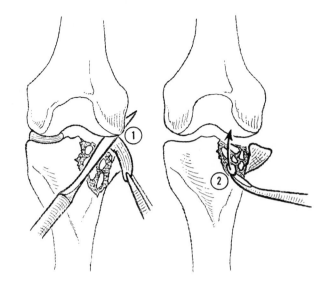

Operative Reduction (Continued)

1. After flushing out the joint cavity with a normal saline solution excise the lateral semilunar cartilage.

2. With a curette elevate the central depressed fragments into their anatomic position.

1. Elevate and compress the marginal fragment into its normal position.

2. While the corrected position is maintained (a compression clamp may be used), traverse the marginal fragment and the opposite tibial tuberosity with two threaded pins (Knowles or Haggie) which are parallel to the articular surface and pierce the cortex of the inner tuberosity.

3. Pack the remaining defect with cortical bone struts long enough to support the overlying articular fragments.

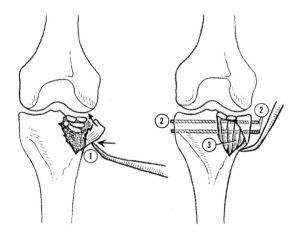

Immobilization

1. Apply a circular cast from groin to toes.
2. The knee is extended.
3. The foot is dorsiflexed 90 degrees.

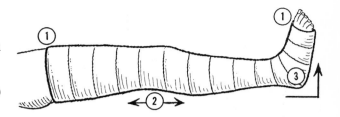

Postreduction X-Ray

1. The central fragments are elevated.
2. The congruity of the articular surface is restored.
3. The pins traverse both tuberosities.

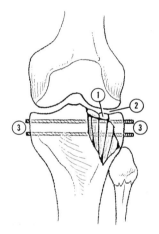

Postreduction Management

Begin quadriceps drill immediately on a regulated schedule, first aided and then unaided, five minutes every hour.

Follow this with straight leg-raising exercises against elastic resistance, then exercises against increasing loads.

After three weeks apply a new plaster cast, maintaining the same position; now permit ambulation on crutches without weight bearing on the affected extremity.

Remove the second cast six weeks after the reduction and institute exercises to restore joint motion.

Permit weight bearing at the end of ten or 12 weeks.

Note: Don't discard crutches until the quadriceps is sufficiently strong to stabilize the knee and protect the ligamentous apparatus during normal function; braces and knee cages should not be worn.

Wires are removed at the end of eight weeks.

T or Y Fractures of the Upper End of the Tibia

REMARKS

These lesions are usually the result of a violent force acting downward on the tibia, as would occur in falling from a height and landing on the feet.

The condyles of the tibia are driven downward and the shaft is displaced upward.

Elevation of the condyles and restoration of the length of the tibia are best achieved by mechanical traction.

Closed methods should be attempted in all cases; if these fail, operative intervention is indicated.

Prereduction X-Ray

1. Both condyles are displaced downward.

2. The shaft of the tibia is displaced upward.

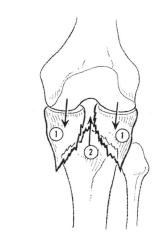

Reduction by Traction, Manipulation and Compression

1. Place the patient on a fracture table.

2. Insert a threaded pin through the lower third of the tibia and attach the pin to a spreader.

3. Make strong mechanical traction on the extended limb until the length of the tibia is restored.

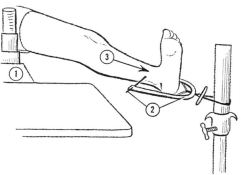

Reduction by Traction, Manipulation and Compression (Continued)

1. Make manual compression on the condyles,

or

2. Use a redresseur to compress the condyles.

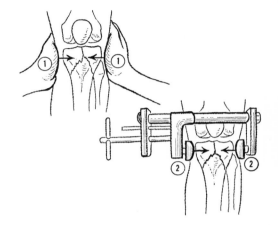

After taking a check x-ray of the fracture and if reduction is acceptable:

1. An assistant maintains traction while

2. The patient is transferred from the fracture table to a fracture bed.

3. Adjust the leg to a Böhler-Braun splint.

4. Apply 10 to 12 pounds of traction.

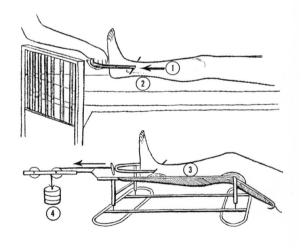

ALTERNATE METHOD

This alternate method is employed if the closed method fails.

Operative Reduction

Apply a tourniquet around the upper third of the thigh.

1. Make two skin incisions, one on each side of the joint, beginning anterior to the collateral ligaments immediately above the joint lines. The incisions curve gently downward and inward to the margins of the patellar tendon 1 cm. below the articular surface of the condyle; then they continue downward parallel to the tendon and terminate at the level of the distal end of the tibial tubercle.

2. Divide the aponeurosis along the lines of the skin incisions.

3. Open the capsule between the collateral ligaments and the margins of the patellar tendon.

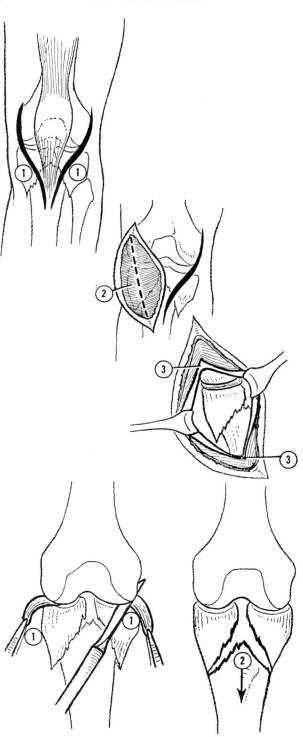

1. After flushing out the joint with a solution of normal saline, excise both menisci.

2. Make downward traction on the tibia to restore length.

Operative Reduction (Continued)

1. Lever and compress the condylar fragments into normal position, using a screw clamp.

2. While compression is maintained, traverse both condyles with two threaded pins (the points of the pins should pierce the cortex of the medial condyle) parallel to the articular surface.

3. Use Knowles or Haggie pins.

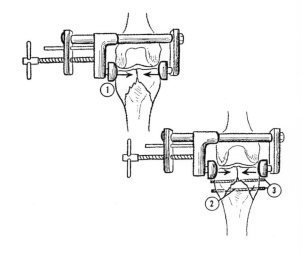

While an assistant maintains traction, transfer the patient to a fracture bed.

1. Place the leg on a Böhler-Braun splint.

2. Apply 10 to 12 pounds of traction.

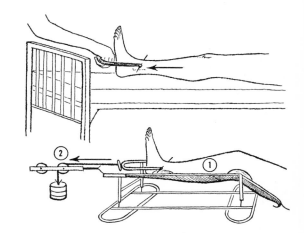

Postreduction Management

Institute quadriceps drill immediately.

No motion at the knee joint is allowed for four or five weeks.

After four or five weeks add active motion at the knee joint while traction is continued.

Eight weeks after the operation remove the traction pin and transfixion pins.

Then institute an intensive program of quadriceps exercises and active exercises to restore knee motion. Ambulation on crutches is now permitted without weight bearing on the affected limb.

Permit weight bearing after 10 to 12 weeks, depending on the strength of the quadriceps apparatus.

FRACTURES OF THE TIBIA AND FIBULA

FRACTURES OF THE SHAFTS OF THE TIBIA AND FIBULA

REMARKS

The lesions are produced by either an angulatory force or a rotational force.

Generally angulatory forces produce transverse or short oblique fractures of both bones at the same level, whereas rotational forces produce spiral fractures at different levels, the fibular fracture being at a higher level than the tibial fracture.

Many fractures are of the open type.

In many instances redisplacement of the fragments occurs after swelling of the soft tissue subsides; always check for this possibility.

Anatomic repositioning of fragments is essential in order to maintain the plane of motion in the knee and ankle in parallel axes; failure to achieve this predisposes these joints to development of osteoarthritis.

Union is notoriously slow, and nonunion is not uncommon.

In treatment, the fibular fracture is disregarded; attention is directed entirely to the tibial fracture.

Remember that fractures of the lower shaft of the fibula are as a rule associated with fracture-dislocation of the ankle joint.

Fractures of the Shafts of the Tibia and Fibula with No Displacement (with or without Angulation)

Prereduction X-Ray

1. Fractures of both bones with no overriding.
2. Mild angulatory deformity; the fragments are in good contact.

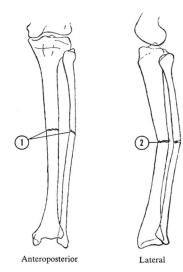

Anteroposterior   Lateral

Manipulative Reduction

1. The patient's leg hangs over the edge of the table.
2. The knee is flexed 90 degrees.
3. The leg lies in the line of gravity.
4. The surgeon with one hand steadies the upper fragment and with the other brings the lower fragment into normal alignment. (The patella and the toe point in the same direction.)

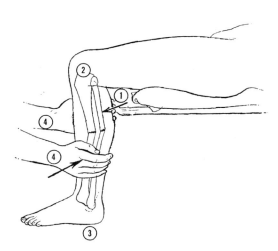

Manipulative Reduction
(Continued)

1. The surgeon steadies the limb with his knee and

2. Applies a plaster cast from the toes to the tibial tubercle, then

3. He holds the fragments in the position of normal alignment until the plaster hardens.

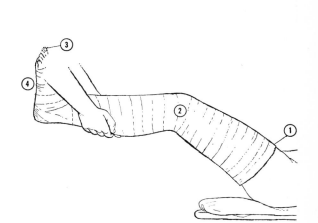

1. The plaster cast is extended to the groin.

2. The knee is flexed 20 to 30 degrees.

3. The toes are free.

4. The metatarsal heads lie in the normal arched position.

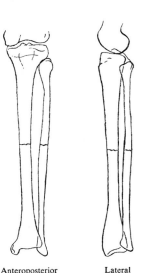

Postreduction X-Ray

The fragments are now in normal alignment.

Anteroposterior   Lateral

Wedging of Cast

Note: If the postreduction x-rays show that angulation of the fragments still exists, the deformity is corrected by wedging the plaster cast.

1. Make a linear cut around one half of the plaster cast at the level of the fracture on the concave side of the angle.

2. From the opposite half of the cast, take out a wedge of plaster $3/4$ to 1 inch centered over the convex side of the angle at the level of the fracture.

3. Leave two hinges of plaster between both cuts.

4. Correct the alignment and place a small block of wood between the cut edges on the concave side of the angle.

Note: If the position of the fragments is acceptable as shown by x-ray, bind the two segments of the cast with plaster bandage.

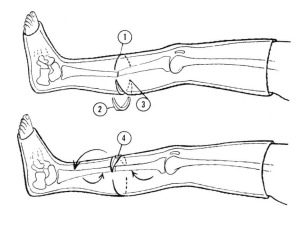

Prewedging X-Ray

Moderate posterior bowing of the leg bones.

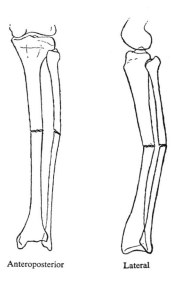

Anteroposterior   Lateral

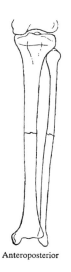
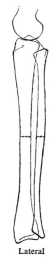

Anteroposterior   Lateral

Postwedging X-Ray

Posterior bowing has been corrected.

Page 1509

Postreduction Management

Make sure that the plaster is well molded under the metatarsal heads, preserving the anterior arch.

Institute full active flexion exercises of the toes on a regulated regimen (five minutes every hour). This prevents rigid clawing of the toes.

Institute quadriceps drill and, later, exercises against increasing loads; continue these throughout the period of convalescence.

After three weeks replace the original cast with an almost unpadded cast from the toes to the groin and with the knee slightly flexed.

Remove the plaster cast after 10 to 12 weeks and check for union clinically and by x-ray.

If union is solid by clinical tests and by x-ray, apply a cotton elastic bandage to the lower leg and foot; permit partial weight bearing with crutches.

Now institute exercises to restore normal knee motion.

Discard the crutches when the quadriceps is sufficiently strong to stabilize the knee while walking.

If the fracture is clinically solid but x-ray evidence of healing is inadequate, apply a plaster walking cast from the toes to the groin with the knee slightly flexed. Reevaluate the state of healing after four to six weeks; the cast is not discarded until union is complete by both clinical and x-ray tests.

If both clinical tests and x-rays reveal that union is not firm, reapply the plaster cast and reevaluate the state of healing after six to eight weeks.

Remember that healing may be slow, especially in the lower half of the shaft of the tibia. Maintain complete immobilization in a long leg cast until bony healing is achieved; it may take up to one year.

Don't rely on braces and short leg casts to promote healing; they do not.

Transverse, Short Oblique, or Mildly Comminuted Fractures of the Tibia and Fibula with Displacement

REMARKS

It is essential to restore the length of the tibia and to correct any lateral displacement and rotational deformity of the fragments.

Most of these fractures can be treated by closed methods provided that pins inserted in the proximal and distal fragments and incorporated in the cast are employed to prevent redisplacement of the fragments.

This method can also be used in open fractures which have been débrided and converted to closed fractures.

If reduction is not achieved by this closed method or if redisplacement of the fragments occurs, open reduction is indicated.

When the fractures occur in the middle third or in the proximal end of the distal third, intra-medullary fixation can be used (see page 1523).

Prereduction X-Ray

1. Transverse fracture of both bones.
2. The distal fragment of the tibia is displaced upward and outward.
3. The limb is bowed outward.

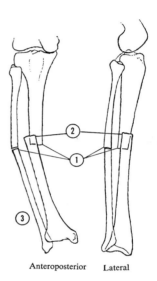

Anteroposterior   Lateral

Prereduction X-Ray

1. Short oblique fracture of both bones.
2. The distal tibial fragment is displaced upward and inward.
3. The limb is bowed inward.

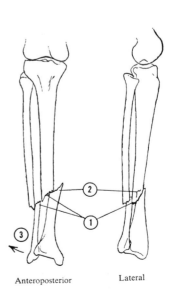

Anteroposterior   Lateral

Page 1511

Reduction by Traction and Manipulation

1. Insert a stout threaded wire through the tibia 1 inch above the ankle joint; the wire must be parallel to the joint line.

2. Insert a second threaded wire through the tibia just below the tibial tubercle.

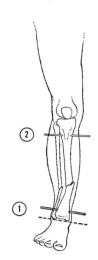

The patient lies on a fracture table.

1. Place a well padded canvas sling under the distal end of the thigh and suspend it from an overhead crossbar on the fracture table.

2. The knee is flexed 45 degrees.

3. Fix a stirrup to the lower wire and secure it to a mechanical traction apparatus at the foot of the table.

4. Correct any rotational deformity by positioning the foot so that the patella and the great toe point in the same direction.

5. Exert steady mechanical traction until the length is restored.

6. Place the palm of one hand on the upper fragment and the palm of the other hand on the lower fragment and exert firm pressure to lock the fragments.

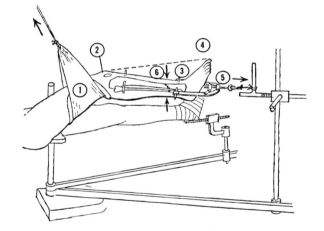

1. Apply one or two turns of sheet wadding around the leg and foot.

2. Apply a plaster slab on the posterior aspect of the leg; pass it through the stirrup and on the sole of the foot.

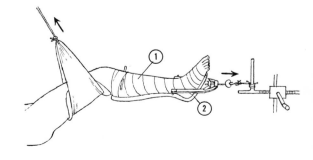

Reduction by Traction and Manipulation (Continued)

1. Apply a circular plaster cast incorporating both wires.

While the plaster is setting,

2. Exert firm lateral pressure on both fragments to maintain contact and alignment.

3. Support and mold the back of the cast to prevent posterior bowing of the leg.

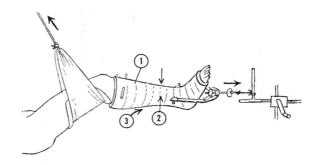

After the plaster has hardened, release the traction and

1. Extend the cast to the groin.

2. The knee is flexed 20 to 30 degrees.

3. The toes are free; the anterior arch of the foot is supported.

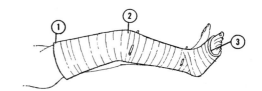

Postreduction X-Ray

1. The length of the tibia has been restored.

2. The fragments are in normal anatomic alignment.

3. Contact between the fragments is complete.

Note: If the x-rays reveal angulation at the fracture site, wedge the cast to correct the deformity, as depicted on page 1509.

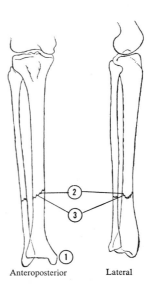

Anteroposterior   Lateral

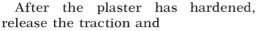

Postreduction Management

Elevate the leg on pillows or place it on a Böhler-Braun frame.

Check the toes frequently for evidence of circulatory embarrassment. If it is present, split the entire length of the cast longitudinally on its anterior aspect.

Immediately institute quadriceps drill and active flexion exercises for the toes on a regulated regimen.

Wires are removed at the end of eight to ten weeks.

After three weeks replace the original cast with an almost unpadded cast from the toes to the groin and with the knee slightly flexed.

Remove the plaster cast after 10 to 12 weeks and check for union clinically and by x-ray.

If union is solid by clinical tests and by x-ray, apply a cotton elastic bandage to the lower leg and foot and permit partial weight bearing with crutches.

Now institute exercises to restore normal knee motion.

Discard the crutches when the quadriceps is sufficiently strong to stabilize the knee while walking.

If the fracture is clinically solid but x-ray evidence of healing is inadequate, apply a plaster walking cast from the toes to the groin with the knee slightly flexed. Reevaluate the state of healing after four to six weeks; the cast is not discarded until union is complete by both clinical and x-ray tests.

If both clinical tests and x-rays reveal that union is not firm, reapply the plaster cast and reevaluate the state of healing after six or eight weeks.

ALTERNATE METHOD FOR TREATMENT OF TRANSVERSE, SHORT OBLIQUE, OR MILDLY COMMINUTED FRACTURES OF THE TIBIA AND FIBULA

REMARKS

Most of these fractures can be reduced and stabilized by the closed method (traction, manipulation, and a transfixion pin in the distal and proximal fragments incorporated in a plaster cast).

However, occasionally some fractures defy all efforts at closed reduction; here open reduction is justifiable.

In the hands of competent surgeons skilled in the techniques of open reduction, the surgical approach to these fractures as a primary method of treatment is justifiable.

Surgeons employing open methods must be cognizant at all times of the responsibility that these methods impose.

Surgical methods should not be employed unless there is definite assurance that infection can be avoided.

Infections are common sequels to operative intervention, especially in the hands of the uninitiated.

Never choose open reduction when there is the slightest doubt that the skin and soft tissues may not tolerate the procedure.

The best method of internal fixation is a massive cortical onlay graft; this provides fixation and stimulates osteogenic activity.

Another excellent method, in the hands of a skillful surgeon, is the application of a compression plate. When properly applied union is assured and the healing time is reduced. In addition to the compression plate, the placing of cancellous bone slabs around the fracture site enhances bony union.

Operative Reduction and Bone Grafting

1. Make a 5 inch incision just lateral to the tibial crest and centered at the fracture site.

2. By sharp dissection expose the tibial crest and incise the periosteum longitudinally.

3. By subperiosteal dissection expose the fragments just sufficiently to effect a reduction and apply the cortical graft; preserve as much of the periosteal attachments on the anteromedial aspect as possible.

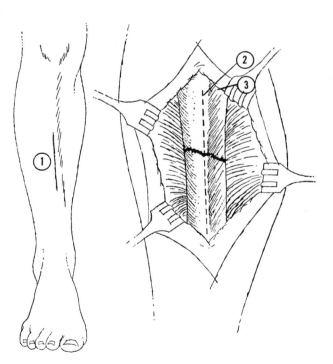

Operative Reduction and Bone Grafting *(Continued)*

1. First correct any rotational deformity; the great toe and the patella should point directly forward.

2. Exert traction on the leg to restore its length.

3. With a curette lever the fragments into normal position.

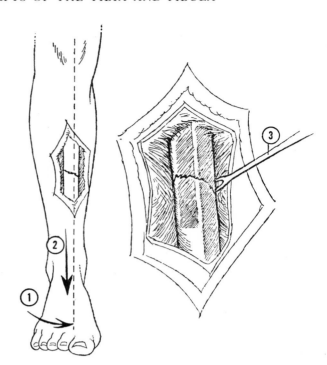

1. Apply a tibial cortical bone graft deep on the lateral aspect of the fragments; the graft is ¾ to 1 inch wide and at least 4 inches long.

2. Hold the graft in position with bone-holding forceps.

Note: Be sure that the fragments are in good contact and impacted.

3. Fix the graft in position with four vitallium or stainless steel screws; the ends of the screws should just pierce the medial cortex of the fragments.

4. Pack cancellous bone (previously obtained from the proximal end of the tibia with a curette through the defect made by removal of the graft) across the fracture site on the medial surface of the tibia.

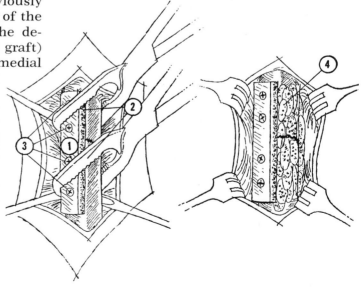

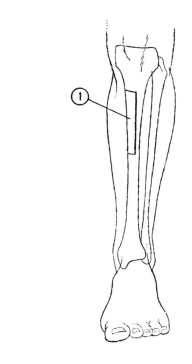

Removal and Preparation of Graft

1. Remove the graft from the upper third of the opposite tibia.

2. Through the defect in the tibia obtain cancellous bone from the proximal end of the tibia.

3. With a bone biter, make the endosteal side of the graft smooth in order to insure maximum contact with a corresponding smooth bed on the lateral aspect of the tibia.

The cancellous bone is laid across the fracture site on the medial aspect of the tibia.

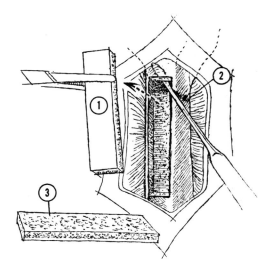

Immobilization

1. Apply a plaster cast from just proximal to the metatarsal heads to the groin.

2. The foot is dorsiflexed 90 degrees.

3. The knee is flexed 30 degrees.

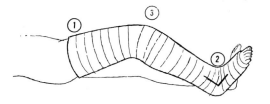

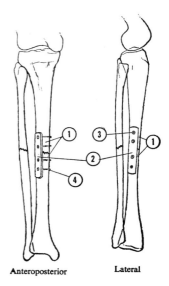

Anteroposterior   Lateral

Postreduction X-Ray

1. The fragments are in normal anatomic position.

2. The graft spans the fracture site.

3. Four screws secure the graft to the tibia.

4. The ends of the screws just perforate the medial cortex.

Postreduction Management

Elevate the leg on pillows.

Immediately institute quadriceps drill and active flexion exercises for the toes on a regulated regimen.

Watch the toes for signs of circulatory embarrassment; if it is present split the full thickness of the entire length of the cast; make a cut in the center of its anterior surface.

After three weeks apply an almost unpadded cast and check the position of the fragments by x-ray; now permit ambulation on crutches.

After eight to ten weeks remove the cast and test the state of union.

If union is solid clinically (no motion or spring is present at the fracture site; the callus is not tender) and by x-ray, apply an elastic cotton bandage from the toes to the lower thigh and permit protected weight bearing with crutches.

Increase the intensity of the quadriceps exercises and institute exercises to restore motion at the knee joint.

The crutches are discarded gradually after two to three weeks.

Long Oblique or Spiral Fractures of the Tibia with Displacement

REMARKS

These fractures are best treated by one or more transfixion screws.

Open reduction is justified only when the condition of the skin and of the soft tissues is such that it will permit surgical intervention with minimal risk of infection.

The incidence of infection following open reduction of the tibia is high; the procedure should be undertaken only by those thoroughly qualified to perform the operation.

Prereduction X-Ray

1. Long oblique fracture of the upper third of the tibia.

2. The distal fragment is displaced upward and outward.

3. The leg is bowed outward.

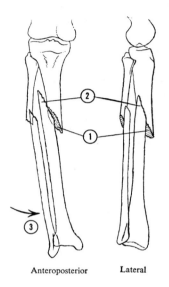

Anteroposterior   Lateral

Prereduction X-Ray

1. Spiral fracture of the tibia through its middle third.

2. Spiral fracture of the upper third of the fibula.

3. The distal fragments are displaced upward.

4. The leg is bowed forward.

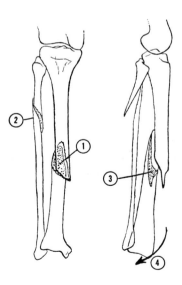

Open Reduction and Screw Fixation

1. Make a 5 inch skin incision centered over the fracture just lateral to the tibial crest.

2. Expose the tibial crest and cut the periosteum longitudinally and by subperiosteal dissection expose the fracture site.

Note: Preserve if possible the periosteal attachments on the anteromedial aspect of the fragments.

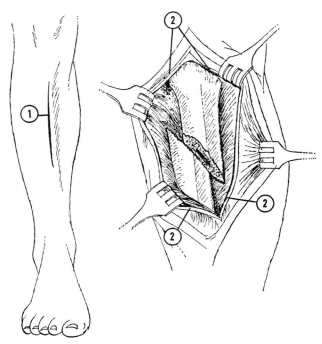

1. Apply traction to the leg and correct any rotational deformity.

2. Lever the fragments into normal anatomic alignment.

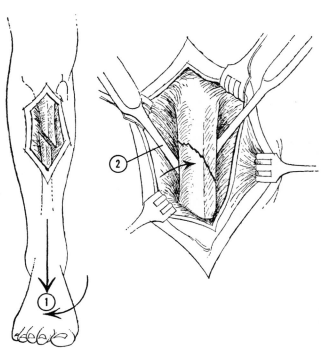

Open Reduction and Screw Fixation (Continued)

1. Grasp the fragments with bone forceps and hold the corrected position.

2. Insert one or preferably two screws across the fracture site at a right angle to the longitudinal axis of the tibia.

Note: The ends of the screws must just pierce the medial cortex of the tibia.

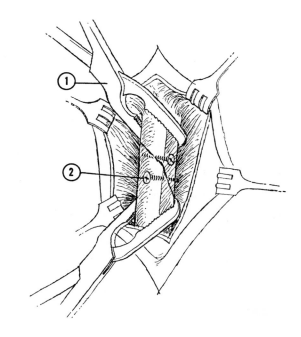

Immobilization

1. Apply a plaster cast from the toes to the groin.

2. The knee is flexed 30 degrees.

3. The toes are free and the anterior arch is supported.

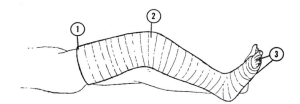

Postreduction X-Ray

1. The length of the tibia is restored.

2. The fragments are in normal anatomic position.

3. Two screws transfix the fracture site.

4. The fibular fragments are in good alignment.

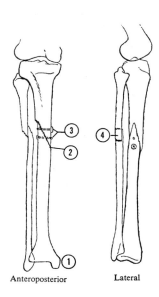

Anteroposterior   Lateral

Page 1521

Postreduction Management

Elevate the limb on pillows or a Böhler-Braun frame.

Check the toes frequently for evidence of circulatory embarrassment.

Immediately institute quadriceps drill and active flexion exercises for the toes on a regulated regimen.

After three weeks remove the cast and apply an almost unpadded plaster cast.

Now allow the patient on crutches with no weight bearing on the affected limb.

After eight to ten weeks remove the cast and check clinically and by x-ray the state of healing.

If union is solid, apply a cotton elastic bandage and permit protected weight bearing on crutches.

Institute exercises to restore normal knee motion.

Crutches can usually be discarded after two to three weeks; be sure that the quadriceps is strong enough to stabilize the knee during walking before discarding the crutches.

Segmental or Severely Comminuted Fractures of the Tibia and Fibula

REMARKS

These fractures readily lend themselves to intramedullary nailing.

This method is especially applicable to fractures of the middle third and the proximal end of the distal third of the tibia.

Intramedullary nailing corrects alignment and permits good contact of the fragments, but it does not prevent rotational stresses from acting at the fracture site, hence external fixation is also necessary.

Blind nailing is usually feasible, but if the fragments cannot be adequately aligned to introduce the nail blindly, then the nail should be introduced under vision.

When the fracture site is opened surgically to introduce the nail, strip as little soft tissue from the fragments as possible and always surround the fracture with slabs of cancellous bone.

The most satisfactory nail is the Lottes nail.

Prereduction X-Ray

Multiple fractures of the tibia and fibula with marked angular and rotational deformities.

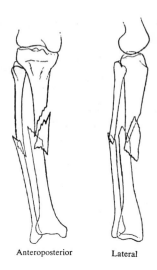

Anteroposterior   Lateral

INTRAMEDULLARY NAILING: BLIND METHOD

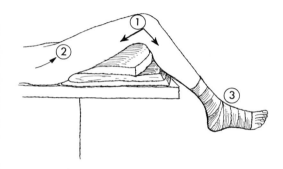

Operative Procedure

The patient lies on a fracture table:
1. The knee is flexed 90 degrees.
2. The hip is flexed 50 degrees.
3. The foot and ankle are draped separately.

1. While an assistant exerts downward traction on the foot,

2. Manipulate the fragments into anatomic alignment.

3. Make a skin incision on the anteromedial aspect of the tibia 2 cm. medial to the most prominent part of the tibial tubercle; extend it proximally to the medial side of the inferior margin of the patella.

4. Deepen the incision to the bone but do not open the knee joint.

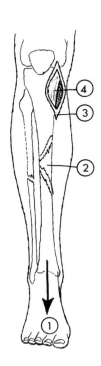

Operative Procedure (Continued)

1. With a ³⁄₈ inch drill make a hole in the tibia at the level of the middle of the tibial tubercle; first perforate the tibial cortex, holding the drill at right angles to the bone.

2. Then aim the top of the drill at the crest of the tibia at the point of juncture of the middle and distal thirds. While drilling the channel, slowly depress the drill handle until it is almost parallel to the shaft of the tibia.

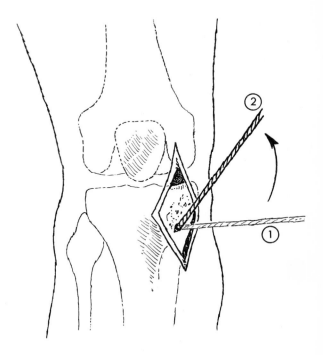

Determination of the Length of the Nail

1. Measure the distance from the medial malleolus to the tibial tubercle of the unaffected side.

2. Use a Lottes nail ³⁄₈ inch in diameter.

Note: Occasionally in young patients use a nail ⁵⁄₁₆ inch in diameter.

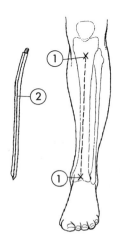

Page 1524

Insertion of the Nail

1. Insert the Lottes nail and align the tip with the juncture of the middle and distal thirds of the tibia.

2. Its dorsal fin points foward.

3. Tap the nail until it strikes the posterior cortex of the tibia.

Note: To prevent maceration of the skin and soft tissues while driving the nail, place a metal shield between the nail and the soft tissues in front of the knee.

4. Then with the palm of the hand depress the middle of the nail so that it almost parallels the longitudinal axis of the tibia. (This advances the tip of the nail forward.) As the nail is driven into the canal, maintain downward pressure until it actually dents the skin over the knee.

5. As the nail advances check its progress from time to time; this is done by comparing the protruding portion of the nail with a nail of equal length.

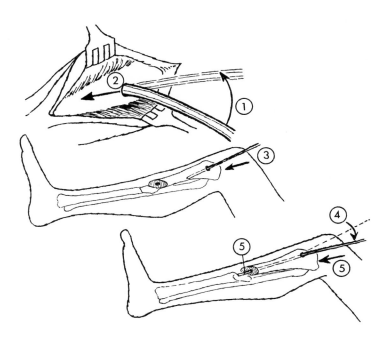

Insertion of the Nail *(Continued)*

1. When the level of the fracture site is reached by the tip of the nail,

2. Check the alignment of the fragments and correct any rotational deformity.

3. Drive the nail across the fracture site for 2 to 3 inches.

Note: Check the stability of the fragments. Obvious instability means that the nail has not engaged the distal fragment. If this is the case, withdraw the nail and reinsert it.

4. Now drive the nail into the distal fragment.

Note: Before seating the nail, take x-rays to determine the position of the fragments and the relationship of the tip of the nail to the ankle joint.

5. If the position of the fragments and the level of the tip of the nail are satisfactory, drive the nail in until the driver strikes the cortex. (The threaded portion of the nail remains above the level of the cortex so that it can be extracted later.)

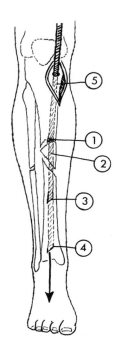

Postreduction X-Ray

1. The fragments are in normal position.

2. The tip of the nail is well above the distal articular surface of the tibia.

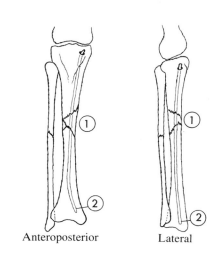

Anteroposterior   Lateral

Immobilization

1. Apply a plaster cast from just proximal to the metatarsal heads to the groin.

2. The foot is dorsiflexed 90 degrees.

3. The knee is flexed 30 degrees.

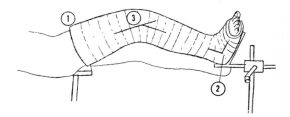

Page 1526

Postreduction Management

Elevate the limb on pillows.

Immediately institute quadriceps drills and active flexion exercises for the toes on a regulated regimen.

Watch the toes for signs of circulatory embarrassment; if it is present split the cast down to its full thickness through its entire length; make a cut in the center of its anterior surface.

After three weeks apply an almost unpadded cast and check the position of the fragments by x-ray; now permit ambulation on crutches.

After eight to ten weeks remove the cast and test the state of union.

If union is solid clinically (no motion or spring is present at the fracture site; the callus is not tender) and by x-ray, apply an elastic cotton bandage from the toes to the lower thigh and permit protected weight bearing on crutches.

Increase the intensity of the quadriceps drills and institute exercises to restore motion at the knee joint.

The crutches are discarded gradually after two to three weeks.

The nail is not removed until the fracture lines are obliterated.

Note: For transverse fractures and short oblique fractures with good, stable contact of the fragments, permit weight bearing with crutches after the second cast is applied.

For comminuted fractures, weight bearing should not be allowed until there is definite x-ray evidence of callus bridging the fragments.

INTRAMEDULLARY NAILING: OPEN OPERATION

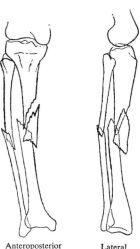

Anteroposterior   Lateral

Prereduction X-Ray

Multiple fractures of the tibia and fibula with marked angular and rotational deformities.

Open Reduction, Intramedullary Nailing and Bone Grafting

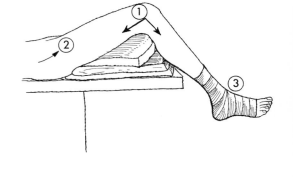

The patient lies on a fracture table.

1. The knee is flexed 90 degrees.
2. The hip is flexed 50 degrees.
3. The foot and ankle are draped separately.

Note: If the levels of the fracture sites are in close proximity to each other, make one incision; if they are at a great distance make two incisions.

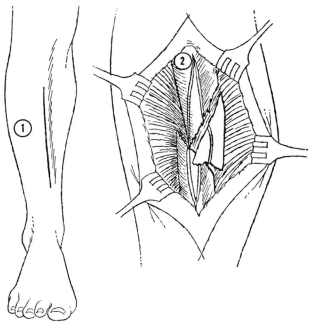

1. Make the incisions just lateral to the tibial crest.
2. By sharp dissection expose the tibial crest and incise the periosteum longitudinally.

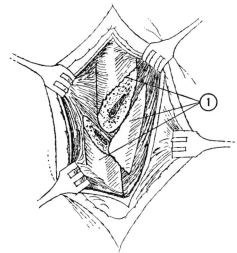

1. By subperiosteal dissection expose the ends of the fragments just enough to permit reduction and application of cancellous bone grafts across the fracture sites.

Page 1528

Open Reduction, Intramedullary Nailing and Bone Grafting (Continued)

1. Make a short longitudinal incision 2 cm. medial to the tibial tubercle; it extends proximally to the inferior margin of the patella.

2. By subperiosteal dissection expose the bone at the inferior portion of the incision.

3. With a ⅜ inch drill for a Lottes nail, first perforate the tibial cortex.

4. Then aim the tip of the drill at the crest of the tibia at the juncture of its middle and lower thirds.

Note: While drilling the channel, depress the drill handle slowly and continuously until it is almost parallel to the shaft of the tibia.

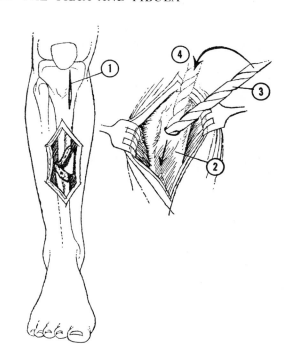

Selection of the Nail and Determination of its Length

1. Measure the distance from the medial malleolus to the tibial tubercle of the unaffected side.

2. Use a Lottes nail ⅜ inch in diameter. (Occasionally in young patients a nail ⁵⁄₁₆ inch diameter is necessary.)

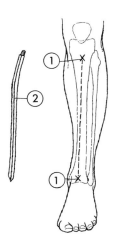

Insertion of the Nail

1. Insert the Lottes nail and align the tip with the juncture of the middle and lower thirds of the shaft.

2. Its dorsal fin points forward.

3. Tap the nail until it strikes the posterior cortex.

4. Then with the palm of the hand depress the middle of the nail so that it lies almost parallel with the longitudinal axis of the tibia.

5. Drive the nail until the tip appears through the medullary canal of the proximal fragment.

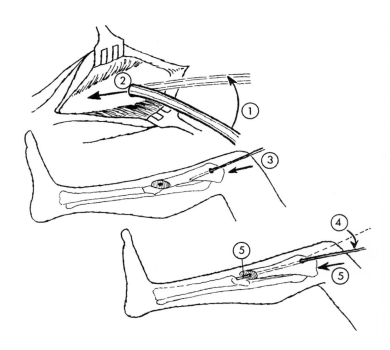

Insertion of the Nail (Continued)

1. An assistant exerts traction on the lower end.

2. He aligns the great toe with the patella.

3. With a curette lever the fragments into their normal anatomic position.

4. Drive the nail into the medullary canal of the middle fragment.

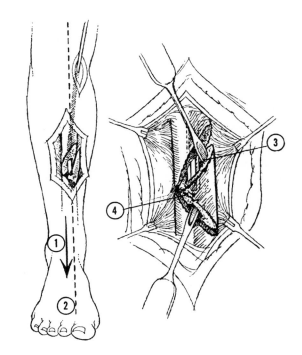

1. Drive the nail until it appears through the medullary canal of the middle fragment.

2. Again exert traction; correct the rotational deformity and with a curette lever the fragments into their normal position; now drive the nail across the fracture site.

3. Finally drive the nail further in until the driver strikes the cortex.

4. Tap the sole of the foot with the palm of the hand to impact all fragments.

Note: At this point check the reduction and the position of the nail by x-ray; if it is satisfactory, proceed.

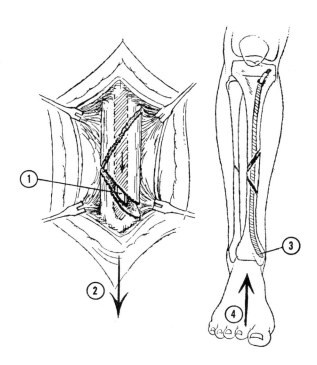

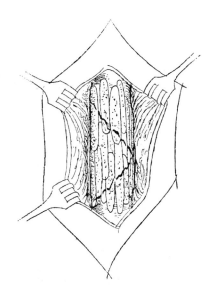

Insertion of the Nail (Continued)

Pack slabs of cancellous bone (previously removed from the anterior crest of the ilium) around the fracture site.

Postreduction X-Ray

1. The nail is in correct position and is of proper length.
2. The fragments are in normal alignment.
3. Cancellous bone slabs surround the fracture site.

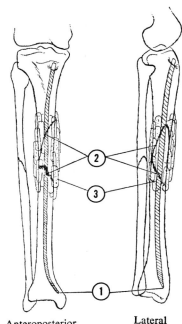

Anteroposterior   Lateral

Immobilization

1. Apply a plaster cast from just proximal to the metatarsal heads to the groin.
2. The foot is dorsiflexed 90 degrees.
3. The knee is flexed 30 degrees.

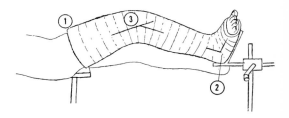

Page 1532

Postreduction Management

Elevate the limb on pillows.

Immediately institute quadriceps drills and active flexion exercises for the toes on a regulated regimen.

Watch the toes for signs of circulatory embarrassment; if it is present split the cast down to its full thickness through its entire length; make a cut in the center of its anterior surface.

After three weeks apply an almost unpadded cast and check the position of the fragments by x-ray; now permit ambulation on crutches.

After eight to ten weeks remove the cast and test the state of union.

If union is solid clinically (no motion or spring is present at the fracture site; the callus is not tender) and by x-ray, apply an elastic cotton bandage from the toes to the lower thigh and permit protected weight bearing with crutches.

Increase the intensity of the quadriceps drills and institute exercises to restore motion at the knee joint.

The crutches are discarded gradually after two to three weeks.

The nail is not removed until the fracture lines are obliterated.

Note: In the case of transverse fractures and short oblique fractures with good, stable contact of the fragments, permit weight bearing with crutches after the second cast is applied.

For comminuted fractures, weight bearing should not be allowed until there is definite x-ray evidence of callus bridging the fragments.

Unstable Fractures of the Tibia and Fibula with Severe Soft Tissue Damage

REMARKS

Severe soft tissue injury or extensive blistering and laceration of the skin may render the fracture unsuitable for treatment by the methods previously described. This applies also to some infected fractures. In these cases continuous skeletal traction is indicated.

Be sure not to distract the fragments; this may lead to delayed union or nonunion.

Traction should be continued just long enough to permit sufficient healing to prevent displacement of the fragments (three to four weeks).

Continuous traction should never be employed if some other method can be used.

Continuous Skeletal Traction

1. Pass a threaded wire through the lower end of the tibia; the wire is parallel to the ankle joint.
2. Apply a plaster cast from the toes to the upper thigh.
3. Place the limb on a Braun frame (or some similar apparatus).
4. Elevate the foot of the bed for counter traction.

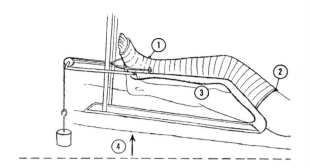

CAUTION

During the first two weeks take repeated x-rays and check for distraction.

Check the toes constantly for any evidence of circulatory embarrassment.

Reduce the weight if there is the slightest evidence of distraction.

Postreduction Management

After four to six weeks discontinue traction and apply a more snugly fitting cast.

After eight to ten weeks remove the threaded wire and the cast. Thereafter the treatment is the same as in the standard method described on page 1533.

Fractures of the Shaft of the Tibia Alone

TREATMENT

The management is the same as for fractures of the tibia and fibula together (see pages 1506 to 1534).

Fractures of the Shaft of the Fibula Alone

REMARKS

Isolated fractures are rare.

Displacement is seldom severe.

Always check the integrity of the medial collateral and cruciate ligaments when the fracture is through the neck or upper shaft of the fibula.

Always check for tibiofibular diastasis when a fracture of the shaft of the fibula is encountered without a fracture of the tibia.

Appearance on X-Ray

Fracture of the shaft of the fibula with slight comminution.

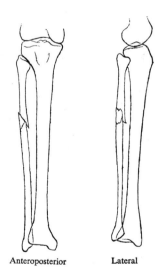

Anteroposterior   Lateral

Management

No reduction is required.

1. Apply a snug-fitting cotton elastic bandage from the toes to the knee and allow walking.

2. If the pain is severe apply a walking plaster cast below the knee for three weeks.

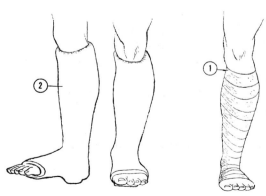

DELAYED UNION AND NONUNION IN FRACTURES OF THE TIBIA AND FIBULA

REMARKS

Many fractures in the lower half of the tibia unite very slowly; some do not unite but develop a false joint at the fracture site (pseudarthrosis).

If the fracture site is still freely mobile after three to four months, surgical intervention is justifiable; this is also true when frank nonunion exists.

The fibula in these instances is disregarded.

Massive onlay or sliding bone grafts reinforced by cancellous bone chips is the treatment of choice.

Occasionally cancellous chip grafting with intramedullary nail fixation is advisable, especially in segmental fractures.

If the fragments can be apposed, a compression plate enhances union and provides rigid fixation. This is an excellent method and should be used more frequently.

Preoperative X-Ray (Delayed Union)

1. Oblique comminuted fracture of the middle of the tibia.

2. Fracture of the lower third of the fibula.

3. The fragments are bowed posteriorly.

Note: The fracture sites were freely mobile four months after the injury.

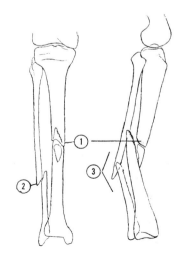

Anteroposterior   Lateral

Preoperative X-Ray (Nonunion)

1. Short oblique fracture of the middle of the tibia.
2. The bone ends are sclerotic and smooth.
3. The medullary canal is closed.

Note: This fracture is 11 months old and exhibited free motion.

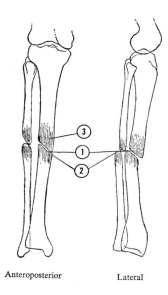

Anteroposterior   Lateral

BONE GRAFTS

Cortical graft material may be obtained from the same tibia or the opposite tibia. For lesions in the lower third of the tibia, grafts can be obtained from the upper portion of the same bone. For lesions in the middle and upper thirds, grafts should be taken from the opposite tibia. Grafts should be ½ to ¾ inch wide and at least 4 inches long.

Cancellous bone chips or slabs are obtained from the anterior iliac crest or from the upper portion of the tibia.

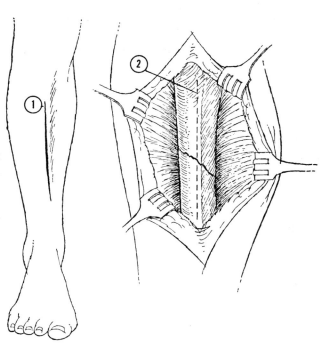

Bone Grafting

1. Make a 5 inch incision just lateral to the tibial crest and centered over the fracture site.
2. By sharp dissection expose the tibial crest and incise the periosteum longitudinally.

Page 1537

Bone Grafting (Continued)

1. By subperiosteal dissection expose the tibial fragments sufficiently to correct any deformity; permit application of an onlay graft at least 4 inches long.

2. Freshen the bone ends and open the medullary canals of both fragments.

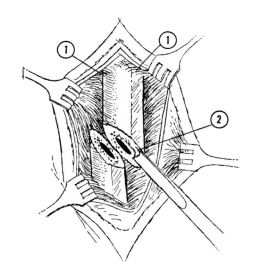

1. With a sharp, thin osteotome prepare a flat surface on the lateral aspect of each fragment.

2. Correct any rotational deformity. (The great toe and patella should point directly forward.)

3. Restore the length (an assistant makes traction on the leg) and

4. With a curette lever the fragments into normal position.

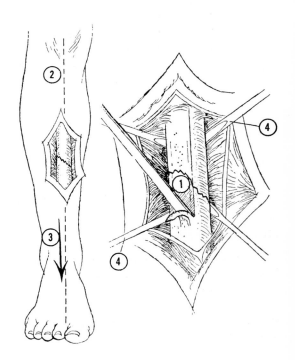

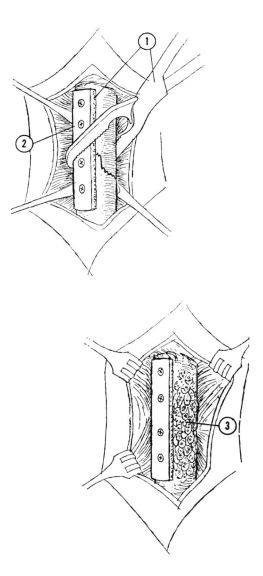

Bone Grafting (Continued)

1. Place the endosteal side of the bone graft across the fracture site and hold it in place with bone-holding forceps.

2. Secure the graft to the tibia with four vitallium or stainless steel screws. Two screws are placed on each side of the fracture site. (The screws must engage the opposite cortex but not beyond it if possible.)

3. Pack cancellous bone chips over the fracture site not covered by the bone graft.

ALTERNATE METHOD (INTRAMEDULLARY NAILING AND CANCELLOUS BONE CHIP GRAFTING)

This method is especially indicated in severely comminuted or segmented fractures with delayed union or nonunion.

The operative method is the same as that described and depicted for the treatment of Segmental or Severely Comminuted Fractures of the Tibia and Fibula (pages 1527 to 1532).

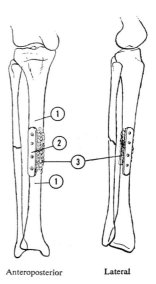

Anteroposterior   Lateral

Postoperative X-Ray

1. The fragments are in normal alignment.

2. The cortical graft spans the fracture site.

3. Cancellous bone chips are reinforcing the fracture line.

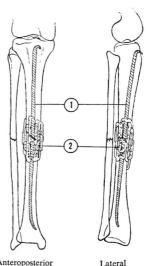

Anteroposterior   Lateral

Postoperative X-Ray

1. An intramedullary nail engages both fragments.

2. Cancellous bone slabs and chips are packed around the fracture site.

Postoperative Immobilization

1. Apply a plaster cast from just proximal to the metatarsal heads to the groin.
2. The foot is dorsiflexed 90 degrees.
3. The knee is flexed 30 degrees.

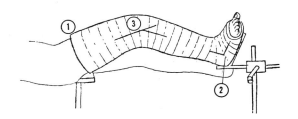

Postoperative Management

Elevate the leg on pillows.

Immediately institute quadriceps drills and active flexion exercises for the toes on a regulated regimen.

Watch the toes for signs of circulatory embarrassment; if it is present split the cast down to its full thickness through its entire length and make the cut in the center of its anterior surface.

After three weeks apply an almost unpadded cast and check the position of the fragments by x-ray; now permit ambulation on crutches.

After eight to ten weeks remove the cast and test the state of union.

If union is solid clinically (no motion or spring is present at the fracture site, the callus is not tender), and by x-ray, apply an elastic cotton bandage from the toes to the lower thigh and permit protected weight bearing with crutches.

Increase the intensity of the quadriceps drills and institute exercises to restore motion at the knee joint.

The crutches are discarded gradually after two to three weeks.

The nail is not removed until the fracture lines are obliterated.

If union is not solid, reapply a circular plaster cast from the groin to just behind the metatarsal heads. After six to eight more weeks, remove the cast and evaluate the state of union.

INJURIES OF THE ANKLE: SPRAINS, DISLOCATIONS AND FRACTURES

ANATOMIC FEATURES AND MECHANISMS OF INJURIES

REMARKS

Injuries to the ankle joint are common injuries; they are the most common injuries of athletes.

In order to institute intelligent and effective treatment, comprehension of the anatomy of the region and of the mechanisms producing the injuries is mandatory.

Because the ankle joint is a weight-bearing joint it is most essential that in all injuries all components of the ankle affected be restored to their normal anatomic status; failure to do so results invariably in serious sequels such as instability and osteoarthritis of the joint.

It is most important in all ankle injuries that a definitive diagnosis be made and that early effective treatment be instituted.

This means that all information bearing on the injury must be carefully searched for and critically evaluated so that a proper assessment of the injury can be made. Such an evaluation requires a history of the mechanism of the injury, determination of the degree of immediate disability, a careful examination of the injured part and the taking of good x-rays to demonstrate the lesion.

X-rays should be taken of the foot before an attempt is made to correct any existing deformity. Such x-rays may provide important information that may not be available if x-rays are taken only after the reduction of an existing deformity. After these preliminary x-rays are taken, then the foot may be positioned to get the following views: (1) anteroposterior view of the ankle, (2) anteroposterior view of the tarsus and (3) lateral view of the foot and ankle. If these views do not provide the desired information take oblique views and anteroposterior views while an abduction or adduction stress is applied to the foot.

Pertinent Anatomic Features of the Ankle Joint

BONY COMPONENTS

The bony configuration of the ankle joint provides inherent stability; essentially it is a hinge joint capable of movement in one plane— flexion and extension.

The mortise of the joint comprises on one side the distal end of the tibia, the internal (medial) malleolus, and on the other side the distal end of the fibula, the external (lateral) malleolus; the moving component projecting into the mortise is the talus, which fits very tightly.

The malleoli which hug the sides of the talus are of unequal length and shape; the medial malleolus is a short, stubby pyramidal structure whose tip extends only halfway down on the body of the talus; the lateral malleolus is rectangular and extends almost to the level of the talocalcaneal joint.

The body of the talus is not symmetrical; its anterior portion is much wider than its posterior, so that when the foot is dorsiflexed the anterior portion abuts firmly against the two malleoli, creating a very stable situation. On the other hand when the foot is plantar-flexed the narrow posterior portion of the talus advances forward into the mortise; this position produces lateral instability.

When the foot is dorsiflexed the talus applies lateral stress to the external malleolus, forcing the fibula outward. When the foot is both dorsiflexed and everted, the side of the talus makes even stronger pressure against the external malleolus.

Bony Configuration of the Ankle Joint

1. Articular surface of tibia forms the top of the mortise.
2. The internal and external malleoli form the sides of the mortise.
3. Note the length of the internal malleolus as compared to
4. The external malleolus which flanks the entire side of the talus.

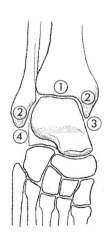

Body of the Talus

1. Anterior portion of the body; it is wider than
2. Posterior portion of the body.

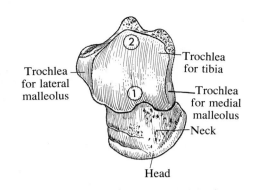

Trochlea for lateral malleolus

Trochlea for tibia

Trochlea for medial malleolus

Neck

Head

When the Foot is Dorsiflexed

1. The anterior portion of the body is gripped firmly by
2. The internal and external malleoli. This creates a stable situation.

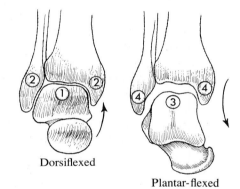

When the Foot is Plantar Flexed

3. The posterior portion advances into the mortise.
4. There is added space between the posterior portion of the talus and the malleoli. This creates lateral instability.

Dorsiflexed

Plantar-flexed

LIGAMENTS

In addition to the stability provided by the bony configuration, the ankle joint is further stabilized by a tough investment of ligaments surrounding the joint and by the anterior and posterior tibiofibular ligaments, which are really thickened portions of the interosseous membrane; these ligaments firmly bind together the distal ends of the tibia and fibula but do allow a certain amount of motion between the two bones.

On either side of the joint are the tibial and fibular collateral ligaments; these strong, thick structures provide excellent stability and protect the ankle joint against lateral stress.

On the anterior aspect of the joint there are no ligaments except the fibrous capsule; posteriorly the ligaments are thin. This arrangement permits free flexion and extension of the joint.

The medial collateral ligament (deltoid ligament) is larger and stronger than the lateral collateral ligament. It is attached to the internal malleolus by a broad base; distally it is attached to the navicular and to the talus. In addition some of its fibers are continuous with the ligaments supporting the arch of the foot. It is also continuous posteriorly with the talotibial ligament.

The lateral collateral ligament comprises many fibrous bands extending anteriorly, posteriorly and distally; there are three distinct, clearly delineated structures: (1) the anterior talofibular, which is attached anteriorly to the talus, (2) the posterior talofibular, which is directed backward to the posterior aspect of the talus, and (3) the calcaneofibular, which extends directly downward and is attached to the calcaneus.

Ligaments on the Posterior Aspect of the Ankle Joint

1. Posterior tibiofibular ligament.
2. Interosseous membrane.
3. Posterior talofibular ligament.
4. Calcaneofibular ligament.
5. Deltoid ligament.
6. Posterior talocalcaneal ligament.

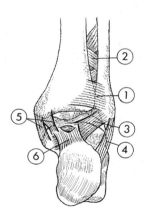

Ligaments on the Anterior Aspect of the Ankle Joint

1. Anterior tibiofibular ligament.
2. Anterior talofibular ligament.
3. Deltoid ligament.
4. Talonavicular ligament.

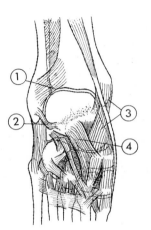

Page 1547

Ligaments on the Medial Aspect of the Ankle Joint

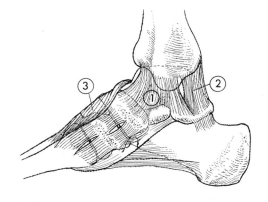

1. Deltoid ligament.
2. Posterior talotibial ligament.
3. Talonavicular ligament.

Ligaments on the Lateral Aspect of the Ankle Joint

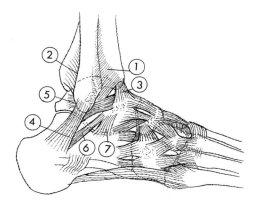

1. Anterior inferior talofibular ligament.
2. Posterior inferior talofibular ligament.
3. Anterior talofibular ligament.
4. Calcaneofibular ligament.
5. Posterior talofibular ligament.
6. Lateral talocalcaneal ligament.
7. Anterior talocalcaneal ligament.

Mechanisms of Sprains, Dislocations and Fractures

The mechanisms producing sprains, dislocations and fractures of the ankle joint are essentially the same; the intensity of the abnormal forces governs the type of lesion produced.

In general most injuries are the result of lateral stresses that force the ankle beyond the normal arcs of motion; to a lesser degree some injuries are produced by stresses forcing the ankle into excessive hyperextension and hyperflexion.

From a clinical point of view the injuries to the lateral structures can be grouped into inversion injuries and eversion injuries.

MECHANISM OF INVERSION INJURIES

The great majority of ankle injuries are of this type and primarily implicate the ligaments; occasionally there may be an avulsion fracture of the tip of the lateral malleolus. In young people the injuries are usually confined to the ligaments; in older people often there is a fracture of the lateral malleolus or of the medial malleolus, or of both malleoli.

With the inversion mechanism, in most instances, there is also an element of internal rotation and plantar flexion of the foot.

As the foot inverts in relation to the leg, the lateral collateral ligament is stretched; if the force continues some of the fibers tear. If the force continues further, part of the ligament tears and finally it ruptures completely. With even further continuation of the force the talus is jammed against the medial malleolus, whose tip now digs into the body of the talus, thus acting as a fulcrum and causing the talus to rotate over the malleolus.

In older people this mechanism may produce a bimalleolar fracture; instead of the lateral ligament rupturing, the lateral malleolus is avulsed and the talus may shear off the medial malleolus, the fracture line being oblique or vertical and beginning at the lateral margin of the medial malleolus.

There may result a rupture of the lateral ligament and a fracture of the medial malleolus. Finally, if the force is violent enough, a fracture of the posterior lip may occur in addition to a fracture of both malleoli.

Inversion Mechanism

1. The foot is forced into inversion.
2. The lateral collateral ligament is stretched and some of its fibers tear.

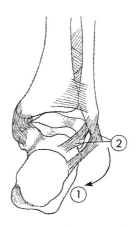

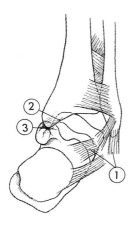

As the force continues:
1. The lateral collateral ligament ruptures.
2. The talus abuts against the tip of the medial malleolus.
3. The tip of the malleolus digs into the side of the talus as the talus rotates over the malleolus.

Page 1549

Inversion Mechanism
(Continued)

This same inversion mechanism may also produce:

1. Tear of the lateral collateral ligament.

2. Oblique fracture of the medial malleolus.

or

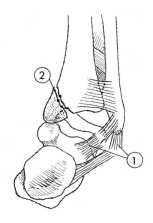

1. Avulsion of the lateral malleolus.

2. Oblique or vertical fracture of the medial malleolus.

or

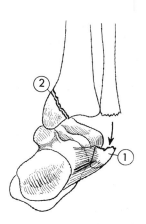

1. Avulsion of the lateral malleolus.

or

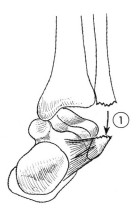

Page 1550

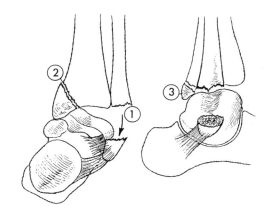

Inversion Mechanism
(Continued)

1. Avulsion of the lateral malleolus.
2. Fracture of the medial malleolus.
3. Fracture of the posterior lip of the tibia.

MECHANISM OF EVERSION INJURIES

The mechanism is the opposite of the inversion mechanism. With an eversion force acting on the foot, the foot is everted, externally rotated and dorsiflexed; the foot is forced outward and the talus abuts against the lateral malleolus. Considerable pressure can be exerted against the lateral malleolus before the medial collateral ligament is stretched beyond its capacity, because the deltoid ligament permits a certain amount of tilting of the talus. Therefore, a fracture of the lateral malleolus may occur without injury to the medial collateral ligament. This is a relatively common injury and the fracture occurs below the level of the articular surface of the tibia.

If the force continues the deltoid ligament may rupture. Also this same mechanism, instead of causing a fracture of the lateral malleolus, may force the fibula away from the tibia by producing a complete rupture of the tibiofibular ligament. As this force continues further, the deltoid ligament ruptures and finally the fibula fractures, usually in its lower third, but it may fracture anywhere along its length. The medial malleolus may be avulsed instead of the medial collateral ligament rupturing.

Fracture of the fibula above the level of the ankle joint always indicates that the tibiofibular ligament is torn and that the stability of the ankle mortise is lost.

Bimalleolar fractures in which both malleoli are fractured below the level of the joint are common.

Whenever a fracture of the lateral malleolus occurs below or at the joint line one should always suspect a tear of the deltoid ligament; these lesions are also common.

Eversion Mechanism

1. The foot is forced into eversion.
2. The talus abuts against the lateral malleolus and causes a fracture below the joint line.
3. The deltoid ligament is stretched but not beyond its limits.

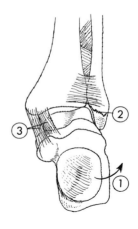

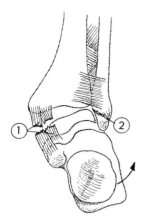

If the force continues:
1. The deltoid ligament ruptures.
2. The lateral malleolus fractures below the joint line.

With greater force:
1. The talus abuts against the lateral malleolus.
2. The tibiofibular ligament ruptures.
3. The shaft of the fibula fractures in its lower third.
4. The deltoid ligament ruptures.

or

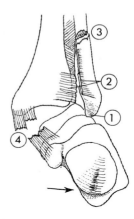

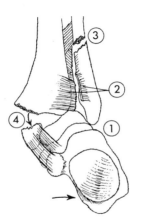

1. The talus abuts against the lateral malleolus.
2. The tibiofibular ligament ruptures.
3. The shaft of the fibula fractures.
4. The medial malleolus is avulsed.

or

Eversion Mechanism
(Continued)

1. The medial malleolus fractures below the joint line.
2. The lateral malleolus fractures below the joint line.

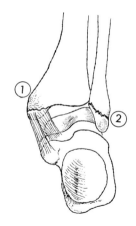

DORSIFLEXION MECHANISM

This mechanism is usually accompanied by some external rotation of the foot.

As the foot is forced into excessive dorsiflexion the anterior portion of the talus, which is wider than the posterior portion, is thrust tightly between the malleoli; if the force continues and if some forced external rotation is also acting, the two malleoli are forced apart, tearing the distal tibiofibular ligament. When the force is expended the two bones spring back into place.

The diagnosis of this lesion is difficult to make early; later the diagnosis becomes apparent as calcification occurs in the tibiofibular ligament.

COMPRESSION FORCES

When compression forces, such as a fall from a height, are added to the inversion and eversion mechanisms, severe disruption of the distal articular surface of the tibia may occur. These are difficult fractures to treat and carry a grave prognosis.

1. Fracture of the lateral malleolus.
2. Fracture of the medial malleolus.
3. Comminution of the distal end of the tibia.

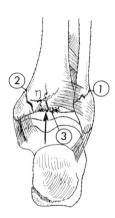

MANAGEMENT OF SPRAINS OF THE LIGAMENTS OF THE ANKLE

REMARKS

The type of treatment instituted is governed by the severity of the sprain. In Grade I sprains only a few fibers of the affected ligament are involved. The ligament is not stretched severely; its continuity is intact and functionally it is not weakened.

In Grade II sprains a portion of the ligament is torn and, although the ligament still retains continuity, it is seriously weakened.

In Grade III sprains the ligament is completely torn and no longer can function.

Obviously the diagnosis between Grade I and Grade II lesions is a subtle one; however, careful clinical examination reveals that there are gradations of findings which permit making the correct diagnosis. In complete ruptures the intensity of the pain may preclude an adequate examination; here do not hesitate to administer local anesthesia, or if necessary general anesthesia, to permit a thorough examination. Always take x-rays of the ankle and tarsus; take stress x-rays if indicated.

LATERAL LIGAMENT — GRADE I SPRAINS

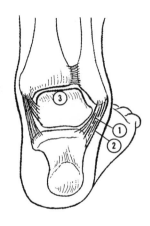

Pathology

1. There is tearing of some of the fibers of the ligament.

2. The continuity of the ligament is intact and its function not affected.

3. The talus occupies its normal position in the mortise.

Clinical Tests

1. There is tenderness over the lateral ligament.

2. Dorsiflexion and plantar flexion are not restricted or painful.

3. Abnormal adduction stress applied to the heel causes some pain.

Note: The disability in these cases is minimal. There is only minimal swelling and ecchymosis over the lateral aspect of the ankle.

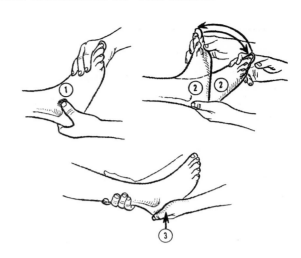

X-Ray Tests for Lesions of the Lateral Ligaments

(These tests should be performed by a surgeon.)

First infiltrate the area with procaine.

1. Take anteroposterior views of the ankle while an adduction stress is applied to the heel.

2. The foot is fully inverted.

3. The talus does not tilt in the mortise (indicating that the lateral ligament is intact). Minor degrees of tilting of the talus may be normal for the individual; therefore always take x-rays of the opposite ankle for comparison.

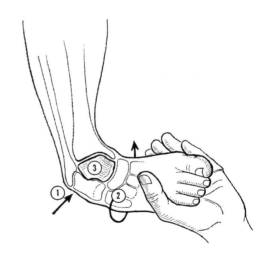

Immobilization

After infiltrating the area with 5 to 10 cc. of 1 per cent procaine, apply an adhesive strapping.

1. The patient holds the foot in a slightly everted position.

2. The foot is at a right angle.

3. Use strips of adhesive tape 1 inch wide; first apply four long longitudinal strips beginning on the inner aspect of the leg at the junction of its middle and lower thirds; the strips pass under the sole of the foot and run up the lateral aspect of the leg; the strips overlap each other.

4. Apply four short longitudinal strips, leaving the front of the ankle and the foot uncovered.

5. Apply five or six overlapping horizontal strips; these extend from well below the malleoli to 2 to 3 inches above them.

6. Reinforce the adhesive strapping with circular turns of 2 inch elastic bandage extending from the metatarsal heads to the upper limits of the adhesive strapping.

Note: Apply the turns of the bandage snugly, not tightly, and always with uniform tension.

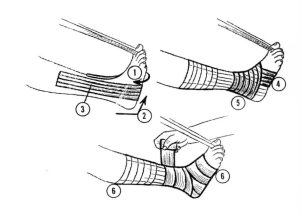

Management

1. Elevate the heel ¼ inch on the side of the ligament involved.

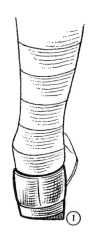

Permit weight bearing.

If the swelling is marked, apply ice packs around the bandaged ankle, and elevate the limb.

Reapply the adhesive strapping every five days.

After two weeks remove all external support.

MEDIAL LIGAMENT – GRADE I SPRAINS

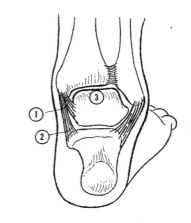

Pathology

1. There is some tearing of the fibers of the deltoid ligament.

2. The ligament is intact and its function not impaired.

3. The talus occupies its normal position in the mortise.

Clinical Tests

1. There is tenderness over the medial ligament.

2. Dorsiflexion and plantar flexion at the ankle are not restricted or painful.

3. Abnormal abduction stress applied to the heel causes some pain.

Note: The disability is minimal. There is only minimal swelling and ecchymosis over the medial aspect of the ankle.

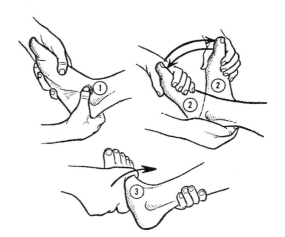

X-Ray Test for Lesions of the Medial Ligament

1. Take anteroposterior views of the ankle while an abduction stress is applied to the heel.

2. The foot is fully everted.

3. The talus does not tilt in the mortise – the ligament is intact.

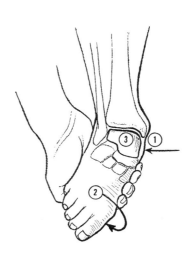

Management

Management is the same as that described for Grade I sprains of the lateral ligament, except that the foot is strapped in slight inversion and if a lift is worn on the shoe it is placed on the inner side of the heel.

LATERAL AND MEDIAL LIGAMENTS – GRADE II SPRAINS

The clinical and x-ray findings are the same as those encountered in Grade I sprains except that in Grade II sprains they are far more severe; also the degree of disability is considerably greater; even normal motion is very painful and swelling may be diffuse over the ankle and foot.

In these lesions the ligaments are partially torn and weakened functionally but their continuity is maintained; hence, x-rays will show no tilt of the talus.

Pathology of Grade II Sprains

1. In lateral lesions the lateral collateral ligament is partially torn.

2. In medial lesions the deltoid ligament is partially torn.

3. Continuity of the ligaments is maintained but the ligaments are weakened.

4. The talus occupies its normal position in the mortise.

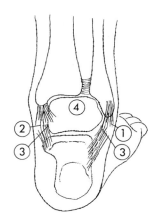

Management

The ligament must be put at complete rest until healing is achieved. Complete rest in bed for 24 hours is necessary.

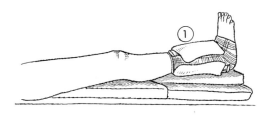

1. Apply a compression bandage and surround the ankle and foot with ice packs; elevate the foot.

2. After 24 hours apply a posterior splint from the toes to the knee, holding the foot in the neutral position, and a compression bandage.

Note: At this time, the patient can be made ambulatory, using crutches without weight bearing on the affected foot.

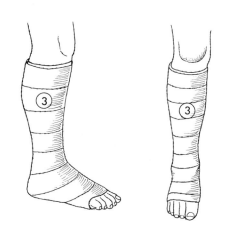

3. After the swelling subsides (five to seven days) apply a nonpadded plaster walking cast.

Note: The nonpadded cast gives the best fixation and is more comfortable than the padded cast. However, the application of a nonpadded cast requires skill, patience and attention to details.

After three weeks remove the cast and institute a program of exercises designed to restore normal motion.

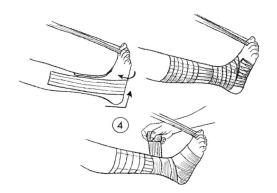

4. After the removal of the cast protect the ankle with an adhesive strapping; this is reapplied at weekly intervals and discarded when the patient is free of pain (four to six weeks).

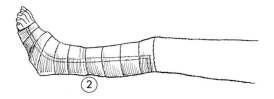

LATERAL AND MEDIAL COLLATERAL LIGAMENTS – GRADE III SPRAINS

REMARKS

These lesions are characterized by complete severance of the ligament and marked disability. The tear may be in the substance of the ligament or at the site of one of its attachments.

Disability is immediate and marked.

Swelling is diffuse and extreme.

All motions at the ankle joint are painful.

Any stress applied to the ligament elicits severe pain.

Abnormal motion is demonstrable, although this test may not be possible if the pain is severe. However, if there is doubt as to the diagnosis the examination should be performed after administering local or general anesthesia.

These lesions are associated with momentary displacement of the talus at the time of injury; subluxation of the talus can always be demonstrated by x-rays taken with stress applied to the ligament.

The great extent of the disability and the soft tissue reaction, such as swelling, edema and ecchymosis, should lead one to suspect a complete rupture of the ligament.

If the ligament is completely ruptured the treatment of choice is immediate surgical repair unless there are contraindications to this approach. This approach is particularly important in young people.

Some complete ruptures heal with conservative management, which is sometimes successful. However, this is not uniformly true and conservative management frequently results in repeated recurrences of the sprain and an unstable ankle joint. Such results occur more frequently following conservative or inadequate management of the lateral collateral ligament.

Moreover, surgical repair reduces the period of convalescence and insures a better functional result.

The lesions that may occur are:

Complete rupture of the lateral collateral ligament.

Complete rupture of the medial collateral ligament.

Complete rupture of the distal tibiofibular ligament.

Complete rupture of the medial collateral and distal tibiofibular ligaments.

COMPLETE RUPTURE OF THE LATERAL COLLATERAL LIGAMENT

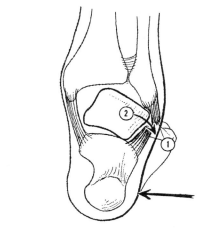

Pathology

1. Complete rupture of the lateral collateral ligament.

2. This allows tilting of the talus in the ankle mortise when an adduction stress is applied to the heel.

Clinical Tests

1. The area of maximum tenderness is over the site of rupture of the ligament, usually just below and in front of the malleolus.

2. Inversion and adduction of the foot elicit severe pain.

3. On inversion of the foot the tilt and migration of the talus are palpable.

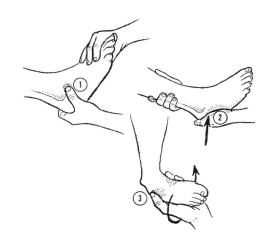

X-Ray Tests

First infiltrate the area with 1 per cent procaine.

1. While adduction stress is applied to the heel take an anteroposterior view.

2. The foot is fully inverted.

3. There is marked tilting of the talus in the mortise. (This shift of the malleolus is possible only when there is a complete tear of the ligament.)

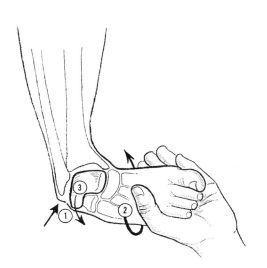

Page 1561

Surgical Repair

1. Begin the skin incision just lateral and distal to the head of the talus, curve the incision around the malleolus 1 inch from its tip and extend it posteriorly and proximally 1 inch posterior to the fibula to a point 2 inches above the tip of the malleolus.

2. Reflect the edges of the wound by sharp dissection. This brings into view the ruptured lateral ligament and the peroneal tendons.

3. Incise the fascia parallel with the peroneal tendons and displace them posteriorly.

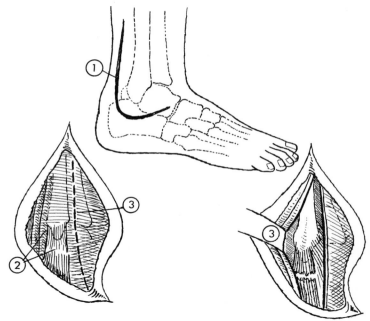

Surgical Repair (Continued)

1. Visualize all three major components of the ligament.

2. By interrupted sutures approximate the edges of the torn ligament.

3. Allow the peroneal tendons to return to their normal position.

4. Approximate the edges of the fascia over the tendons.

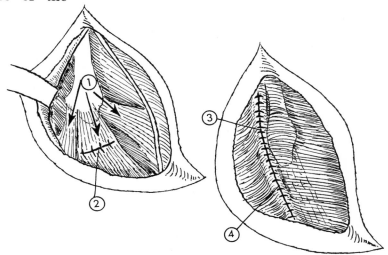

Immobilization

Apply a compression bandage and a posterior plaster splint.

1. The foot is at a right angle with the leg.

2. The foot is slightly everted.

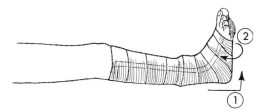

Postoperative Management

After 7 to 10 days remove the splint and apply a nonpadded plaster walking cast.

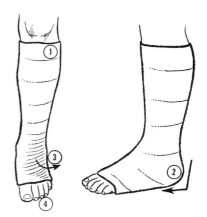

1. The cast extends from the toes to just below the knee.

2. The foot is at a right angle to the leg.

3. The heel is slightly everted.

4. The toes are free.

After three more weeks remove the cast and apply an adhesive strapping (see page 1556).

Institute a program of intensive active exercises to restore normal joint motion.

The ankle should be protected until all symptoms subside, usually in four to six more weeks.

Conservative Method

If the conservative method is chosen:

Put the limb at complete rest for 24 to 48 hours.

Apply a compression bandage and ice and elevate the limb.

After some of the swelling has subsided (24 to 48 hours), apply a posterior plaster splint and a compression bandage; the foot is fixed in the neutral position.

After 7 to 10 days, when most of the swelling has subsided, apply a nonpadded plaster walking cast.

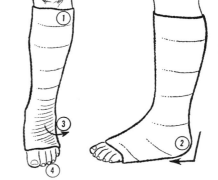

1. The cast extends from below the knee to the toes.

2. The foot is at a right angle to the leg.

3. The heel is slightly everted.

4. The toes are free.

Now apply a heel to the cast and permit weight bearing.

Reapply the cast every three weeks.

Maintain plaster immobilization for eight to ten weeks.

During this period insist on active exercises (flexion and extension) of the knee and toes.

After removal of the plaster cast institute physical therapy and active exercises to restore normal ankle motion.

Protect the ankle with an adhesive strapping as long as there is pain.

Elevate the outer side of the heel 3/16 inch.

COMPLETE RUPTURE OF THE MEDIAL COLLATERAL LIGAMENT AND OF THE INFERIOR TIBIOFIBULAR LIGAMENT

REMARKS

Ruptures of the medial and the inferior tibiofibular ligaments without fracture are very rare, but they do occur and are frequently overlooked.

The lesion is the result of violent eversion of the ankle joint.

Fracture of the lateral malleolus or of the shaft of the fibula is so common in severe eversion injuries that it should be suspected and looked for in all such injuries.

Rupture of these ligaments permits widening of the ankle mortise with lateral displacement of the tibia; this is readily demonstrable by x-ray.

This lesion is difficult to treat by conservative measures; operative intervention is the procedure of choice.

Pathology

1. The medial ligament is ruptured.
2. The inferior tibiofibular ligament is ruptured.
3. The ankle mortise is widened.
4. The talus has shifted laterally.

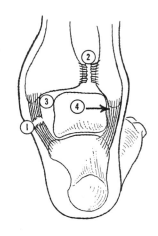

X-Ray Test

First infiltrate the area with 1 per cent procaine.

1. While abduction stress is applied to the heel take anteroposterior views.
2. The foot is fully everted.
3. The talus is tilted in the mortise, and has shifted laterally. There is diastasis of the inferior tibiofibular joint.

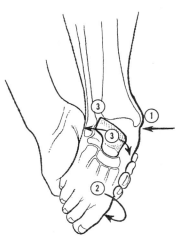

Preoperative X-Ray

1. Tibiofibular diastasis.
2. Lateral displacement of the talus.
3. Lateral displacement of the lateral malleolus.
4. Widening of the interval between the talus and the medial malleolus.

Operative Procedure

1. Make a 3½ inch long incision directly over and parallel to the anterior margin of the distal end of the fibula.
2. Reflect the skin flaps and divide the deep fascia and transverse crural ligament.
3. By subperiosteal dissection expose the anterior and lateral surfaces of the fibula and the lateral surface of the tibia. Visualize the ruptured ligament and diastasis of the joint.

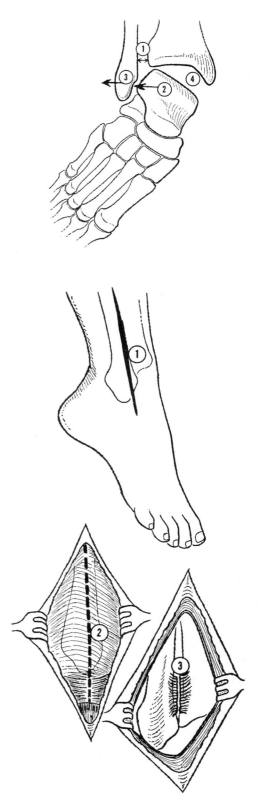

Operative Procedure (Continued)

1. Make firm pressure on the lateral surface of the fibula to reduce the diastasis and hold the fibula snugly against the tibia.

2. Secure the fibula to the tibia with a long screw driven transversely through the fibula to the opposite cortex of the tibia.

Note: The screw should penetrate the cortex enough so that it can be removed from the opposite side if the screw should break.

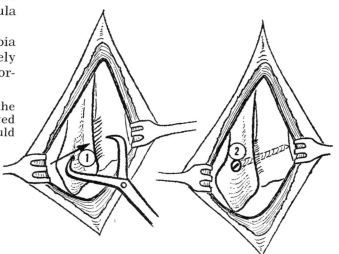

Repair of the Medial Collateral Ligament

1. Make a 4 inch curved incision beginning posterior to the malleolus, extend it distally and anteriorly about 2 cm. distal to the malleolus and end it at the tuberosity of the navicular.

2. Reflect the skin flaps and

3. Visualize the tear in the deltoid ligament.

After washing away blood clots and other tissue debris,

4. Approximate the edges of the tear with interrupted sutures.

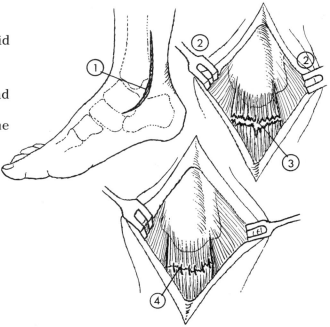

Postoperative X-Ray

1. The fibula fits snugly against the tibia.

2. The talus is in its normal position (the lateral displacement is corrected).

3. The interval between the medial malleolus and the fibula is of normal width.

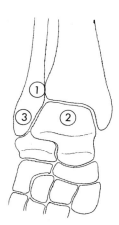

Immobilization

1. Apply a short leg, unpadded plaster cast.

2. The toes are free.

3. The foot is at a right angle to the leg.

4. Mold the plaster well around the malleoli.

5. The foot is in a neutral position as to inversion and eversion.

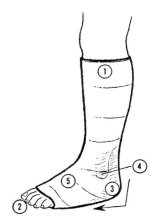

Management

Immediately institute active flexion and extension exercises for the toes.

Apply a new plaster cast every two to three weeks.

After eight weeks apply a walking cast and permit weight bearing.

Remove the last plaster cast ten weeks after the operation.

This lesion must be protected in plaster for a long time (ten weeks) in order to prevent redisplacement of the talus and widening of the ankle mortise.

Remove the screw after 10 to 12 weeks. (The screw should be removed because it may break as a result of normal motion in the distal tibiofibular ligament.)

COMPLETE RUPTURE OF THE MEDIAL COLLATERAL LIGAMENT ALONE

As an isolated lesion this is rare but does occur. It usually occurs in combination with a rupture of the distal tibiofibular ligament or a fracture of the external malleolus.

Pathology

1. The medial collateral ligament is ruptured (an isolated lesion).
2. All other ligaments are intact.

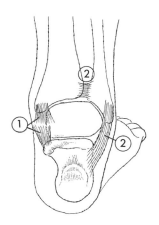

Management

The treatment of this lesion should be surgical repair; the technique and postoperative management are the same as when the lesion occurs together with a rupture of the distal tibiofibular ligament (see page 1567).

TEAR OF THE DISTAL TIBIOFIBULAR LIGAMENT

REMARKS

This lesion rarely occurs as an isolated lesion; however, it may be produced by extreme dorsiflexion of the ankle.

The wide anterior portion of the body of the talus forces the fibula away from the tibia, especially when an external rotation force is acting.

The clinical findings are mild. There is no abnormal lateral motion and no pain when the lateral ligaments are stressed.

Motion is not painful.

There is some pain on extreme dorsiflexion of the foot.

Pressure in the interval between the tibia and fibula, anteriorly and posteriorly, causes pain.

X-ray examinations are negative.

Management

1. Apply an adhesive dressing to prevent dorsiflexion.

2. Elevate the heel on the shoe of the affected side to prevent dorsiflexion movements.

Maintain the strapping for four to six weeks.

Note: Old untreated cases will show calcification of the ligament.

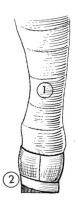

FRACTURES OF THE MALLEOLI

In discussing the inversion and eversion mechanisms responsible for injuries to the ligaments it became clear that fractures and fracture-dislocations of the ankle joint and of the malleoli and injuries to the ligaments are inseparable since they are caused by the same mechanisms. Whether the ligaments or the bones are implicated depends on the age of the patient, the strength of the ligaments and bones and the degree of violence.

Young people are more likely to sustain purely ligamentous injuries while the elderly are more apt to sustain fractures.

In evaluation of any fracture of the malleoli it is essential to analyze the mechanism producing the lesion and to determine whether or not ligaments have been ruptured.

The ankle is a weight-bearing joint. Whenever its component parts have been violated it is most important that the normal anatomy be restored, or marked dysfunction will ensue.

The ankle joint will not tolerate any incongruity of its articular surfaces or disalignment of its mortise.

The mortise must be restored to normalcy and must be stable; fractured malleoli must be returned to their anatomic position without the slightest incongruity of the articular surface. Anything short of these goals will invariably result in dysfunction.

What has been recorded for purely ligamentous injuries also holds true for ligamentous injuries associated with malleolar fractures.

The diagnosis of the character of the injury must be made early; the best treatment for complete rupture of ligaments is immediate surgical repair.

Fracture of the Lateral Malleolus (without and with Lateral Displacement)

REMARKS

The lateral malleolus is most commonly fractured by an eversion mechanism; if the force is not too great, little or no displacement occurs and the medial collateral ligament is not ruptured.

If the lateral malleolus is displaced significantly the medial collateral ligament is always ruptured or the medial malleolus is avulsed.

With this mechanism the fracture is more or less spiral in nature and starts at the level of the tibiofibular joint.

The lateral malleolus may also be fractured by an inversion mechanism; here, instead of the lateral ligament rupturing, the lateral malleolus is avulsed; the medial malleolus may or may not be fractured.

FRACTURE OF THE LATERAL MALLEOLUS WITHOUT LATERAL DISPLACEMENT

Pathology

A. 1. Oblique or spiral fracture of the lateral malleolus at the line of the tibiofibular joint.
  2. The lesion is produced by an eversion force.
  3. All ligaments are intact.
B. 1. Avulsion of the lateral malleolus (transverse fracture).
  2. Lesion is produced by an inversion force.
  3. All ligaments are intact.

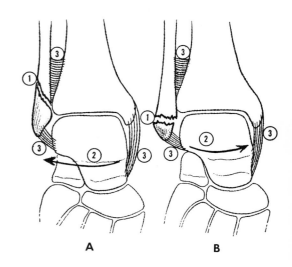

A   B

X-Ray

A. 1. Spiral fracture of the lateral malleolus (displacement is insignificant).
　 2. The talus has not shifted.
　 3. The tibiofibular joint is not widened.
B. 1. Avulsion of the lateral malleolus (transverse fracture).
　 2. No shift of the talus.
　 3. No tibiofibular diastasis.

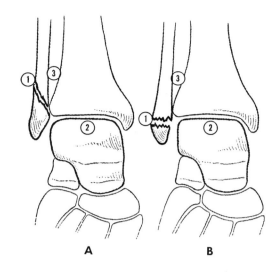

A　　　　**B**

Management

1. Apply a below-the-knee, well-fitting, nonpadded plaster walking cast.
2. The toes are free.
3. The foot is at a right angle to the leg.
4. The foot is in a neutral position.

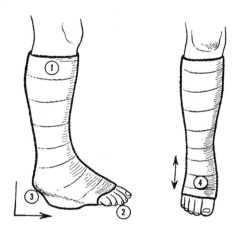

Permit weight bearing at once.
Remove the plaster cast after four to six weeks.
Institute active exercises to restore ankle and foot movements.

FRACTURE OF THE LATERAL MALLEOLUS WITH LATERAL DISPLACEMENT

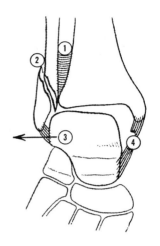

Pathology

1. The tibiofibular ligament is intact.
2. Spiral fracture of the lateral malleolus.
3. The talus shifts laterally.
4. The medial ligament is ruptured.

Prereduction X-Ray

1. Spiral fracture of the lateral malleolus.
2. Widening of the interval between the medial malleolus and the talus.
3. Lateral shift of the talus.

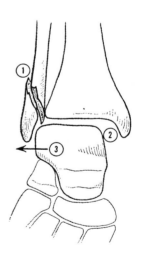

SURGICAL TREATMENT

This is the treatment of choice.

Reduction and Fixation of the Fracture of the Lateral Malleolus

1. Make a vertical incision beginning just distal to the top of the lateral malleolus and extending directly upward on the center of the bone.
2. Divide the deep fascia and retract its margins with the skin flaps.
3. Divide the periosteum longitudinally, and by subperiosteal dissection expose the fibula and the fracture site.

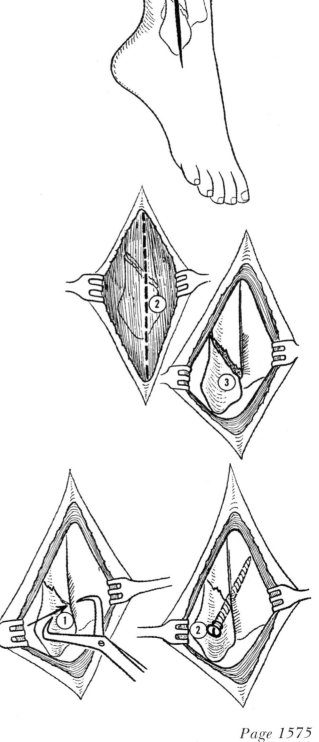

1. Push the lateral malleolus snugly against the tibia.
2. Secure the lateral malleolus in position with a long screw driven obliquely upward from its lateral surface and across both cortices of the tibia.

Page 1575

Repair of the Medial Collateral Ligament

1. Make a 4 inch curved incision beginning posterior to the malleolus, extend it distally and anteriorly about 2 cm. distal to the tip of the malleolus and terminate it on the tuberosity of the navicular.

2. Reflect the skin flaps and

3. Visualize the tear in the deltoid.

After washing out blood clots and other tissue debris,

4. Approximate the edges of the tear in the deltoid ligament.

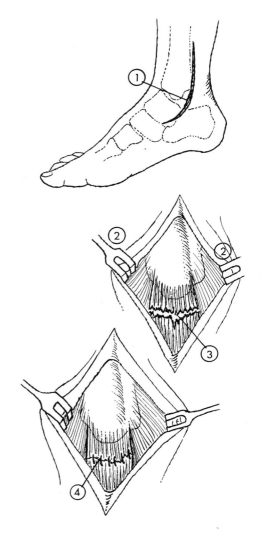

Postreduction X-Ray

1. The anatomic position of the lateral malleolus is restored.

2. A transfixion screw traverses the fracture line and both cortices of the tibia.

3. The talus is in its normal position in the mortise.

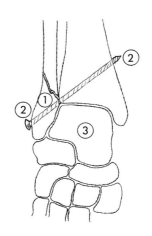

Immobilization

1. Apply a short leg, unpadded plaster cast.
2. The toes are free.
3. The foot is at a right angle to the leg.
4. Mold the plaster well around the malleoli.
5. The foot is in a neutral position as to inversion and eversion.

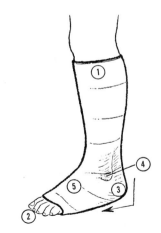

Postreduction Management

Institute immediately active flexion and extension exercises for the toes.

Apply a new plaster cast every two or three weeks.

After eight weeks apply a walking cast and permit weight bearing.

Remove the last plaster cast ten weeks after the operation.

This lesion must be protected in plaster for a long time (ten weeks) in order to prevent redisplacement of the talus and widening of the ankle mortise.

Remove the screw after 10 to 12 weeks.

CONSERVATIVE MANAGEMENT

REMARKS

This should not be the primary choice of treatment. It should be employed only if there are definite contraindications precluding surgical treatment.

Manipulative Reduction (Under General Anesthesia)

1. The limb hangs over the end of the table.
2. Place one hand over the medial aspect of the leg and
3. The other over the lateral aspect of the foot and the lateral malleolus.
4. Push the foot strongly inward.

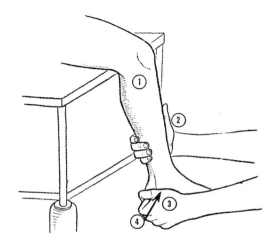

Manipulative Reduction (Under General Anesthesia) (Continued)

1. While the foot rests on the surgeon's knee,
2. Apply an unpadded below-the-knee plaster cast..

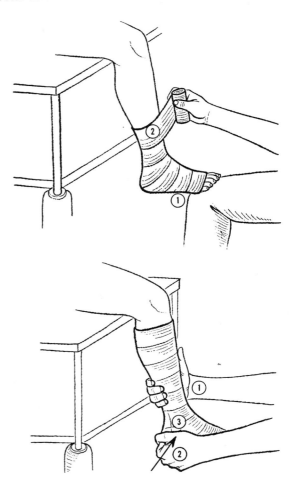

1. While the plaster is setting, steady the limb with one hand on the medial aspect of the leg.
2. The other hand makes steady strong pressure inward over the lateral malleolus and foot.
3. Mold the plaster well over and around the malleoli.

Note: Maintain inward pressure until the plaster has set.

Postreduction X-Ray

1. The talus occupies its normal position in the mortise.
2. The lateral displacement of the lateral malleolus is corrected.

Note: If the reduction is not satisfactory another attempt should be made.

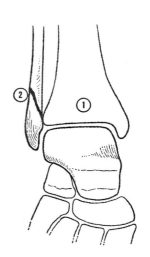

Postreduction Management

Reapply the cast every two or three weeks.

After four weeks apply a plaster walking cast and permit weight bearing.

Remove the last cast eight weeks after reduction of the fracture.

Now institute active exercises and physical therapy to restore ankle and foot movements.

Fracture of the Medial Malleolus

REMARKS

Fracture of the medial malleolus may be produced by an inversion or an eversion mechanism. If caused by an inversion mechanism the lateral collateral ligament must be ruptured. If caused by an eversion mechanism there is either an associated fracture of the lateral malleolus at the level of the ankle joint or a dissolution of the distal tibiofibular ligament. In the latter instance, if the force continues, the fibula is driven far from the tibia and sustains a fracture above the joint line, usually in its lower third.

The amount of displacement varies from no displacement to marked displacement. In the former instance it may be difficult to assess the true nature of the lesion; the x-rays may fail to indicate the degree of ligamentous injury.

In inversion injuries the medial malleolus is avulsed from the tibia and a periosteal flap may drop between the fractured surfaces, preventing reduction. Always anticipate this complication; this situation demands open reduction.

Only rarely does a fracture of the medial malleolus occur as an isolated lesion, but it may happen.

ISOLATED FRACTURE OF THE MEDIAL MALLEOLUS

REMARKS

This lesion can be treated by conservative methods, but if total anatomic reduction is not achieved open operation is indicated.

Always suspect a ligamentous injury and take stress x-rays to determine its presence or absence.

Pathology

A. 1. Transverse fracture of the medial malleolus.
2. The ligaments are intact.
3. The lesion is produced by an eversion stress.
B. 1. Oblique fracture of the medial malleolus.
2. The ligaments are intact.
3. The lesion is produced by an inversion stress.
4. The malleolus is displaced slightly upward and outward.

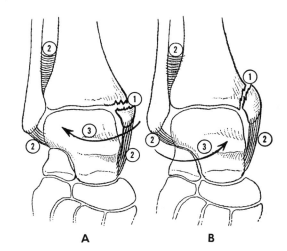

A   **B**

Appearance on X-Ray

1. Transverse fracture of the medial malleolus.
2. Oblique fracture of the medial malleolus.
3. The talus is in its normal position.
4. There is wide separation of malleolar fragments.

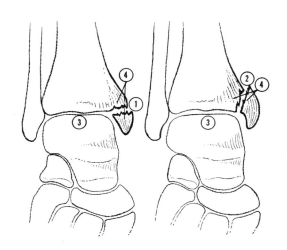

Manipulative Reduction

1. The limb hangs over the end of the table.

2. With both thumbs the surgeon manipulates the fragments into normal position.

3. Then with the heels of the hands he compresses firmly both malleoli.

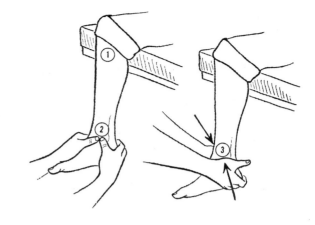

While the foot rests on the surgeon's knee:

1. Apply an unpadded plaster cast.

2. The foot is at a right angle to the leg.

3. The foot is in a neutral position as to inversion and eversion.

4. While the plaster is setting make firm pressure over the medial malleolus, pushing it inward.

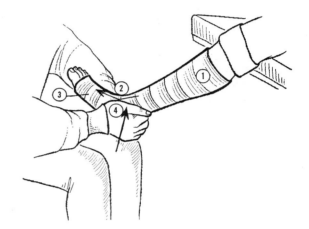

Postreduction X-Ray

1. The malleolus is restored to its normal position.

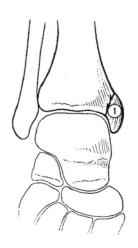

Immobilization

1. A plaster cast extends from below the knee to behind the metatarsal heads.
2. The foot is at a right angle to the leg.
3. The foot is in a neutral position.
4. Heel for walking.

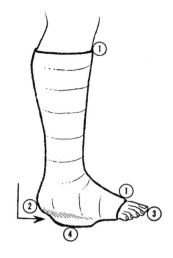

Management

Allow weight bearing.
Insist on active exercises for the toes.
Remove the cast at the end of six weeks.
Institute active exercises to restore ankle and foot movements.

ALTERNATE METHOD

REMARKS

Failure to restore the malleolar fragment to its anatomic position justifies surgical intervention.

In some instances a periosteal flap lying between the fragments precludes manipulative reduction; it must be removed under direct vision.

Always check for evidence of injury to the tibiofibular ligament; if there is a diastasis of the tibiofibular joint fix it with a transfixion screw.

Preoperative X-Ray

1. Wide separation of malleolar fragments (manipulative measures failed in this case).

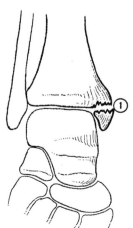

Operative Reduction

In general this method must be resorted to for most displaced fractures.

1. Make a 3 inch incision beginning 1 inch distal to the tip of the malleolus; the incision extends directly upward over the center of the bone.

2. Reflect the skin flaps and divide the deep fascia.

3. Visualize the fracture site and the displaced malleolar fragment.

4. Remove the periosteal flap interposed between the fractured surfaces.

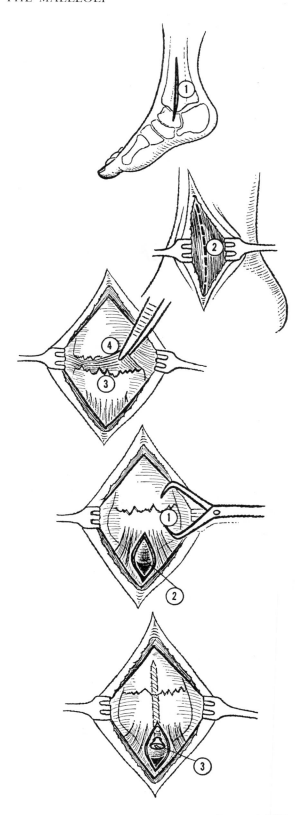

After cleaning out the fracture site with a fine curette:

1. Grasp the malleolar fragment with a towel clip and secure it in its anatomic position.

2. Make a small longitudinal incision through the fibers of the deltoid ligament to expose the tip of the malleolus.

3. Drive a long screw obliquely through the malleolar fragment and the lower end of the tibia.

Postoperative X-Ray

1. The malleolar fragment is in perfect anatomic position.
2. There is a transfixion screw across the fracture in the medial malleolus.

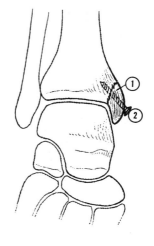

Immobilization

1. Apply a short leg unpadded cast.
2. The toes are free.
3. The foot is at a right angle to the leg.
4. Mold the plaster well around the malleolus.
5. The foot is in a neutral position as to inversion and eversion.

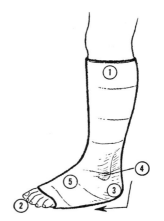

Postoperative Management

Apply a new cast every two or three weeks.

After the fourth week permit weight bearing on a plaster walking cast.

Remove the last plaster cast eight weeks after the operation.

Throughout this period insist on active flexion and extension exercises of the toes.

FRACTURE OF THE MEDIAL MALLEOLUS WITH RUPTURE OF THE LATERAL LIGAMENT

REMARKS

This is an inversion injury.

This lesion, preferably, should be treated surgically; the lateral ligament should be repaired and the medial malleolus fixed by a screw. However, it can also be treated conservatively; but in so doing one must realize that the lateral ligament may heal with considerable elongation, which will cause recurrent subluxations of the ankle.

Pathology

1. Oblique fracture of the medial malleolus.
2. The lesion is produced by an inversion force.
3. The lateral ligament is torn completely.

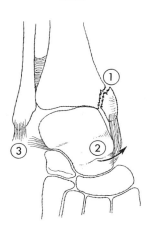

Appearance on X-Ray

1. Oblique fracture of the medial malleolus.
2. The talus is tilted and displaced.
3. Widening of the lateral side of the joint space.

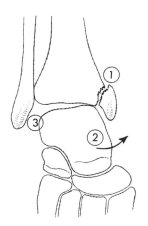

Conservative Management

The reduction and immobilization is the same as that described for isolated fractures of the medial malleolus (see page 1580).

Operative Management

1. The medial malleolus is fixed with a screw. (For technique see page 1582.)

2. The lateral ligament is repaired. (For technique see page 1561.)

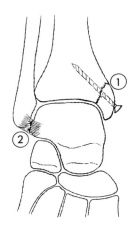

FRACTURE OF THE MEDIAL MALLEOLUS WITH RUPTURE OF THE DISTAL TIBIOFIBULAR LIGAMENT

REMARKS

This is an eversion injury.

The resulting diastasis of the tibiofibular joint must be closed.

There may or may not be a fracture of the fibula above the level of the tibiofibular joint.

These lesions must be treated surgically.

In a variation of this lesion a rupture of the medial collateral ligament combines with a fracture of the fibular shaft.

Pathology

1. Transverse fracture of the medial malleolus.
2. Rupture of the tibiofibular ligament.
3. Lateral displacement of the talus.
4. Separation of the mortise.

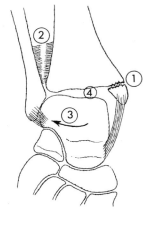

or

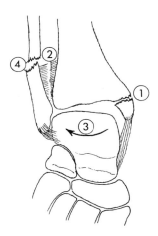

1. Transverse fracture of the medial malleolus.
2. Rupture of the tibiofibular ligament.
3. Lateral displacement of the talus.
4. Fracture of the shaft of the fibula.

or

1. The medial ligament is ruptured.
2. The tibiofibular ligament is ruptured.
3. The talus is tilted and displaced laterally.
4. Fracture of the shaft of the fibula above the tibiofibular joint.

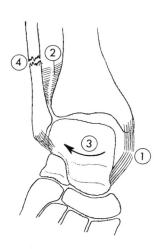

Appearance on X-Ray (First Example)

1. Transverse fracture of the medial malleolus.
2. Lateral displacement and tilting of the talus.
3. Widening of the ankle mortise.
4. Widening of the tibiofibular joint.

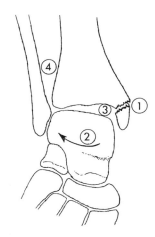

Appearance on X-Ray (Second Example)

1. Transverse fracture of the medial malleolus.
2. Lateral displacement and tilting of the talus.
3. Widening of the mortise.
4. Fracture of the shaft of the fibula.

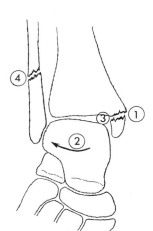

When the Medial Ligament is Ruptured

1. Widening of the interval between the talus and medial malleolus.
2. Lateral displacement of the talus.
3. Diastasis of the tibiofibular joint.
4. Fracture of the shaft of the fibula.

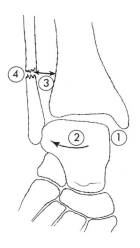

Operative Reduction and Internal Fixation

1. Make a 3½ inch long incision directly over and parallel to the anterior margin of the distal end of the fibula.

2. Reflect the skin flaps and divide the deep fascia and transverse crural ligament.

3. By subperiosteal dissection expose the anterior and lateral surfaces of the fibula and the lateral surface of the tibia. Visualize the ruptured ligament and diastasis of the joint.

1. Make firm pressure on the lateral surface of the fibula to reduce the diastasis and hold the fibula snugly against the tibia.

2. Secure the fibula to the tibia with a long screw driven transversely through the fibula to the opposite cortex of the tibia.

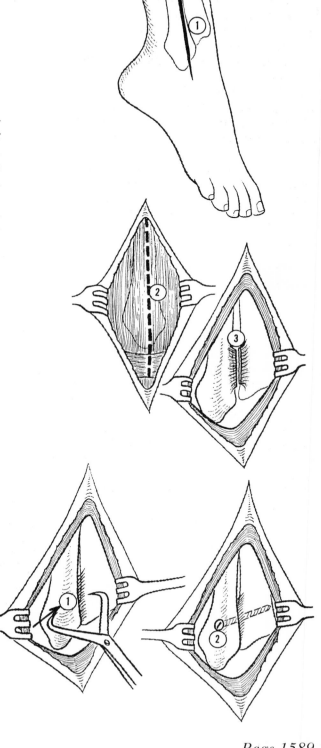

Operative Reduction and
Internal Fixation (Continued)

1. Make a 3 inch incision beginning 1 inch distal to the tip of the malleolus and extending directly upward over the center of the bone.

2. Reflect the skin flaps and divide the deep fascia.

3. Visualize the fracture site and the displaced malleolar fragment.

4. Remove the periosteal flap interposed between the fractured surfaces.

Note: If only rupture of the ligament without a fracture of the malleolus is found, repair the ligament by approximating the edges of the ligament with interrupted sutures.

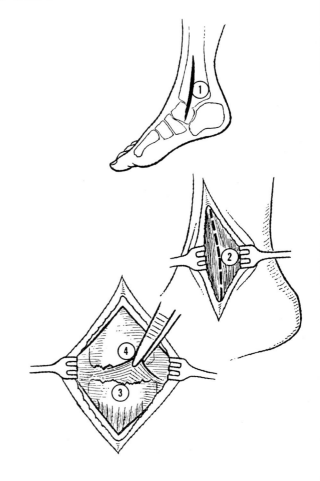

After cleaning out the fracture site with a fine curette,

1. Grasp the malleolar fragment with a towel clip and secure it in its anatomic position.

2. Make a small longitudinal incision through the fibers of the deltoid ligament to expose the tip of the malleolus.

3. Drive a long screw obliquely through the malleolar fragment and the lower end of the tibia.

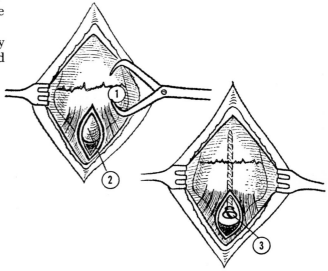

Postreduction X-Ray

(When the medial ligament is ruptured.)

1. A screw driven transversely across the fibula and the tibia has reduced the diastasis.

2. The talus sits squarely in the ankle mortise.

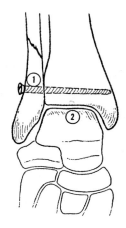

Postreduction X-Ray

(When the tibiofibular ligament ruptures, the fibula is intact and the medial malleolus is avulsed.)

1. The fibula is secured to the tibia with a screw driven transversely.

2. The medial malleolus is anchored with a screw driven obliquely.

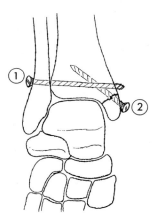

Postreduction X-Ray

(When the medial malleolus is avulsed and the shaft of the fibula is fractured.)

1. The fibula is secured to the tibia with a screw driven transversely.

2. The medial malleolus is fixed to the tibia with a screw driven obliquely.

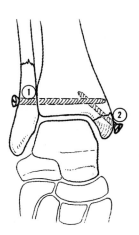

Immobilization

1. Apply a short leg, unpadded plaster cast.

2. The toes are free.

3. The foot is at a right angle to the leg.

4. Mold the plaster well around the malleoli.

5. The foot is in a neutral position as to inversion and eversion.

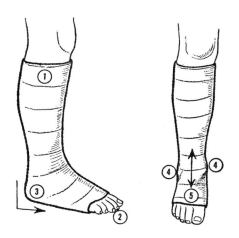

Postreduction Management

Institute immediately active flexion and extension exercises for the toes.

Apply a new plaster cast every two or three weeks.

After eight weeks apply a walking cast and permit weight bearing.

Remove the last plaster cast ten weeks after the operation.

These lesions must be protected in plaster for a long time (ten weeks) in order to prevent redisplacement of the talus and widening of the ankle mortise.

Remove the screw across the tibiofibular joint after 10 to 12 weeks.

Bimalleolar Fractures

REMARKS

These lesions may be produced by either an inversion or eversion mechanism.

The treatment of choice is internal fixation of both malleoli; the exception to this is when the lateral malleolus can be anatomically reduced and remains stable after internal fixation of the medial malleolus.

FRACTURES OF BOTH MALLEOLI WITH LATERAL DISPLACEMENT OF THE TALUS

REMARKS

This lesion is produced by an eversion mechanism.

The medial ligament remains intact but the medial malleolus is avulsed.

The talus is displaced laterally.

There is an oblique fracture of the lateral malleolus at the level of the tibiofibular joint.

Pathology

1. Spiral or oblique fracture of the lateral malleolus.

2. The inferior tibiofibular ligament is intact.

3. Avulsion of the medial malleolus.

4. The collateral ligaments are intact.

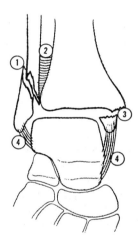

Prereduction X-Ray

1. Spiral fracture of the lateral malleolus.

2. Avulsion of the medial malleolus.

3. Lateral displacement of the talus.

4. Widening of the ankle mortise.

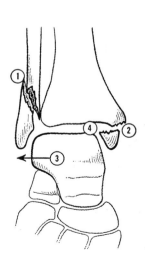

Page 1593

FRACTURE OF BOTH MALLEOLI WITH MEDIAL DISPLACEMENT OF THE TALUS

REMARKS

This lesion is produced by an inversion mechanism.

The talus is displaced medially.

The ligaments are intact; there is a shearing fracture of the medial malleolus and an avulsion of the lateral malleolus.

In some instances the articular surface of the tibia may be crushed; in children the medial portion of the epiphyseal plate may be injured. The prognosis in these lesions must be guarded: if the articular surface of the tibia is crushed osteoarthritis may ensue; in children premature arrest of growth on the medial side will produce an angular deformity of the ankle.

Pathology

1. The talus is displaced medially.
2. There is an oblique fracture of the medial malleolus.
3. The lateral malleolus is avulsed.
4. The ligaments are intact.
5. The lesion is produced by an adduction stress.

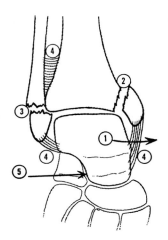

Prereduction X-Ray (First Example)

1. The talus is tilted and displaced medially.
2. There is a shearing fracture of the medial malleolus.
3. The lateral malleolus is avulsed.

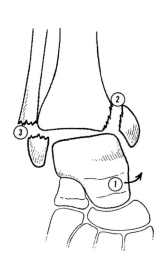

Prereduction X-Ray (Second Example)

This type of lesion carries a poor prognosis.

1. The talus is tilted and displaced medially.

2. There is a crushing of the medial side of the articular surface of the tibia.

3. A large medial malleolar fragment is sheared off the tibia.

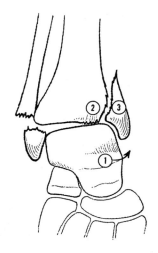

Prereduction X-Ray (Third Example)

This lesion may cause premature arrest of growth on the medial side of the tibial epiphysis.

1. The talus is displaced medially.

2. The medial side of the epiphyseal plate is crushed.

3. The lateral malleolus is avulsed.

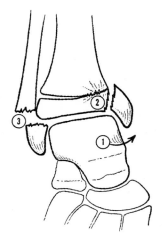

Operative Reduction

1. Make a 3 inch incision beginning 1 inch distal to the tip of the medial malleolus and extending directly upward over the center of the bone.

2. Reflect the skin flaps and divide the deep fascia.

3. Visualize the fracture site and the displaced malleolar fragment.

4. Remove the periosteal flap interposed between the fractured surfaces.

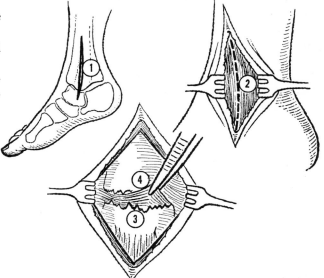

After cleaning out the fracture site with a fine curette:

1. Grasp the malleolar fragment with a towel clip and secure it in its normal anatomic position.

2. Make a small longitudinal incision through the fibers of the deltoid ligament to expose the tip of the malleolus.

3. Drive a long screw obliquely through the malleolar fragment and the lower end of the tibia.

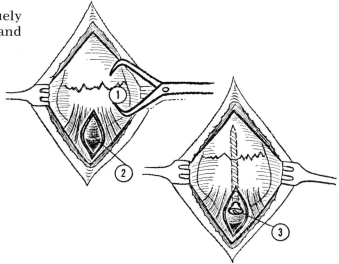

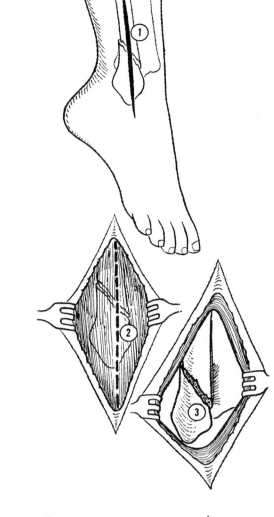

Operative Reduction *(Continued)*

1. Make a vertical incision beginning just distal to the top of the lateral malleolus and extending directly upward on the center of the bone.

2. Divide the deep fascia and retract its margins with the skin flaps.

3. Divide the periosteum longitudinally, and by subperiosteal dissection expose the fibula and the fracture site.

1. Push the lateral malleolus snugly against the tibia.

2. Secure the lateral malleolus in position with a long screw driven obliquely upward from its lateral surface and across both cortices of the tibia.

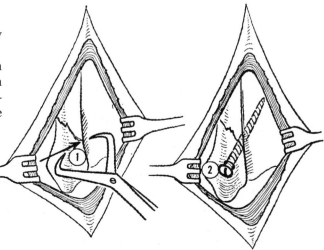

Postreduction X-Ray

1. The medial malleolus is in its normal position and transfixed with a screw.

2. The lateral malleolus is in its normal anatomic position and secured to the tibia with a screw.

3. The talus occupies its normal position in the ankle mortise.

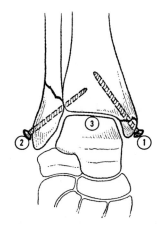

Immobilization

1. Apply a short leg, unpadded plaster cast.

2. The toes are free.

3. The foot is at a right angle to the leg.

4. Mold the plaster well around the malleoli.

5. The foot is in a neutral position as to inversion and eversion.

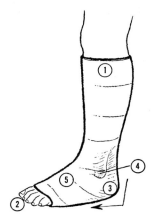

Postreduction Management

Immediately institute active flexion and extension exercises for the toes.

Apply a new plaster cast every two or three weeks.

After eight weeks apply a walking cast and permit weight bearing.

Remove the last plaster cast ten weeks after the operation.

This lesion must be protected in plaster for a long time (ten weeks) in order to prevent redisplacement of the talus and widening of the ankle mortise.

Remove the screw after 10 to 12 weeks.

POSTERIOR DISLOCATION OF THE FOOT WITH POSTERIOR MARGINAL FRACTURE OF THE TIBIA

REMARKS

This lesion may be associated with an eversion injury or an inversion injury; always check these injuries for this complication.

The posterior margin of the tibia is sheared off as the momentum of the body forces the tibia forward on the foot.

In some instances the dislocation is spontaneously reduced; in others it is only partially reduced.

Accurate replacement of the talus in relation to the articular surface of the tibia is mandatory in order to obtain normal movements of the ankle.

As a rule the posterior fragment is displaced upward.

Small fragments, even if not accurately reduced, are of no significance.

Large fragments must be reduced perfectly; surgical intervention is required to achieve this reduction.

These are serious injuries and should be treated surgically.

Pathology (When Caused by an Eversion Stress plus Forward Displacement of the Tibia on the Talus)

1. Lateral displacement of the talus.
2. Avulsion of the medial malleolus.
3. Diastasis of the tibiofibular joint.
4. Fracture of the shaft of the fibula.
5. Posterior dislocation of the talus.
6. Posterior marginal fracture of the tibia.

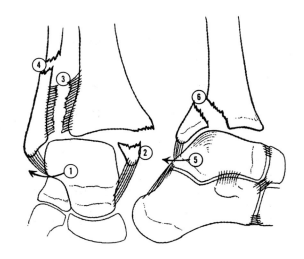

Pathology (When the External Rotational Stress is Dominant)

1. Avulsion of the medial malleolus.
2. Spiral fracture of the lateral malleolus.
3. Intact tibiofibular joint.
4. Posterior dislocation of the talus.
5. Posterior marginal fracture of the tibia.

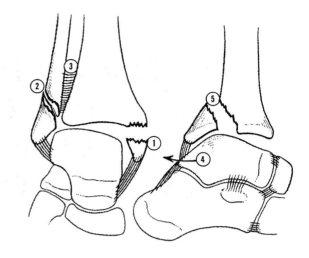

Prereduction X-Ray (External Rotation Stress is Dominant)

1. Spiral fracture of the lateral malleolus.
2. Avulsion of the medial malleolus.
3. The talus is tilted and displaced laterally.
4. Posterior marginal fracture of the tibia.
5. Posterior displacement of the talus.
6. Articular surfaces of the talus and the tibia are not congruous.

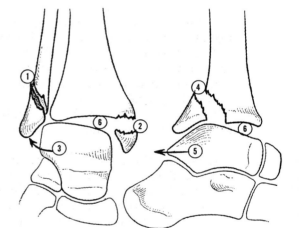

Prereduction X-Ray (Eversion Stress is Dominant)

1. Avulsion of the medial malleolus.
2. Fracture of the shaft of the fibula.
3. Lateral displacement of the talus.
4. Diastasis of the tibiofibular joint.
5. Posterior marginal fracture of the tibia.
6. Incongruous articular surfaces of the tibia and the talus.

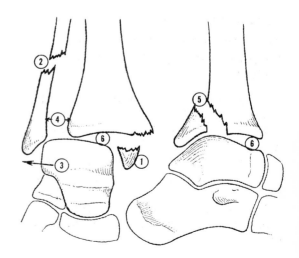

Prereduction X-Ray (Caused by an Inversion Mechanism)

1. Avulsion of the lateral malleolus.
2. Shearing of the medial malleolus.
3. The talus is displaced medially.
4. Posterior marginal fracture of the tibia.
5. Posterior displacement of the talus.

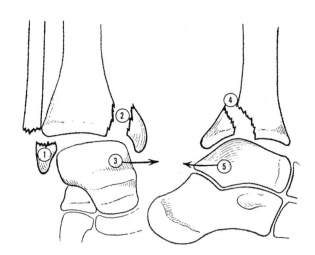

Operative Reduction

The technique to fix internally the medial and lateral malleoli is described on pages 1574 and 1582.

OPERATIVE REDUCTION OF THE POSTERIOR MARGINAL FRAGMENT

REMARKS

Posterior fragments comprising one-third or less of the articular surface of the tibia can, as a rule, be replaced by closed methods; if not accurately reduced the residual displacement is of no significance.

Posterior fragments comprising more than one-third of the articular surface must be accurately reduced in order to prevent posterior displacement of the talus; reduction by open operation is the procedure of choice.

Prereduction X-Ray

1. The posterior fragment comprises more than one-third of the articular surface.
2. The fragment is displaced upward.
3. The talus is displaced backward.

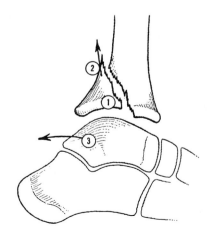

Page 1601

Operative Procedure

The patient lies in a prone position. Place a sandbag under the foot.

1. Make a 3½ inch incision just lateral to the Achilles tendon; begin the incision at the level of the lateral malleolus.

2. Divide the fascia and retract it with skin flaps, exposing the peroneal tendons and the flexor hallucis longus muscle.

3. Divide longitudinally the fascia covering the flexor hallucis longus muscle.

4. Make a longitudinal incision through the lateral fibers of the flexor hallucis longus and the periosteum of the tibia.

5. By subperiosteal dissection expose the distal end of the tibia and the fracture site.

6. Retract the tendon of the flexor hallucis longus and the Achilles tendon medially.

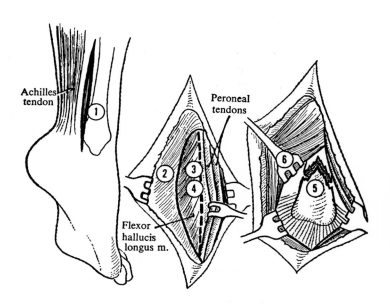

Operative Procedure (Continued)

1. Reduce the posterior dislocation of the talus by forward traction on the foot.

2. Grasp the posterior marginal fragment with a towel clip and pull it into its normal position.

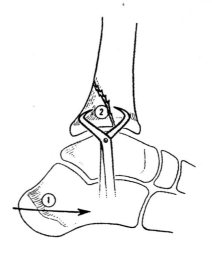

1. Hold the fragment in position with a pressure bar.

2. Drive a screw through the fragment and the shaft of the tibia.

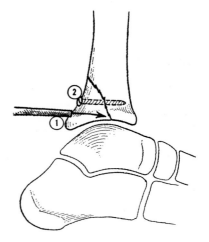

Postreduction X-Ray

LATERAL VIEW

1. The posterior fragment is restored to its anatomic position.

2. The talus fits accurately under the tibia.

3. The articular surfaces of the talus and the tibia are congruous.

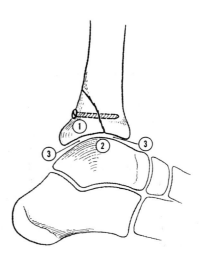

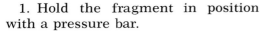

Postreduction X-Ray *(Continued)*

ANTEROPOSTERIOR VIEW

1. The medial malleolus is reduced and fixed by a screw.
2. The lateral malleolus and the tibiofibular joint are transfixed by a screw.
3. The tibiofibular joint is closed.

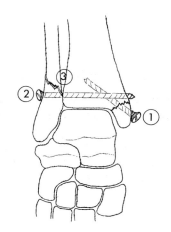

Immobilization

1. Apply a short leg, unpadded plaster cast.
2. The toes are free.
3. The foot is at a right angle to the leg.
4. Mold the plaster well around the malleoli.
5. The foot is in a neutral position as to inversion and eversion.

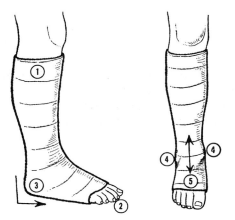

Postoperative Management

Immediately institute active flexion and extension exercises for the toes.

Apply a new plaster cast every two to three weeks.

After eight weeks apply a walking cast and permit weight bearing.

Remove the last plaster cast ten weeks after the operation.

These lesions must be protected in plaster for a long time (ten weeks) in order to prevent redisplacement of the talus and widening of the ankle mortise.

Remove the screw transfixing the tibiofibular joint after 10 to 12 weeks.

Page 1604

VERTICAL COMPRESSION FRACTURES OF THE DISTAL END OF THE TIBIA

REMARKS

These lesions are usually the result of a fall from a height.

Fractures of the calcaneus and the spine are frequent concomitant injuries; always check for these complications.

In general two types of injuries are encountered:
1. Fracture of the anterior margin of the tibia with forward displacement of the foot.
2. Severe comminution of the whole inferior articular surface of the tibia.

The prognosis in the first type is good with correct treatment; in the second type the prognosis is poor regardless of the method of management.

Fracture of the Anterior Surface of the Tibia with Forward Displacement of the Talus

REMARKS

Manipulative methods occasionally effect a reduction; however, in most instances open reduction and internal fixation is necessary.

Accurate replacement of the talus in relation to the articular surface of the tibia is mandatory.

Anything short of a perfect reduction will produce a weak ankle and later osteoarthritis.

These injuries may be complicated by fractures of one or both malleoli.

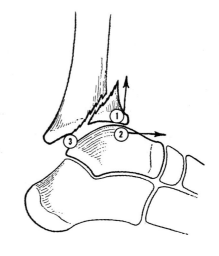

Prereduction X-Ray

1. The anterior marginal fragment is displaced upward.

2. The talus is displaced forward.

3. The articular surfaces of the talus and the tibia are not congruous.

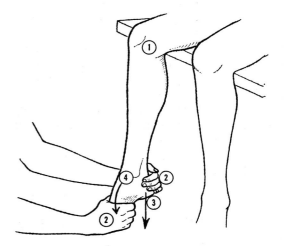

Manipulative Reduction

1. The patient's leg hangs over the edge of the table.

2. The operator grasps the forefoot with one hand and the heel with the other.

3. Make strong traction downward and at the same time,

4. Forcibly plantar flex the foot.

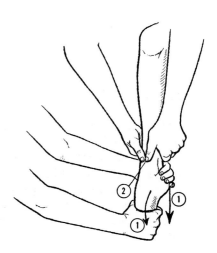

1. While the operator maintains downward traction and plantar flexion of the foot,

2. An assistant makes direct pressure on the fragment with both thumbs molding the fragment into place.

Manipulative Reduction
(Continued)

1. While the position of plantar flexion is maintained,

2. Apply an unpadded below-the-knee plaster cast.

3. Mold the plaster well over the front of the ankle and around both malleoli.

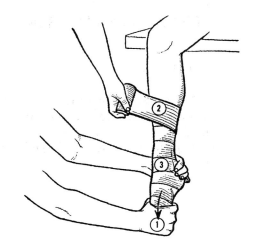

Postreduction X-Ray

1. The anterior marginal fragment is restored to its anatomic position.

2. The articular surfaces of the talus and the tibia are congruous.

3. The forward displacement of the talus is corrected.

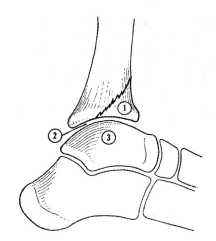

Postreduction Management

Take check x-rays immediately after the application of the plaster cast.

After three weeks apply a new cast and reduce the amount of plantar flexion.

Six weeks after the reduction remove the second cast and bring the foot to a right angle with the leg.

Permit weight bearing in plaster at the end of 10 weeks.

Remove the last cast at the end of 12 weeks.

Now institute active exercises and physical therapy to restore normal movements of the ankle and tarsal joints.

ALTERNATE METHOD (OPERATIVE REDUCTION)

REMARKS

Operative intervention is justified when accurate replacement of the anterior marginal fragment cannot be achieved or when redisplacement occurs in plaster.

In practice most of these lesions require open reduction and internal fixation.

Prereduction X-Ray

(This fracture could not be accurately reduced by manipulative methods.)

1. The anterior marginal fragment is displaced upward.

2. The talus is displaced forward.

3. The articular surfaces of the talus and the tibia are not congruous.

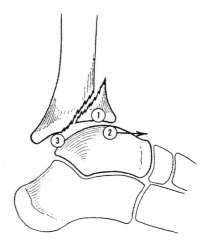

Operative Reduction and Internal Fixation

1. Make a vertical incision on the anterior aspect of the ankle; it begins 3½ inches above and terminates 1 inch below the ankle joint.

2. Divide the deep fascia on the line of the skin incision and develop the interval between the extensor hallucis longus and the extensor digitorum longus tendons.

3. Identify the neurovascular bundle and retract it medially with the extensor hallucis longus.

4. Incise the periosteum and the capsule in the line of the skin incision.

5. Expose the anterior surface of the tibia and the ankle joint by sharp subperiosteal and subcapsular dissection.

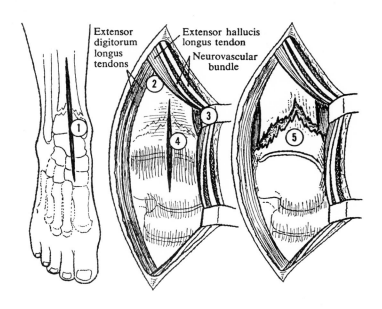

Operative Reduction and
Internal Fixation *(Continued)*

1. Remove all small loose fragments of bone.

2. Reduce the anterior subluxation of the ankle by plantar flexion of the foot.

3. Grasp the fragment with a towel clip and pull it into its anatomic position.

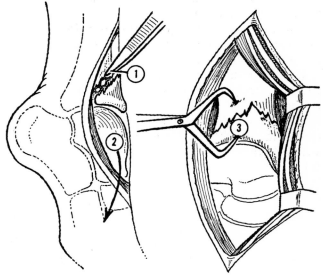

1. Hold the fragment in place with a pressure bar.

2. Drive a screw through the fragment and into the shaft of the tibia.

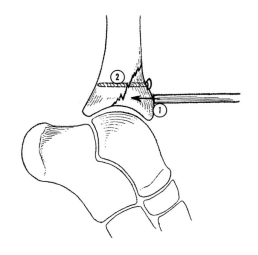

Immobilization

1. Apply a plaster cast from behind the metatarsal heads to below the knee.

2. The foot is in a neutral position of inversion and eversion.

3. The foot is dorsiflexed 90 degrees.

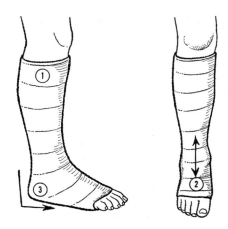

Note: If concomitant malleolar fractures are present, reduce these by manipulative methods previously described.

Check the reduction of the malleolar fractures by x-ray after application of the cast.

If the reduction is unsatisfactory, open reduction and internal fixation is performed as described on pages 1574 and 1582.

Postreduction X-Ray

1. The anterior marginal fragment is restored to its anatomic position and is secured with a screw.

2. The articular surfaces of the talus and the tibia are congruous.

3. The talus fits accurately under the tibia.

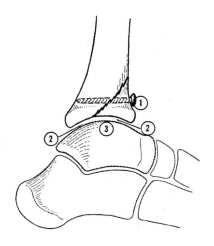

WHEN CONCOMITANT FRACTURES OF THE MALLEOLI ARE PRESENT

These lesions require open reduction and internal fixation (*see pages* 1574 and 1582).

Postreduction X-Ray

1. The medial malleolus is fixed with a screw.

2. The lateral malleolus is fixed with a screw.

3. The anterior marginal fragment is secured with a screw.

4. The articular surfaces of the talus and the tibia are congruous.

Note: Internal fixation of the malleolar fragments is performed if conservative closed methods fail.

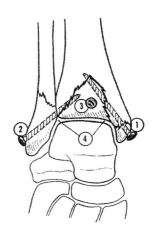

Postoperative Management

Immediately institute active flexion and extension exercises for the toes.

Apply a new plaster cast every two or three weeks.

After eight weeks apply a walking cast and permit weight bearing.

Remove the last plaster cast 10 weeks after the operation.

This lesion must be protected in plaster for a long time (10 weeks) in order to prevent redisplacement of the talus and widening of the ankle mortise.

Remove the screw across the distal tibiofibular joint after 10 weeks.

Severe Comminution of the Inferior Articular Surface of the Tibia (Explosion Fracture)

REMARKS

With severe compression violence the entire lower end of the tibia may be disrupted. A fracture of the fibula also may occur.

The talus is driven into the substance of the lower end of the tibia.

Fracture of one or both of the malleoli may be concomitant lesions.

Restoration of a smooth articular surface is impossible by either closed or open methods.

Fusion of the ankle joint is the procedure of choice.

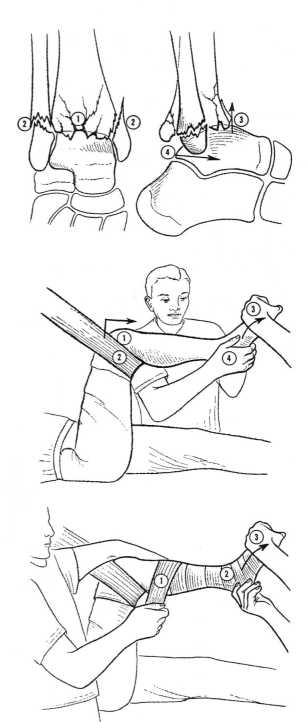

Prereduction X-Ray

1. Severe comminution of the articular surface of the tibia.
2. Fracture of both malleoli.
3. The talus is displaced upward.
4. The talus is displaced forward.

Initial Treatment

Place the patient on a fracture table.

1. The leg is flexed at the knee 90 degrees.
2. Counter traction is made by a strap passing under the lower end of the thigh and suspended from an overhead cross bar.
3. An assistant makes steady traction with the foot slightly plantar flexed.
4. The surgeon molds the fragments into the best possible position.

1. Apply a circular cast from behind the metatarsal heads to just below the knee.
2. The foot is in a neutral position as to inversion and eversion.
3. The foot is slightly plantar flexed.

Arthrodesis of the Ankle Joint

(After a period of four to six weeks sufficient coalescence of the fragment will have occurred and the soft tissues will have recovered sufficiently to permit surgical fusion of the ankle joint with safety.)

1. Make a vertical incision on the anterior aspect of the ankle joint; it begins 4 inches above and terminates 1½ inches below the ankle joint.

2. Divide the deep fascia longitudinally and develop the interval between the extensor hallucis longus and the extensor digitorum longus tendons.

3. Identify the neurovascular bundle and retract it medially with the extensor hallucis longus.

4. Incise the periosteum and capsule.

5. Expose the anterior surface of the tibia and the ankle joint by sharp subperiosteal and subcapsular dissection.

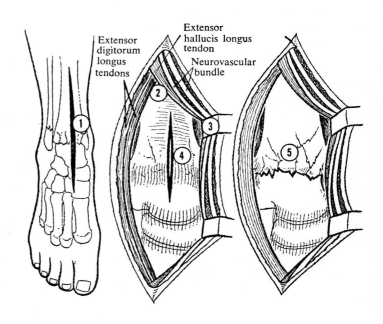

Arthrodesis of the Ankle Joint
(Continued)

1. Plantar flex the foot.

2. With a thin-bladed osteotome and a fine curette remove the cartilage of the articular surface of the tibia and of the superior articular surface of the talus.

3. Remove the cartilage from the articular surfaces of the medial and lateral malleoli and the lateral surfaces of the talus.

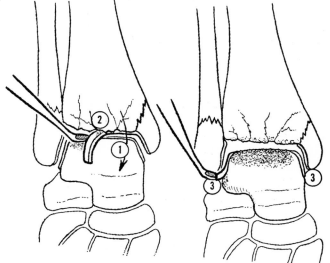

1. Align the talus accurately under the tibia.

2. With a motor saw remove a full thickness of cortical graft 1 inch wide and 3 inches long from the tibia immediately above the joint surface.

3. With a thin-bladed osteotome make a slot of suitable dimensions on the anterior portion of the body and on the superior surface of the neck of the talus.

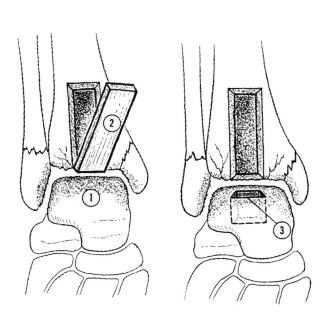

Page 1615

Arthrodesis of the Ankle Joint
(Continued)

1. Slide the tibial graft into the slot in the talus and impact it firmly in position with an impactor.

2. Fill the spaces between the lateral surfaces of the talus and the malleoli and between the talus and the tibia with cancellous bone chips. (Obtain them from the anterior crest of the ilium.)

Note position of foot in relation to the tibia:

In males the position of the foot should be at a right angle to the leg.

In females the position of the foot should be in 95 to 100 degrees plantar flexion.

Note: The compression arthrodesis described on page 1639 is the preferred surgical procedure.

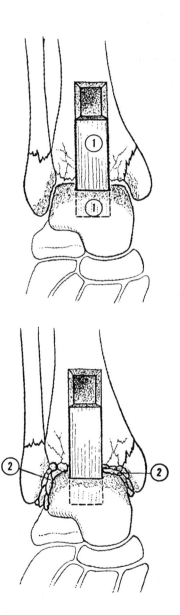

Immobilization

1. Apply a circular cast from behind the metatarsal heads to the midthigh.

2. The knee is flexed 30 degrees.

3. In males the foot is at a right angle.

4. In females the foot is plantar flexed 95 to 100 degrees.

5. The foot is in a neutral position as to inversion and eversion.

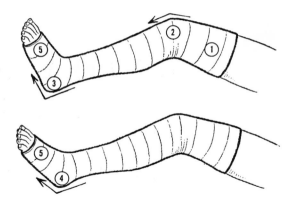

Postoperative Management

Apply a snug-fitting, long leg plaster cast at the end of three weeks.

Apply a walking, non-padded, below-the-knee cast at the end of eight weeks.

Now permit weight bearing with crutches.

The cast immobilization is discontinued only when x-ray examinations reveal complete consolidation.

It may require four to six months before consolidation is complete.

DISLOCATIONS OF THE ANKLE JOINT

Posterior Dislocation of the Ankle Joint

REMARKS

Although this lesion is rare it is the most common of all dislocations of the ankle joint.

The lesion is the result of severe plantar flexion of the foot with a strong forward thrust of the leg.

In most instances the dislocation is accompanied by a fracture of one or both malleoli or a posterior marginal fracture of the tibia.

Prereduction X-Ray

1. The tibia and the fibula are displaced forward.

2. The talus, with the foot, is displaced backward.

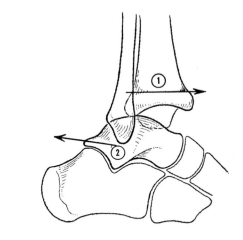

Manipulative Reduction (Under General Anesthesia)

1. The knee is flexed.

2. The assistant makes counter traction on the leg.

3. The operator grasps the forefoot with one hand and the heel with the other.

4. The foot is slightly plantar flexed.

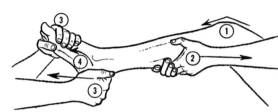

Manipulative Reduction (Under General Anesthesia) (Continued)

1. Make straight downward traction on the plantar flexed foot, then,
2. Pull the foot forward while
3. A second assistant makes counter pressure on the front of the lower leg.

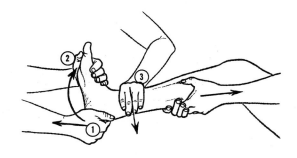

Postreduction X-Ray

1. The talus is in accurate relation to the tibia.
2. The articular surfaces of the talus and the tibia are congruous.

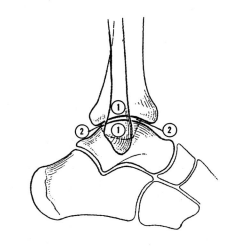

Immobilization

1. Apply a circular plaster cast from the base of the toe to just below the knee.
2. The foot is dorsiflexed 90 degrees.
3. The foot is in a neutral position as to inversion and eversion.
4. Mold the plaster well around the heel and the front of the foot and the malleoli.

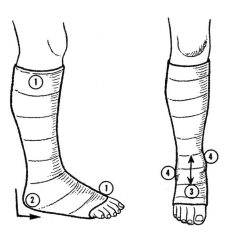

Postreduction Management

The patient can be ambulatory on crutches immediately.

Reapply the cast at the end of three weeks.

Remove the second cast six weeks after reduction and permit weight bearing, at first on crutches.

Institute physical therapy and active exercises to restore normal ankle and foot movements.

Note: If associated fractures of the malleoli are present, the dislocation is first reduced and then the fractures are treated as previously described, by open reduction and internal fixation.

Anterior Dislocation of the Ankle Joint

REMARKS

This lesion is indeed rare and when it occurs it is frequently accompanied by a fracture of the anterior margin of the tibia.

The lesion is produced by forcible dorsiflexion of the foot or a fall on the heel with the foot in dorsiflexion.

Fracture of one or both malleoli may be concomitant lesions.

In this lesion the anterior capsule may be separated from the neck of the talus.

Prereduction X-Ray

1. Backward displacement of the tibia and the fibula.

2. Forward displacement of the talus.

3. Small marginal fracture of the anterior tip of the tibia.

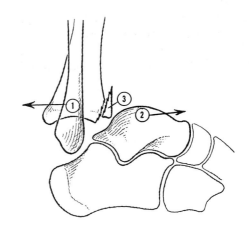

Manipulative Reduction (Under General Anesthesia)

1. The knee is flexed.
2. The operator grasps the forefoot with one hand and the heel with the other.
3. Dorsiflexion of the foot is slightly increased (to disengage the talus).
4. An assistant makes counter traction on the leg.

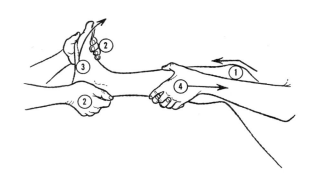

1. Make straight downward traction.
2. Then push the foot directly backward while
3. A second assistant makes counter pressure on the back of the lower leg.

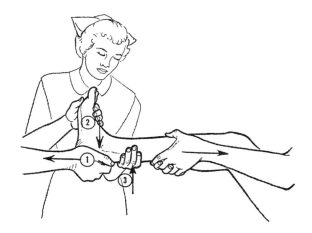

Postreduction X-Ray

1. The talus is in normal relation to the tibia.
2. The articular surfaces of the talus and the tibia are congruous.
3. The small anterior marginal fragment is in its anatomic position.

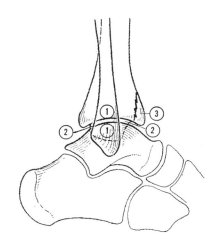

Page 1621

Immobilization

1. Apply a circular plaster cast from the base of the toes to just below the knee.

2. The foot is slightly plantar flexed.

3. The foot is in a neutral position as to inversion and eversion.

4. Mold the plaster well around the heel, the front of the foot, and the malleoli.

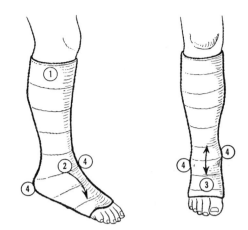

Postreduction Management

The patient should be ambulatory on crutches immediately without weight bearing on the affected limb.

Reapply the plaster cast at the end of three weeks and place the foot in 90 degrees dorsiflexion.

Remove the second cast six weeks after reduction and permit weight bearing on crutches.

Institute physical therapy and active exercises to restore normal movements of the ankle and foot.

Note: If concomitant fractures of the malleoli are present, reduce the dislocation and then treat the fracture as previously described, by open reduction and internal fixation.

Upward Dislocation of the Talus

REMARKS

This rare lesion is frequently complicated by marked comminution of the lower end of the tibia and a fracture of the fibula.

There is complete disruption of the distal tibiofibular joint with upward displacement of the talus between the tibia and the fibula.

Internal fixation of the tibiofibular joint and repair of the deltoid ligament is the procedure of choice.

Prereduction X-Ray

1. Wide separation of the tibiofibular joint.

2. Upward displacement of the talus.

3. Slight comminution of the lateral portion of the tibial articular surface.

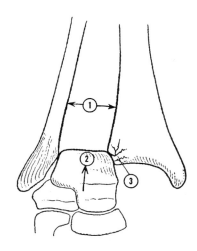

Treatment and Postoperative Management

After reduction of the dislocation by strong downward traction on the foot and counter traction on the leg, the diastasis of the ankle joint is reduced and stabilized by a screw driven through the fibula and the tibia, and the deltoid ligament is repaired.

Employ the same technique described for avulsion of the medial ligament and diastasis of the inferior tibiofibular joint (pages 1566 and 1567).

Postreduction X-Ray

1. The talus fits accurately under the tibia and in the ankle mortise.

2. The fibula is secured to the tibia with a transfixion screw.

3. The fibula fits snugly against the tibia.

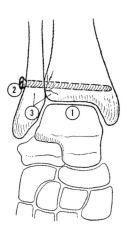

Lateral Dislocation of the Ankle Joint

REMARKS

This lesion is always associated with fractures of the malleoli and may be the result of violent inversion or eversion mechanisms.

Often the lesion is an open one.

Prereduction X-Ray

1. Fracture of the medial and lateral malleoli.

2. Lateral and upward displacement of the talus.

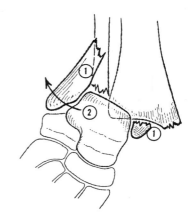

Treatment and Postreduction Management

After reduction by traction and manipulation the subsequent plan of treatment is the same as for fractures of the malleoli with lateral or medial displacement of the talus; these techniques have been described previously (pages 1596 and 1597).

Postreduction X-Ray

1. The talus is in its normal position in the mortise.

2. The lateral malleolus is secured by a screw.

3. The medial malleolus is secured by a screw.

4. The articular surfaces of the talus and the tibia are congruous.

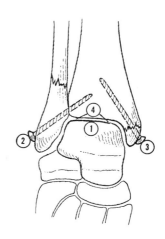

Irreducible Fractures of the Lateral Malleolus

REMARKS

In rare instances widening of the ankle mortise is not the result of diastasis of the inferior tibiofibular joint.

It may be the result of rupture of the medial ligament or avulsion of the medial malleolus with displacement of the posterior tibial tendon or posterior tibial artery and nerve between the intact portion of the medial malleolus and the talus.

Always suspect such a possibility when, in a fracture of the lateral malleolus with lateral displacement of the talus, the talus cannot be accurately reduced.

Pathology

1. The posterior tibial tendon is trapped between the medial malleolus and the talus.
2. The talus is displaced laterally.
3. There is a fracture of the lateral malleolus.
4. There is an avulsion of the tip of the medial malleolus.

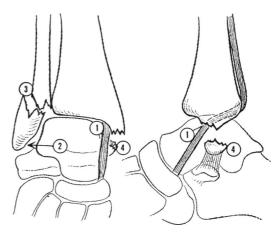

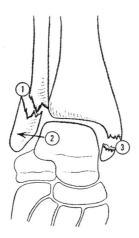

Prereduction X-Ray

1. Fracture of the lateral malleolus.
2. Lateral shift of the talus.
3. Avulsion of the tip of the medial malleolus.

Operative Reduction

1. Make a 3 inch incision along the posterior margin of the medial malleolus; the incision curves forward just below the tip of the malleolus for 2 inches more.

2. Divide the deep fascia, exposing

3. The avulsed medial malleolus and

4. The medial ligament.

5. Identify the posterior tibial tendon between the intact portion of the malleolus and the talus.

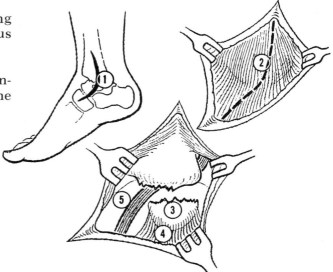

1. With a hook replace the posterior tibial tendon in its normal position.

2. Secure the avulsed tip of the medial malleolus to the tibia with a screw.

Note: Treatment of a fracture of the lateral malleolus with displacement is now given as previously described on page 1597.

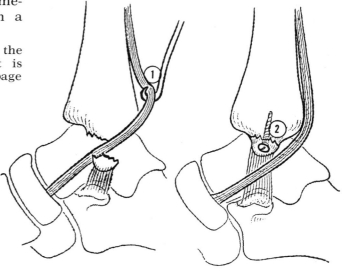

IRREDUCIBLE POSTERIOR FRACTURE-DISLOCATION OF THE ANKLE JOINT

REMARKS

Occasionally in posterior fracture-dislocations the proximal end of the fractured fibula is displaced behind the tibia and locked there by the posterolateral ridge of the tibia (Bosworth).

Closed manipulative maneuvers will not effect a reduction.

Failure to achieve an adequate reduction of the fibula and to restore the talus to its normal position results in severe disability and later in osteoarthritis.

This lesion must always be suspected when manipulative methods fail to reduce the fracture-dislocation.

Prereduction X-Ray

1. Posterior displacement of the talus.

2. Spiral fracture of the distal end of the fibula.

3. Widening of the ankle mortise.

4. Displacement of the talus laterally.

5. The proximal fibular fragment is locked on the posterolateral aspect of the tibia.

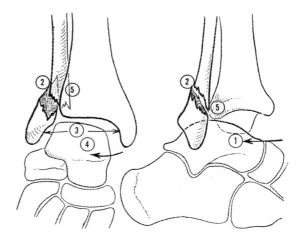

Operative Reduction

1. Make a 4 to 5 inch incision on the lateral aspect of the leg beginning just distal to the tip of the lateral malleolus.

2. Divide the deep fascia; retract the flaps and expose the fractured end of the distal fragment.

3. Locate the distal end of the proximal fibular fragment behind the tibia.

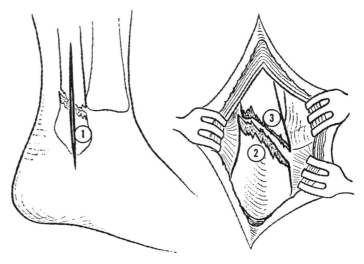

1. Place a pry or curette between the fibular fragment and the tibia and apply strong leverage on the displaced fragment.

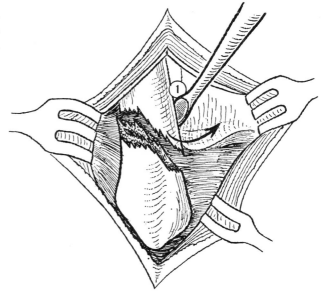

Operative Reduction (Continued)

1. The fibular fragments are in alignment.

2. Transfix the fragments with a small screw or

3. Pass a wire through the distal fragment and into the medullary canal of the proximal fragment.

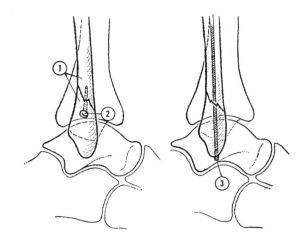

Treatment and postreduction management of the fracture of the lateral malleolus and lateral displacement of the talus is described on page 1598.

If a medullary wire is used in the fibula it is usually removed at the end of six weeks.

OPEN FRACTURES AND FRACTURE-DISLOCATIONS OF THE ANKLE JOINT

REMARKS

Because of the superficial position of the malleoli marked displacement of the foot to one side or the other frequently causes rupture of the soft tissues and skin on the side opposite the displacement.

Falls from a height may drive the ends of the tibia and the fibula through the skin.

Direct violence may puncture, lacerate and macerate the soft tissue.

These lesions should be given immediate definitive attention just as soon as the patient's condition permits. Delay in treatment may mean a serious infection.

Every effort should be made to treat these lesions in the first 12 hours—preferably in the first six hours.

The goal is to convert an open wound to a closed wound which will heal by first intention.

Don't inflict any more surgical trauma than is necessary to achieve your goal.

Don't sacrifice skin needlessly; it is essential to be able to approximate the skin edges without tension.

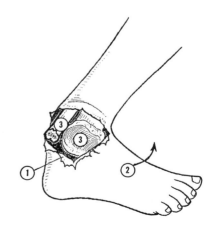

Typical Case

1. Ragged open wound on the outer aspect of the ankle.

2. The foot is markedly inverted.

3. The fractured end of the fibula and the articular surface of the tibia are exposed.

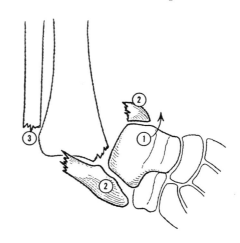

Prereduction X-Ray

1. The talus is displaced upward and inward.
2. The medial and lateral malleoli have followed the talus.
3. Exposed end of the proximal fragment of the fibula.

Preparation of the Area

(The surgeon is in sterile attire.)
1. Cover the wound with sterile gauze.
2. After shaving the area around the wound, cleanse the area first with benzine and ether, then with Septisol.

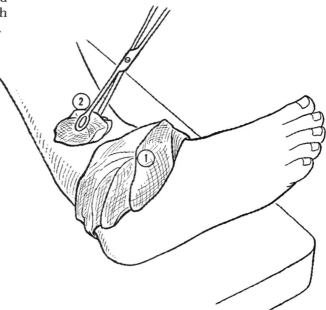

Preparation of the Area
(Continued)

1. While the wound is being flushed with copious quantities of normal saline solution,

2. Scrub the wound with Septisol using cotton balls. (Don't traumatize the soft tissues.)

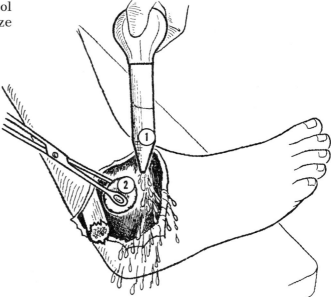

1. Paint the leg, the foot and the wound area with tincture of Zephiran (0.1 per cent solution), then,

2. Drape the field.

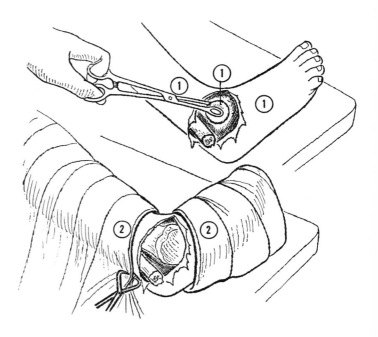

Preparation of the Area
(Continued)

(Surgeon and assistant change gowns and gloves.)

1. Excise the skin edges but spare as much skin as possible.

2. Excise all devitalized soft tissue.

3. Remove all detached loose fragments of bone and other foreign material.

4. Remove contaminated dirty ends of bone with a rongeur or a sharp curette.

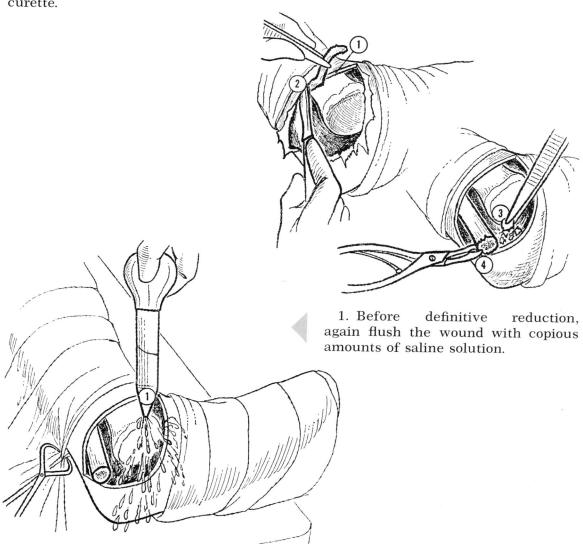

1. Before definitive reduction, again flush the wound with copious amounts of saline solution.

Reduction

Depending on the type of dislocation or fracture dislocation employ
the same methods depicted for the
closed lesions of the same types.

Always give preference to methods
without use of internal fixation if at
all possible.

After reduction:
1. Close the wound edges loosely
with interrupted fine stainless steel
sutures.

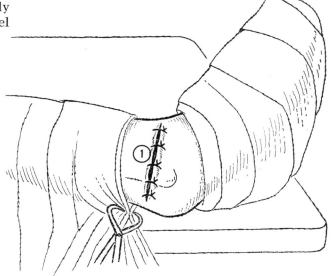

Immobilization

1. Apply a circular cast from behind the metatarsal heads to the upper thigh.
2. The foot is in a neutral position
and at a right angle to the leg.
3. The knee is flexed 30 degrees.

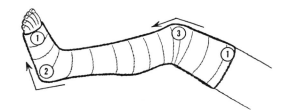

Postoperative Management

Elevate the limb on pillows.
Surround the operative site with ice bags.
Prescribe a wide-spectrum antibiotic; continue the drug until the
danger of infection is past.
Check constantly for evidence of circulatory embarrassment or infec-
tion.
If no complications arise, the subsequent treatment is the same as
for closed lesions of the same type.

MALUNITED FRACTURE-DISLOCATIONS OF THE ANKLE JOINT

REMARKS

Traumatic arthritis is the inevitable sequel of incongruity of the articular surfaces of the talus and diastasis of the tibiofibular mortise.

This is the penalty the patient pays when an inadequate reduction is attained following any type of fracture-dislocation of the ankle joint.

Arthrodesis of the ankle joint is the procedure of choice in order to assure the patient a painless, weight-bearing limb.

Be sure that the foot is so positioned that following arthrodesis it is in a neutral position as to inversion and eversion.

In males, place the foot at a right angle; in females, in 10 degrees of equinus.

Some Types of Malunited Fracture-Dislocations Requiring Arthrodesis

X-RAY (FIRST EXAMPLE)

1. Lateral displacement of the talus.
2. Diastasis of the tibiofibular joint.
3. Eversion of the talus and the foot.
4. Widening of the mortise.

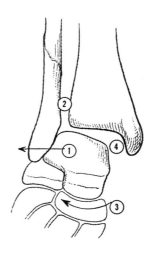

Some Types of Malunited Fracture-Dislocations Requiring Arthrodesis (Continued)

X-RAY (SECOND EXAMPLE)

1. Lateral displacement of the talus.
2. Healed unreduced fracture of the external malleolus.
3. Incongruity of the articular surfaces of the talus and the tibia.
4. Widening of the mortise.

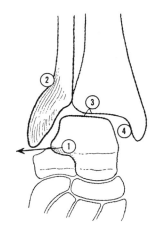

X-RAY (THIRD EXAMPLE)

1. Healed fracture of the posterior margin of the tibia.
2. The talus is displaced posteriorly.
3. Incongruity of the articular surfaces of the talus and the tibia.

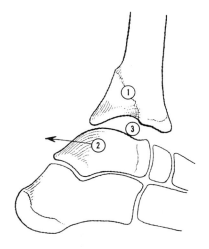

X-RAY (FOURTH EXAMPLE)

1. Marked incongruity of the articular surfaces of the talus and the tibia.
2. Marked irregularity of the articular surface of the tibia.
3. Thinning of the joint space.
4. Posterior displacement of the talus.

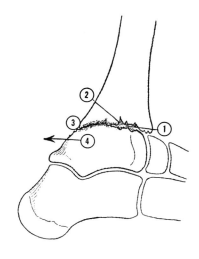

Arthrodesis of the Ankle Joint
(Anterior Method)

1. Make an incision on the anterior aspect of the ankle joint beginning 4 inches above and terminating 2 inches below the ankle joint.

2. Divide the deep fascia in the line of the skin incision and develop the interval between the extensor hallucis longus and the extensor digitorum longus tendons.

3. Retract the neurovascular bundle medially.

4. Incise the periosteum, capsule, and synovium in the line of the skin incision.

5. By subperiosteal dissection expose the anterior surface of the tibia, the talus and both malleoli.

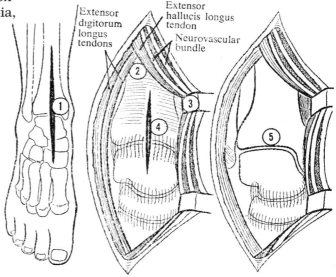

Extensor digitorum longus tendons

Extensor hallucis longus tendon

Neurovascular bundle

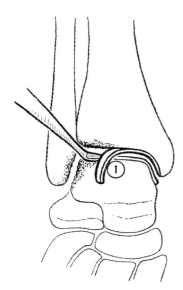

1. With a thin-bladed, sharp osteotome remove the articular cartilage of the tibia, the talus and the fibula.

Note: Correct any medial or lateral deviation of the talus by removing a larger wedge of bone from the inner or outer side of the talus or tibia.

Page 1637

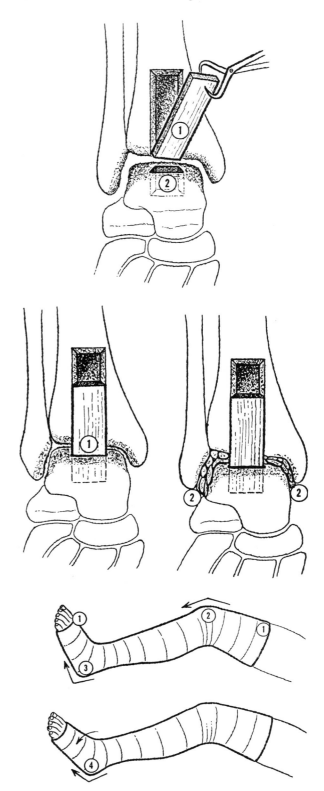

Arthrodesis of the Ankle Joint (Anterior Method) (Continued)

1. Remove a full thickness cortical graft 1 by 3 inches from the anterior surface of the tibia immediately above the joint.

2. Cut a slot in the anterior portion of the body and the superior surface of the neck of the talus.

After aligning the talus in the desired position in relation to the tibia,

1. Slide the cortical graft into the slot in the talus and countersink its distal end into the slot.

2. Pack bone chips into the space between the talus and the tibia and fibula.

Note: In males, place the foot at a right angle; in females, in 10 degrees plantar flexion.

Immobilization

1. Apply a circular plaster cast from behind the metatarsal heads to the midthigh.

2. The knee is slightly flexed.

3. In males the foot is at a right angle.

4. In females the foot is plantar flexed 10 degrees.

Postoperative Management

Elevate the limb on pillows.

Apply ice bags around the operative site.

After four weeks remove the long leg cast and apply a short leg, skin-tight plaster cast with a walking heel.

Now permit weight bearing with crutches.

Take check x-rays every four weeks.

Discontinue the plaster immobilization when consolidation is complete (usually 12 to 16 weeks).

Alternate Arthrodesis

I prefer the compression arthrodesis for these cases.

Compression Arthrodesis of the Ankle (Charnley)

REMARKS

This arthordesis is by far the procedure of choice.

I prefer to use the transfibular approach rather than the transverse incision across the front of the ankle as described by Charnley.

Operative Procedure

1. Make a 4 inch longitudinal incision over the subcutaneous surface of the distal end of the fibula ending ½ inch distal to the lateral malleolus.

2. Expose the fibula at the upper end of the wound and, with a sharp osteotome, divide it.

3. By sharp dissection free the fibula from all soft tissue attachment except along its posterior aspect.

4. Reflect the fibula downward.

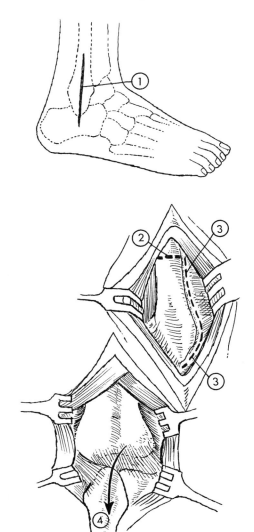

Operative Procedure (Continued)

1. Divide the capsule and ligaments on the anterior and lateral aspect of the ankle joint and expose the articular surfaces of the tibia and talus.

2. Open up the ankle joint like a book with the hinge medially.

3. Resect the articular surfaces of the tibia and talus so that there is good contact between the raw surfaces when the ankle is in 5 to 10 degrees of plantar flexion.

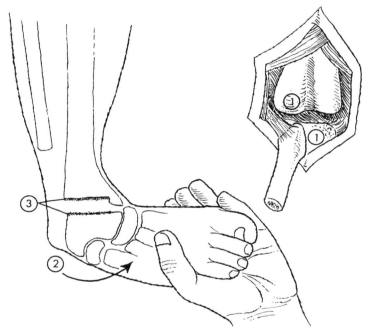

1. Split the fibula longitudinally; the medial half can now be used for chips to pack around the site of arthrodesis.

2. With a sharp osteotome make a level surface on the lateral aspect of the tibia and talus.

3. Pass a Steinmann pin through the talus anterior to its transverse axis.

4. Apply the compression clamps to the distal pin.

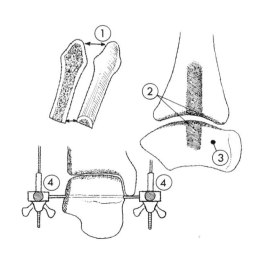

Operative Procedure *(Continued)*

1. Using the arms of the clamp as a guide, insert the proximal pin through the tibia.

2. Tighten the clamps.

Note: At this time correct any rotary deformities.

3. Allow the raw medial surface of the fibula to make contact with the tibia and talus.

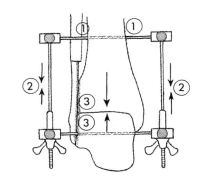

Immobilization

1. Apply a well-padded cast from the toes to just below the knee.

2. The foot is in 5 to 10 degrees of plantar flexion.

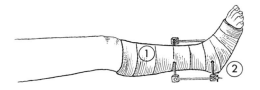

Postoperative Management

After 6 weeks remove the pins and cast.

Apply a walking cast and allow weight bearing.

After four more weeks remove the cast and allow unrestricted activity.

FRACTURES AND FRACTURE-DISLOCATIONS OF THE BONES OF THE FOOT

DISLOCATIONS OF THE TALUS

Subtalar Dislocation of the Talus

REMARKS

Subtalar dislocation is the result of a combination of forces acting simultaneously on the foot, namely, inversion-adduction and forced plantar flexion.

These forces rupture the interosseous ligaments of the subtalar joint and permit inward dislocation of the foot at the subtalar and talonavicular joints.

The talus is still in the ankle mortise but it is forced into a position of equinus.

Always check for associated fractures of the head of the talus or of the navicular.

Prereduction X-Ray

1. The talus is held in the tibiofibular mortise.
2. The foot is displaced inward at the subtalar and talonavicular joints.
3. The talus is in equinus.

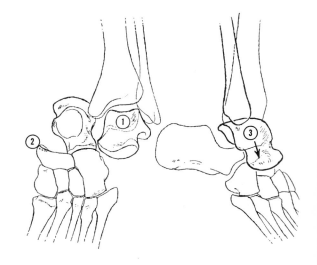

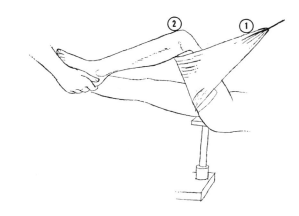

Manipulative Reduction (Under General Anesthesia)

1. Place a well-padded canvas sling under the distal end of the thigh and suspend it from an overhead cross bar on the fracture table.
2. The knee is flexed 90 degrees.

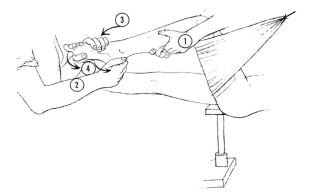

1. The assistant holds and steadies the lower leg.
2. The operator grasps the heel with one hand and the forefoot with the other.
3. The foot is first strongly plantar flexed, then
4. The foot is everted and abducted.

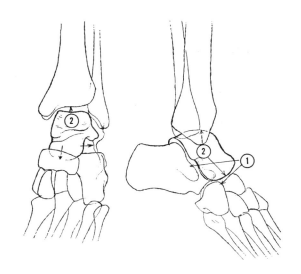

Postreduction X-Ray

1. The subtalar and talonavicular dislocations are reduced.
2. The talus is in its normal relation to the navicular, calcaneus and tibia.

Immobilization

1. Apply a circular plaster cast from behind the toes to the midthigh.
2. The knee is flexed 30 degrees.
3. The foot is at 90 degrees dorsiflexion.
4. The foot is in slight eversion.

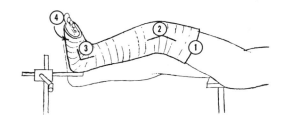

Postreduction Management

Elevate the limb on pillows.

Surround the foot with ice bags.

Frequently check the circulation of the foot.

Apply a short leg plaster cast with a walking heel at the end of three weeks and place the foot in a neutral position as to inversion and eversion.

Remove the plaster cast eight weeks after reduction.

Institute physical therapy and active exercises to restore normal motion in all joints of the foot.

Total Dislocation of the Talus

REMARKS

This lesion is produced by forceful inversion-adduction and plantar flexion of the foot.

Both the lateral ligaments of the ankle joint and the interosseous ligaments of the subtalar joint are ruptured.

The talus is projected out of its anatomic position and assumes a position with its body in front of the lateral malleolus; its head points medially and its inferior articular surface is directed posteriorly.

Frequently the overlying soft tissues and skin are ruptured from within, producing an open dislocation.

Occasionally in open lesions the talus is ejected out of the wound.

Frequently the circulation of the talus is markedly embarrassed, predisposing it to development of avascular necrosis.

Closed and open dislocations must be reduced at once to prevent further circulatory disturbance.

Prereduction X-Ray

1. The body of the talus is in front of the external malleolus.

2. The head of the talus is directed medially.

3. The talus is rotated in its longitudinal axis so that its inferior articular surface faces posteriorly.

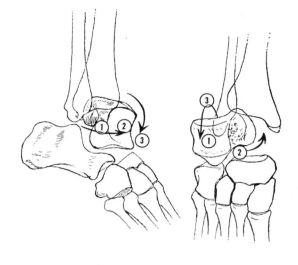

Manipulative Reduction

1. Place the limb in a padded canvas sling suspended from an overhead cross bar on a fracture table.

2. The knee is flexed 90 degrees.

3. An assistant grasps the heel with one hand and the forefoot with the other.

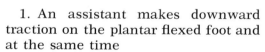

1. An assistant makes downward traction on the plantar flexed foot and at the same time

2. The foot is forcefully inverted.

3. While the position of inversion and plantar flexion is maintained the surgeon's thumbs make firm pressure on the posterior portion of the talus.

4. The pressure is directed inward, backward, and at the same time

5. The talus is rotated around its longitudinal axis.

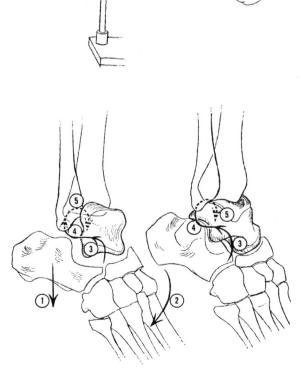

Page 1647

Postreduction X-Ray

1. The talus is in normal relation to the navicular.

2. The talus is accurately seated in the tibiofibular mortise.

3. The talus is in normal relation to the tibia, calcaneus and navicular.

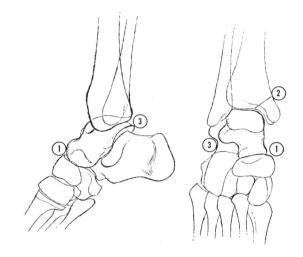

Immobilization

1. Apply a circular plaster cast from behind the metatarsal heads to the midthigh.

2. The knee is flexed 30 degrees.

3. The foot is at a right angle.

Note: The foot is in a neutral position as to inversion and eversion.

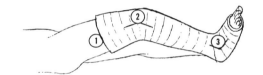

Postreduction Management

Elevate the limb on pillows.

Surround the foot with ice bags.

Reapply a long leg cast after three weeks.

After six weeks apply a short leg cast.

Allow ambulation on crutches without weight bearing on the affected foot for at least 12 weeks.

Take check x-rays each time the plaster cast is changed.

At the end of 12 weeks permit weight bearing only if x-ray shows no evidence of avascular necrosis as demonstrated by an increase in relative density of the talus.

If evidence of avascular necrosis is demonstrable, reapply a short leg cast and maintain immobilization without weight bearing until the talus is revascularized; this may take many months.

ALTERNATE METHOD (SKELETAL TRACTION)

REMARKS

This method is employed when manipulative measures fail to achieve a reduction.

Reduction by Skeletal Traction and Manipulation

1. Place the distal end of the thigh in a canvas sling suspended from a cross bar on the fracture table.
2. The knee is flexed 90 degrees.
3. Pass a Steinmann pin through the calcaneus and secure it to the mechanical traction apparatus at the foot of the table.
4. Make steady downward traction to open the interval between the tibia and the calcaneus.

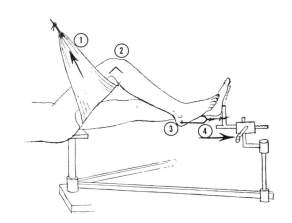

1. An assistant makes strong inversion on the plantar flexed foot while
2. The surgeon with both thumbs pushes the posterior portion of the talus inward and backward; at the same time
3. The surgeon attempts to rotate the talus around its longitudinal axis.

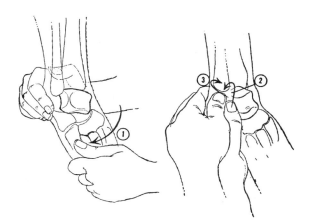

Immobilization and postreduction management are the same as described on page 1648.

Remove the pin from the calcaneus before the plaster cast is applied.

Note: In the event that the lesion is an open dislocation, excise the wound edges, flush the wound with copious quantities of saline solution, then proceed to reduce the dislocation as previously depicted (page 1647). Close the skin edges loosely and without tension after reduction is achieved.

Don't needlessly sacrifice skin.

Handle all soft tissues with great gentleness.

Don't sever the soft tissue attachments of the talus—its blood supply is already severely compromised.

FRACTURES OF THE TALUS

Fracture of the Posterior Process of the Talus

REMARKS

This lesion is usually the result of forcible plantar flexion of the foot.
Don't misinterpret the os trigonum, an anomalous bone, as a fracture of the posterior process.

Prereduction X-Ray

The posterior process of the talus is displaced slightly upward.

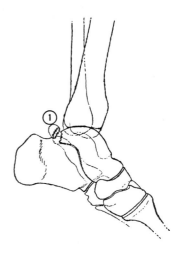

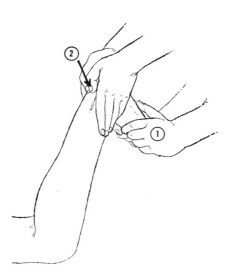

Manipulative Reduction

The patient is in the prone position with the knee flexed 90 degrees.

1. An assistant strongly dorsiflexes the foot while

2. The operator makes deep downward pressure on either side of the Achilles tendon directly over the displaced fragment.

Postreduction X-Ray

1. The posterior process of the talus is in apposition to the body of the talus.

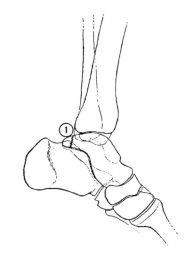

Immobilization

1. Apply a circular plaster cast from behind the toes to midthigh.
2. The foot is slightly dorsiflexed.
3. The knee is flexed 30 degrees.

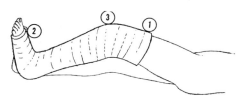

Postreduction Management

Allow immediate ambulation on crutches without weight bearing on the affected foot.

Remove the cast at the end of four weeks.

Now permit weight bearing.

Fracture of the Body of the Talus

REMARKS

This is a rare lesion and is the result of falls from a height; the talus is compressed between the tibia and the calcaneus.

Generally a vertical fracture is sustained; occasionally the inferior or superior surfaces of the talus are disrupted.

Prereduction X-Ray

1. Vertical fracture through the body of the talus with no displacement.

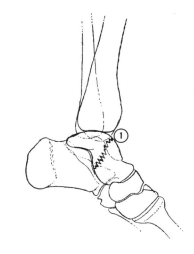

Immobilization

1. Apply a circular plaster cast from behind the metatarsal heads to the midthigh.
2. The knee is flexed 30 degrees.
3. The foot is in slight dorsiflexion.

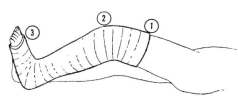

Management

Ambulate patient immediately on crutches without weight bearing on affected limb.

Change the cast every three or four weeks.

Discard plaster immobilization after eight weeks, but don't allow weight bearing on the limb.

Institute exercises to restore normal motion in the ankle and joints of the foot

Permit weight bearing at the end of 12 weeks.

Fracture of the Neck of the Talus
without Displacement

REMARKS

A vertical fracture through the neck of the talus is produced by forcible dorsiflexion of the foot.

This mechanism forces the neck of the talus against the anterior margin of the tibia.

Always check for possible backward displacement of the body of the talus; in this lesion displacement of the body is the rule rather than the exception.

Appearance on X-Ray

1. Fracture through the neck of the talus without displacement.

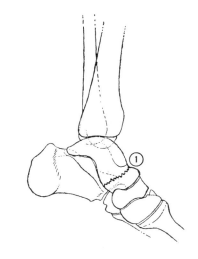

Immobilization

Apply a circular plaster cast from behind the metatarsal head to the midthigh.
1. The knee is flexed 30 degrees.
2. The foot is at a right angle.
3. The foot is in a neutral position as to inversion and eversion.

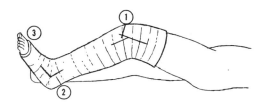

Management

Ambulate patient immediately on crutches without weight bearing on the affected limb.

Change the cast every three or four weeks.

Discard plaster immobilization after eight weeks, but don't allow weight bearing on the limb.

Institute exercises to restore normal motion in the ankle and joints of the foot.

Permit weight bearing at the end of 12 weeks.

Page 1653

Fracture of the Neck of the Talus with Subluxation of the Subtalar Joint

REMARKS

Forcible dorsiflexion of the foot may result in fracture of the talus with dislocation of the body of the talus.

The body is displaced slightly forward and into the equinus position.

The normal relationship of the body to the calcaneus must be restored in order to obtain a normally functioning foot without pain.

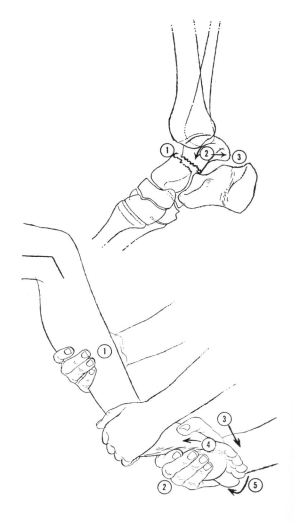

Prereduction X-Ray

1. Vertical fracture through the neck of the talus.

2. The body is displaced slightly forward and is in equinus.

3. There is incongruity of the articular surface of the body and the calcaneus.

Manipulative Reduction

1. The leg hangs over the end of the table with the knee flexed 45 degrees; an assistant steadies the lower leg.

2. The operator grasps the heel with one hand and the forefoot with the other hand.

3. The operator strongly plantar flexes the foot and at the same time

4. Pushes the foot backward; also

5. The foot is everted.

Postreduction X-Ray

1. The neck and body are in normal position.
2. The articular surfaces of the body and the calcaneus are now congruous.

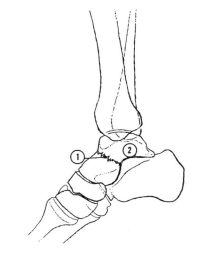

Immobilization

1. Apply a circular cast from behind the metatarsal heads to the midthigh.
2. The knee is flexed 30 degrees.
3. The foot is plantar flexed and everted.

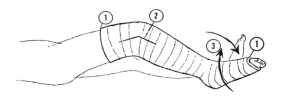

Postreduction Management

Allow the patient up on crutches without weight bearing on the affected foot.

Change the cast every three to four weeks.

At the end of eight weeks apply a cast with the foot at a right angle and neutral to inversion and eversion.

At the end of 12 weeks if bony healing is complete, remove the cast and permit weight bearing.

Check for avascular necrosis of the body. Warn the patient that such a sequel may develop.

ALTERNATE METHOD

This alternate method is employed if subluxation recurs or is not reducible or if there is displacement between the body and the neck of the talus.

Prereduction X-Ray

1. Vertical fracture of the neck of the talus.

2. Subluxation of the body of the talus.

3. The articular surfaces of the body and the calcaneus are incongruous.

Note: In this instance manipulative methods failed to achieve a reduction.

Operative Reduction

1. Make a 3 inch incision on the anteromedial aspect of the ankle; it begins in front and above the medial malleolus, curves forward, then downward and terminates on the inner aspect of the navicular.

2. By sharp dissection expose the head and neck of the talus.

3. Retract the posterior tibial tendon out of the field.

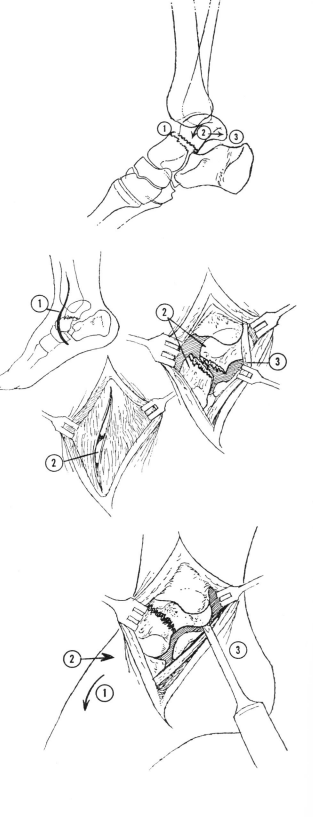

Reduce the fracture-dislocation by

1. Plantar flexion of the foot.

2. Push the foot backward.

3. Lever (if necessary) the body into apposition with the neck of the talus.

Operative Reduction (Continued)

1. Grasp and hold both fragments with a towel clip.

2. On the medial aspect of the neck just proximal to the articular surface drill a hole directed obliquely posteriorly and laterally through the neck and body and secure the fragments with a screw of proper length.

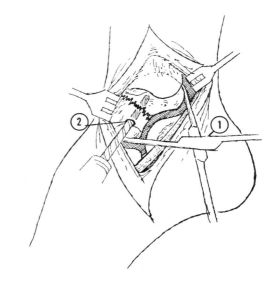

Postreduction X-Ray

1. The body and calcaneus are in normal relationship.

2. A screw is transfixing both fragments.

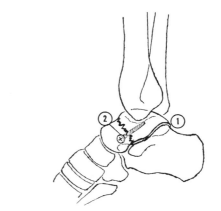

Immobilization

1. Apply a circular cast from behind the toes to the midthigh.

2. The knee is flexed 30 degrees.

3. The foot is at a right angle.

4. The foot is neutral as to inversion and eversion.

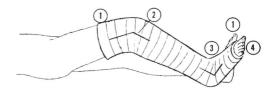

Postreduction Management

This is the same as for fractures treated by manipulative methods (page 1655).

Note: During the exposure of the fracture preserve, as much as is possible, all soft tissue attachments to the neck and body of the talus; the circulation of this bone is already severely compromised.

Fracture of the Neck of the Talus with Total Posterior Dislocation of the Body

REMARKS

With extreme violence which forces the foot into marked dorsiflexion the neck of the talus is fractured and the calcaneus is displaced and locked under the body of the talus; when the foot returns to plantar flexion the body is ejected out of the tibiofibular mortise.

The body comes to lie on the medial aspect of the tuber calcanei with its fractured surfaces directed laterally.

The lesion may be complicated by severe soft tissue injury; avascular necrosis of the body is a frequent sequel.

Reduction of the talus must be achieved promptly in order to avoid soft tissue sloughs and irreversible damage to the neurovascular structures (posterior tibial artery and nerve) from excessive pressure.

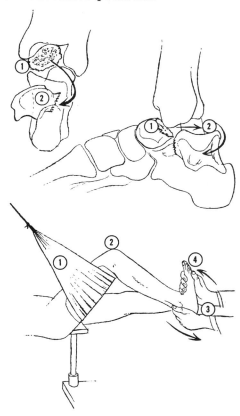

Prereduction X-Ray

1. Vertical fracture through the neck of the talus with some comminution.

2. The body of the talus is displaced backward and is rotated.

Manipulative Reduction (Under General Anesthesia)

1. Place a canvas sling around the distal end of the thigh; the sling is suspended from an overhead cross bar on the fracture table.

2. The knee is flexed 90 degrees.

3. The operator grasps the heel with one hand and the forefoot with the other.

4. Pull the foot forward and force it into marked dorsiflexion.

Manipulative Reduction (Under General Anesthesia) (Continued)

While the forward pull on the foot and dorsiflexion are maintained,

1. Strongly evert the foot; this maneuver unlocks the sustentaculum tali.

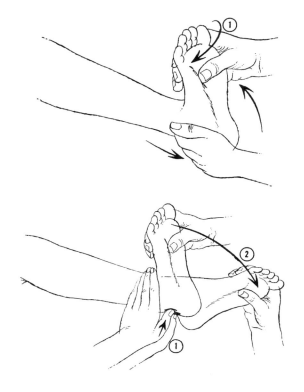

1. While an assistant makes firm pressure behind the ankle on either side of the Achilles tendon,
2. Plantar flex the foot.

ALTERNATE METHOD (OPEN REDUCTION)

This method is used when the manipulative maneuvers fail to achieve a perfect reduction of the dislocation or when the neck and body are not in perfect apposition.

Operative Procedure

1. Make a 3½ inch vertical incision over the posterior medial aspect of the ankle joint.
2. Expose the body of the talus and the posteromedial aspect of the calcaneus.

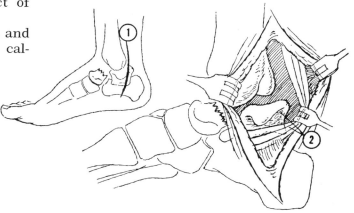

Page 1659

Operative Procedure (Continued)

1. With the foot pulled forward and dorsiflexed lever the body into the tibiofibular mortise.

2. Finally, plantar flex the foot to complete the reduction.

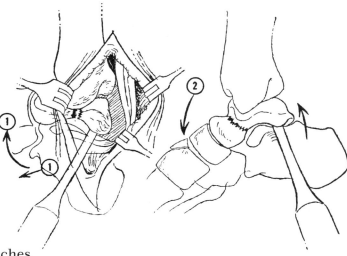

1. Make a second incision 3 inches long on the anteromedial aspect of the ankle; it begins anterior to and above the medial malleolus, curves forward, then downward, and ends on the medial aspect of the navicular.

2. Expose the neck and body of the talus.

3. With the foot plantar flexed grasp the body and neck with a towel clip, holding both fragments in accurate anatomic position.

4. Transfix the fragments with a screw passing obliquely posteriorly and laterally; the screw enters the neck just posterior to the articular surface on the medial aspect of the neck.

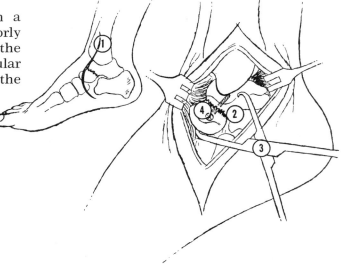

Postreduction X-Ray

1. The body of the talus is in normal relation to the neck of the talus and to the calcaneus.

2. A transfixion screw holds the fragments in accurate position and good apposition.

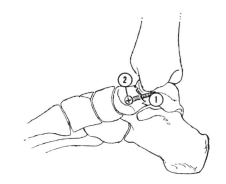

Immobilization

1. A circular cast is applied from behind the toes to the midthigh.
2. The knee is flexed 30 degrees.
3. The foot is at a right angle.
4. The foot is neutral to eversion and inversion.

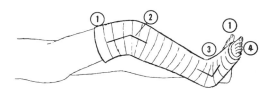

Postoperative Management

Elevate the limb on pillows and apply ice bags around the foot and ankle.

Check the limb constantly for evidence of circulatory embarrassment.

Allow the patient up on crutches without weight bearing on the affected foot.

Change the cast every three to four weeks.

If healing is complete and there is no evidence of avascular necrosis of the body, discontinue plaster fixation after 12 to 14 weeks and permit weight bearing on the affected limb.

Avascular necrosis is the rule when the body is completely dislocated; this complication is manifested by the relative increased density of the body.

In the presence of avascular necrosis, protect the talus for two to three more months in a short leg plaster cast and defer weight bearing during this period.

AVASCULAR NECROSIS OF THE BODY OF THE TALUS AND DEGENERATIVE ARTHRITIS OF THE ANKLE AND SUBTALAR JOINTS

REMARKS

Degenerative arthritis is the inevitable sequel to avascular necrosis of the body of the talus.

In some instances the changes are manifested early—in a few months; in others they appear later, requiring several years.

The associated disability is great and can be remedied only by a tibio-calcaneal fusion.

In comminuted fractures of the body of the talus incongruity of the articular surfaces between the talus, tibia and calcaneus is the rule, and avascular necrosis is a certainty. Here tibiocalcaneal fusion as a primary procedure is indicated.

Operative Procedure
(Talocalcaneal Fusion)

1. Make a 5 inch vertical skin incision centered on the fibula beginning 1 inch below the tip of the lateral malleolus.

2. Divide the deep fascia and periosteum in the line of the skin incision and expose the fibula by sharp subperiosteal dissection.

3. Divide the fibula by an osteotomy directed medially and downward.

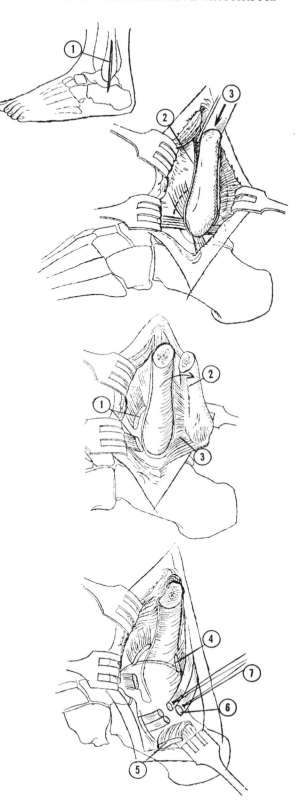

1. Cut the anterior lateral malleolar ligaments and the anterior talofibular ligaments.

2. Rotate the fibular fragment outward.

3. Divide the posterior lateral malleolar and posterior talofibular ligaments.

4. Complete detachment of the fibular fragment is achieved by cutting the calcaneofibular ligament.

5. Divide the superior peroneal retinaculum.

6. Deliver and divide the peroneus longus and the peroneus brevis tendons.

7. Place retention sutures in the proximal ends of both tendons.

Page 1663

Operative Procedure
(Talocalcaneal Fusion)
(Continued)

1. Incise the periosteum over the lateral aspect of the tibia and expose the surface by subperiosteal dissection.

2. Expose the lateral aspect of the calcaneus by subperiosteal dissection.

3. With a fine osteotome remove the lateral surface of the talus.

4. Remove the articular cartilage from both the ankle and the subtalar joints.

5. Cut a trough ½ inch wide on the lateral aspect of the calcaneus.

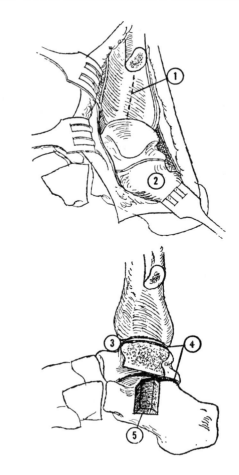

1. Remove the articular cartilage from the distal end of the fibular fragment.

2. Cut and shape the distal end of the fibular fragment to fit the trough in the calcaneus.

3. Correct any inversion or eversion deformity; then place the foot at a right angle to the leg.

4. Apply the fibular fragment as a free graft on the lateral side of the tibia, bridging both joints.

5. Counter-sink the distal end of the fibular fragment in the calcaneal trough.

6. Secure the graft with two screws, one through the tibia and the other through the calcaneus.

7. Pack bone chips in any remaining defects.

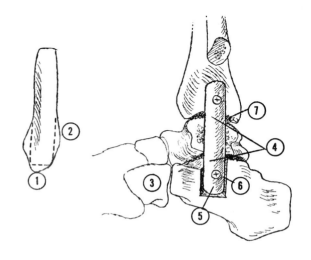

Page 1664

Operative Procedure (Talocalcaneal Fusion) (Continued)

1. Join the ends of the peroneal tendons with fine interrupted sutures.

2. Approximate the edges of the superior peroneal retinaculum.

3. In men, the foot is placed at a right angle to the tibia; in women, allow 10 degrees plantar flexion.

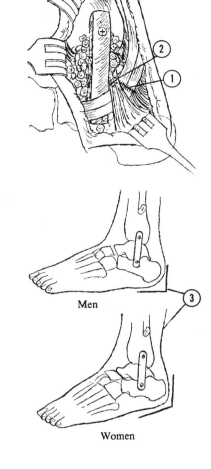

Men

Women

Postoperative X-Ray

1. The fibular graft bridges both joints.

2. The foot is at a right angle to the tibia (for men).

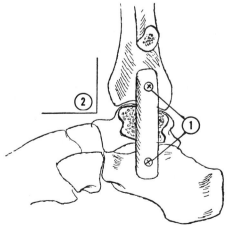

Immobilization

1. Apply a circular plaster cast from behind the metatarsal heads to the midthigh.

2. The knee is flexed 30 degrees.

3. The foot is at a right angle and neutral as to inversion and eversion.

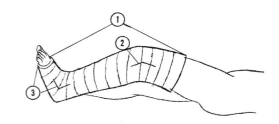

Postoperative Management

Elevate the limb on pillows.

Surround the foot and ankle with ice bags.

Allow the patient up on crutches after seven days without weight bearing on the affected limb.

Change the cast every three to four weeks.

After eight weeks apply a short leg cast with a walking heel.

Fusion of the ankle should be complete at the end of 12 to 14 weeks; now remove the cast.

FRACTURES OF THE CALCANEUS

REMARKS

Fractures of the spine are frequent concomitant lesions of fractures of the calcaneus; always check the spine.

Comprehension of the numerous varieties of fractures of the calcaneus is essential in order to institute intelligent treatment.

In addition to lateral x-ray views always take axial views of the calcaneus; such views reveal the true pattern of the fracture and the severity of the injury.

Whenever possible always try to restore displaced fragments to their anatomic position.

In some types with severe comminution of all of the articular surfaces, reduction by any method is impossible. Accept these deformities and institute early mobilization of implicated joints. Many of these feet will require some form of surgical arthrodesis at a later date.

Remember that some severe fracture-dislocations will heal with minimal dysfunction regardless of the type of treatment; however, such a result may require three to five years. This period is too long and should be decreased by surgical intervention.

The classification and some of the methods of treatment of fractures involving the subtalar joint depicted herein adhere closely to those advocated by Essex-Lopresti.

Isolated Fractures of the Calcaneus without Implication of the Subtalar Joint

REMARKS

Most of these fractures exhibit minimal or no displacement.

Vertical fractures occasionally show displacement of the medial tuberosity and some horizontal fractures show upward displacement of the fragment; these require manipulative reduction.

ISOLATED FRACTURES OF THE CALCANEUS REQUIRING NO REDUCTION

Appearance on X-Ray (First Example)

1. Vertical fracture of the tuberosity without displacement.

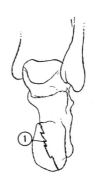

Appearance on X-Ray (Second Example)

1. Fracture of the sustentaculum tali with minimal displacement.

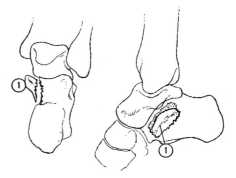

Appearance on X-Ray (Third Example)

1. Horizontal fracture of the tuberosity without displacement.

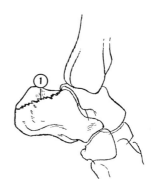

Immobilization

1. Apply a below-the-knee plaster cast with
2. Walking heel.
3. The foot is at a right angle to the leg and in a neutral position as to in-·version and eversion.

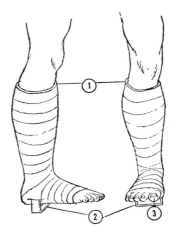

Management

Permit weight bearing immediately.

Reapply the cast at the end of three weeks.

Remove the second cast six weeks after the injury.

Now apply an elastic cotton bandage around the foot and ankle for several more weeks.

Institute exercises to restore normal motion at the ankle, subtalar and other joints of the foot.

ISOLATED FRACTURES OF THE CALCANEUS REQUIRING REDUCTION

Prereduction X-Ray

1. Vertical fracture of the tuberosity with medial displacement of the medial process.

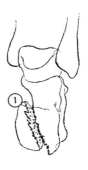

Manipulative Reduction

1. The patient's leg hangs over the edge of the table.

2. The forefoot rests on the operator's knee.

3. The operator compresses the heel firmly with both hands, or

4. Compresses the heel with a Böhler clamp.

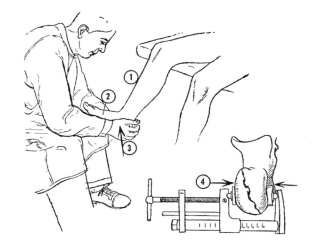

Immobilization

1. Apply a below-the-knee plaster cast with

2. Walking heel.

3. The foot is at a right angle to the leg and in a neutral position as to inversion and eversion.

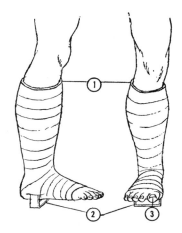

Management

Permit weight bearing immediately.

Reapply the cast at the end of three weeks.

Remove the second cast six weeks after the injury.

Now apply an elastic cotton bandage around the foot and ankle for several more weeks.

Institute exercises to restore normal motion at the ankle, subtalar and other joints of the foot.

Prereduction X-Ray

1. Horizontal fracture of the tuberosity with upward displacement of the fragment.

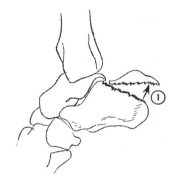

Manipulative Reduction

1. The patient is in the prone position.
2. The knee is flexed 70 degrees.
3. The foot is plantar flexed.
4. The operator places his thumbs on both sides of the Achilles tendon and makes firm downward pressure on the displaced fragment.

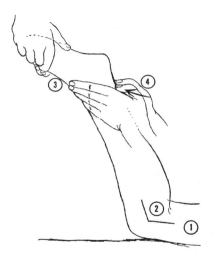

Immobilization

1. Apply a below-the-knee plaster cast with
2. Walking heel.
3. The foot is in slight plantar flexion.

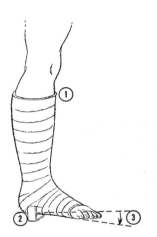

Page 1671

Management

Permit weight bearing immediately.

Reapply the cast at the end of three weeks.

Remove the second cast six weeks after the injury.

Now apply an elastic cotton bandage around the foot and ankle for several more weeks.

Institute exercises to restore normal motion at the ankle, subtalar and other joints of the foot.

ALTERNATE METHOD

This alternate method is employed if the fragment is large or if manipulative methods fail.

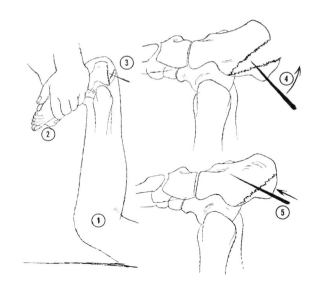

1. The knee is flexed.
2. The foot is dorsiflexed.
3. Drive a Steinmann pin through the posterior fragment.
4. Lever it into apposition, then
5. Drive it into the body of the calcaneus.

Postreduction X-Ray

1. The fragment is in normal apposition to the rest of the calcaneus.
2. The Steinmann pin is transfixing both fragments.

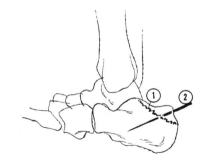

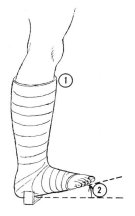

Immobilization

1. Apply a below-the-knee plaster cast incorporating the pin.
2. The foot is in slight dorsiflexion.

Management

After four weeks remove the Steinmann pin and reapply the plaster cast with a walking heel.

Six weeks after reduction remove the second cast and apply a cotton elastic bandage to the foot and ankle.

Allow weight bearing.

Institute exercises to restore motion in the ankle and all other joints of the foot.

Fracture of the Calcaneus with Implication of the Subtalar Joint

REMARKS

Essex-Lopresti recognized two principal types:
1. Tongue type fracture.
2. Joint depression type fracture.

The former lends itself to simpler methods of treatment; the latter requires repositioning of the fragments under vision. In some instances comminution of the articular surfaces is so severe that restoration of the anatomic configuration of the calcaneus is impossible by any method.

Varying gradations of each type are encountered, depending on the intensity of the downward forces.

TONGUE TYPE FRACTURES OF THE CALCANEUS

Mechanism of Injury

1. Downward force is transmitted by the talus to the subtalar joint.

2. The calcaneus is everted.

3. Spur on the lateral surface of the talus drives into the crucial angle of the calcaneus.

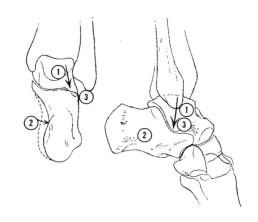

When downward force is minimal:

1. Spur of the talus digs into the crucial angle.

2. Fracture of the lateral wall of the calcaneus.

3. Note that the remaining portion of the calcaneus is not disrupted. This degree of involvement needs no reduction; simply immobilize in a short leg cast for six to eight weeks.

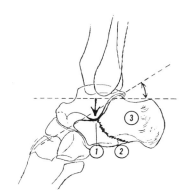

When downward force is moderate:

1. Fracture of the lateral wall of the calcaneus.

2. Shearing off of the sustentaculum tali with a medial portion (one-half to one-third) of the posterior articular surface of the calcaneus.

3. Secondary fracture line runs directly backward to the posterior border of the tuberosity.

4. The anterior end of the tongue-shaped fragment is displaced downward into the cancellous bone of the body and its posterior end is displaced upward.

5. Step between medial and lateral portions of the subtalar joint.

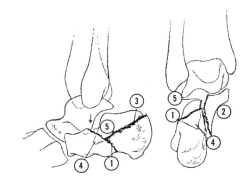

Page 1674

Mechanism of Injury
(Continued)

When downward force is severe:
1. The tuberosity is forced upward.
2. Primary fracture line opens up from below.
3. Step between medial and lateral elements of the posterior subtalar joint.

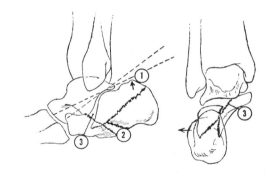

Prereduction X-Ray

1. Primary fracture through the lateral wall of the calcaneus.
2. Tongue-shaped fragment is depressed anteriorly and elevated posteriorly.
3. Secondary fracture line through the body of the calcaneus.
4. Loss of tuber angle. (*Note:* The normal angle is 35 to 40 degrees.)

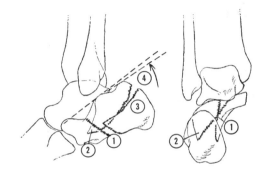

Manipulative Reduction and Pin Fixation

1. The patient is in a prone position.
2. Make a small incision over the calcaneus lateral to the Achilles tendon.
3. Insert a heavy Steinmann pin into the tongue fragment; the pin is directed in a longitudinal direction slightly to the lateral side.

Note: At this point check the position of the pin by x-rays.

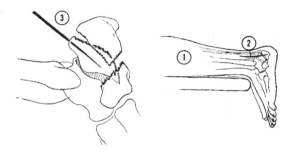

Manipulative Reduction and Pin Fixation (Continued)

1. Flex the knee 45 degrees.
2. Lift upward on the pin until the knee clears the table.

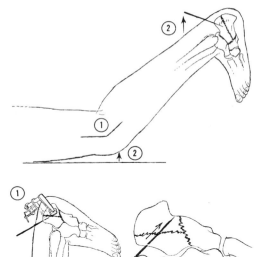

1. After measuring the exact thickness of the calcaneus of a normal foot with a Böhler clamp, quickly compress the lateral walls of the fractured calcaneous with a Böhler clamp to the measurements of a normal calcaneus.
2. Drill the pin across the fracture site and into the anterior calcaneal fragment.

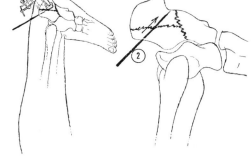

Note: Don't leave the clamp on too long because the skin may slough!

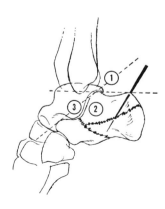

Postreduction X-Ray

1. The tuber angle has been restored.
2. The tongue fragment is elevated into normal position.
3. Articular surfaces of the subtalar joint are congruous.

Immobilization

1. While the position is maintained by downward pressure on the pin,
2. Apply a below-the-knee plaster cast incorporating the pin.

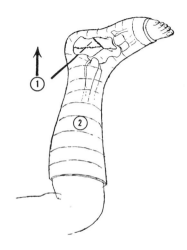

Postreduction Managememt

Elevate the foot on pillows.

Surround the foot and ankle with ice bags.

Within two to three days allow ambulation without weight bearing.

Remove the pin at the end of four weeks and apply another plaster cast.

Remove the second cast eight weeks after reduction.

Institute an intensive program to restore motion in the ankle and all other joints of the foot.

Permit weight bearing, at first with crutches, 10 to 12 weeks after the fracture.

Apply a cotton elastic bandage to control or prevent excessive swelling.

FRACTURES OF THE CALCANEUS WITH JOINT DEPRESSION

Mechanism of Injury

1. Downward force is transmitted by the talus to the subtalar joint.

2. The calcaneus is everted.

3. Spur in the lateral side of the talus drives into the crucial angle of the calcaneus.

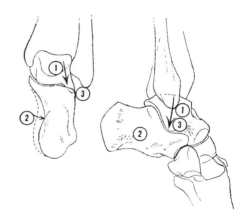

When downward force is minimal:

1. Spur of the talus digs into the calcaneus.

2. Fracture of the lateral wall of the calcaneus.

3. Secondary fracture line passes immediately around the subtalar joint. (The fragment comprises the outer one-half to two-thirds of the posterior articular surface; displacement is minimal or none.)

Note: This fracture needs no reduction and is treated by simple immobilization for six to eight weeks.

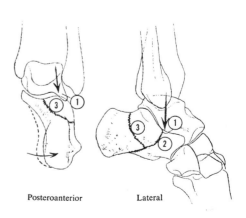

Posteroanterior   Lateral

Page 1677

Mechanism of Injury
(Continued)

When downward force is moderate:

1. The joint fragment is slightly displaced into the lateral aspect of the body of the calcaneus.

2. The sustentaculum tali is sheared off together with one-half to one-third of the medial portion of the posterior articular surface.

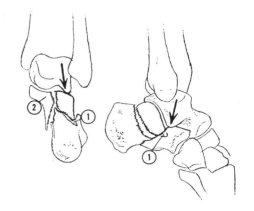

When downward force is severe:

1. The joint fragment is displaced deep into the lateral portion of the body of the calcaneus, causing bulging of the lateral wall.

2. Primary fracture line opens up from below.

3. The tuberosity is forced upward.

4. Reduction of tuber angle.

Note: In some instances the calcaneocuboid joint may be totally disrupted and the posterior articular surface of the calcaneus markedly comminuted.

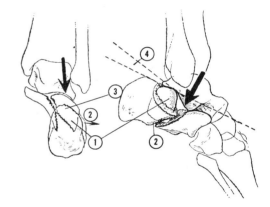

Prereduction X-Ray

1. The tuber angle is reduced.

2. The tuberosity is displaced upward.

3. The joint fragment is driven into the body.

4. The lateral wall bulges.

5. The sustentaculum tali is sheared from the body.

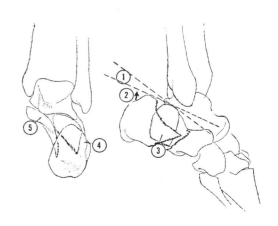

Operative Reduction

1. The patient is in the lateral position and the foot rests on a sandbag.

2. Make a slightly oblique incision beginning 1 inch behind the tip of the external malleolus, extending downward and forward to the second cuneiform bone.

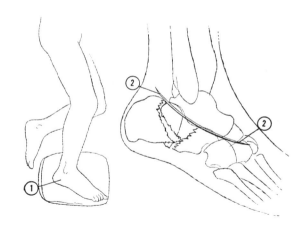

1. Divide the deep fascia in the line of the skin incision.

2. Excise the fatty tissue from the sinus tarsi.

3. Retract the peroneal tendons posteriorly.

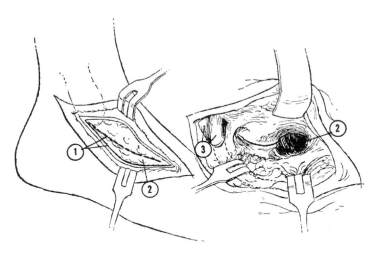

Operative Reduction (Continued)

1. By sharp periosteal dissection expose the lateral surfaces of the calcaneus and talus.

2. Place a periosteal elevator inside the lateral wall under the depressed joint fragment and elevate the fragment to its normal position.

3. While the elevated position of the fragment is maintained.

4. Place three or four struts of cancellous bone under the fragment.

Note: Bone grafts are obtained from the ilium.

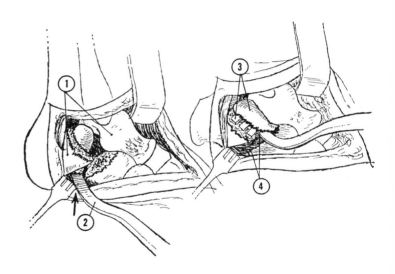

1. Pack any remaining defects with cancellous bone chips.

2. With an impactor correct any lateral bulge of the lateral wall.

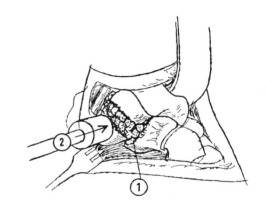

Postoperative X-Ray

1. The tuber angle is restored.
2. There are struts holding the joint fragment elevated.
3. The articular surfaces of the sub-talar joint are congruous.

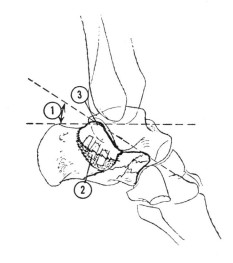

Immobilization

1. Apply a circular cast from be-hind the metatarsal heads to just be-low the knee.
2. The foot is at a right angle.
3. The foot is neutral as to inver-sion and eversion.

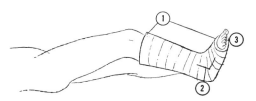

Postreduction Management

Elevate the foot on a pillow.

Surround the foot and ankle with ice bags.

Within two or three days allow ambulation without weight bearing.

Another plaster cast is applied after four weeks.

Remove the second cast eight weeks after reduction.

Institute an intensive program to restore motion in the ankle and all other joints of the foot.

Permit weight bearing, at first with crutches, 10 to 12 weeks after the fracture.

Apply a cotton elastic bandage to control or prevent excessive swelling.

ALTERNATE METHOD

This alternate method is employed when there is severe comminu-tion and depression of the articular surface of the calcaneus and dis-ruption of the calcaneocuboid joint.

Appearance on X-Ray

1. Severe comminution and tele-scoping of the articular surface of the calcaneus.

2. The tuber angle is reversed.

3. The tuberosity is displaced up-ward.

4. Comminution of the calcaneocu-boid joint.

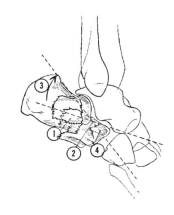

Immobilization

Apply a compression bandage to the foot and leg.

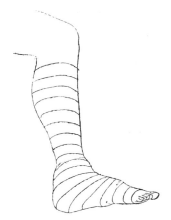

Management

Elevate the foot on pillows.

Surround the foot and ankle with ice bags.

Immediately institute active exercises at the ankle, subtalar and mid-tarsal joints.

Exercise program should be on a regulated regimen under super-vision if possible.

The patient is confined to bed for eight to ten weeks.

After this the patient may be ambulatory on crutches with partial weight bearing on the affected extremity; the crutches are discarded when weight bearing on the affected foot is painless.

During this period exercises are continued.

If after six months pain is still of such severity that marked dysfunc-tion results, arthrodesis of the implicated joints is justifiable; this means either a subtalar or a triple arthrodesis.

FRACTURES AND FRACTURE-DISLOCATIONS OF THE NAVICULAR BONE

REMARKS

Fractures and fracture-dislocations are usually the result of forcible dorsiflexion of the foot.

Fracture of the tuberosity of the navicular is really an avulsion fracture produced by pull of the tibialis posterior.

Isolated fractures rarely exhibit marked displacement of the fragments.

In fracture-dislocations the dorsal fragment is displaced upward.

Aseptic necrosis and osteoarthritis are common sequels to these lesions and may require arthrodesis of the implicated joints.

Fracture of the Navicular without Displacement

Appearance on X-Ray (First Example)

1. Small fracture of the dorsal lip of the navicular; displacement is minimal. (No reduction is needed.)

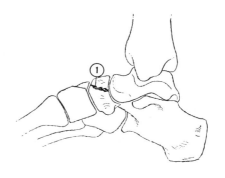

Appearance on X-Ray (Second Example)

1. Fracture of the tuberosity of the navicular with minimal displacement.

Note: Distinguish this lesion from an accessory center of ossification frequently encountered at this site.

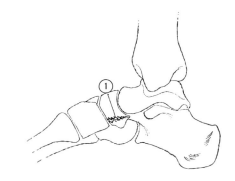

Immobilization

1. Apply a circular cast from behind the metarsal heads to the tibial tubercle.
2. The foot is slightly plantar flexed.
3. The foot is in a neutral position as to inversion and eversion.

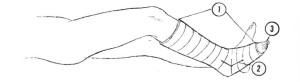

Management

1. Apply a walking heel and permit weight bearing.
2. Exercise the toes actively.

For fractures of the dorsal lip of the navicular remove the cast after four weeks.

For fractures of the tuberosity remove the cast after eight weeks.

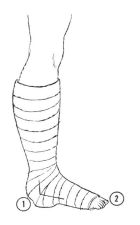

Fracture-Dislocation of the Navicular Bone

Prereduction X-Ray

1. Fracture of the body of the navicular.

2. The dorsal fragment is displaced upward and medially.

Note: This fragment is prone to develop aseptic necrosis.

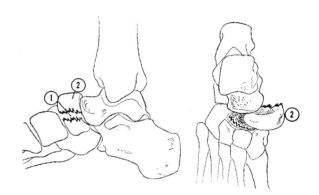

Manipulative Reduction (Under General Anesthesia)

1. The first assistant steadies the leg.

2. The second assistant makes strong traction while

3. The foot is plantar flexed and

4. The foot is everted.

5. With the thumbs on the fragment the surgeon makes strong pressure downward.

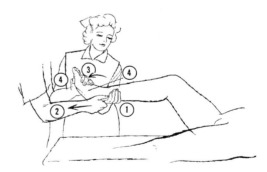

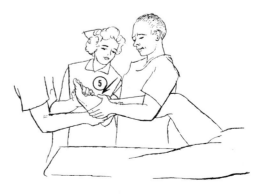

Immobilization

1. Apply a circular cast from behind the metatarsal heads to the tibial tubercle.

2. The foot is slightly dorsiflexed.

3. The foot is in a neutral position as to inversion and eversion.

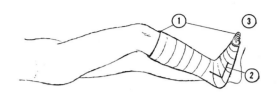

Management

Allow the patient up on crutches without weight bearing on the affected foot after two to three days.

Change the cast at the end of three weeks; now add a walking heel and permit weight bearing.

At the end of six weeks again change the cast and bring the foot to a right angle position.

Remove the last cast 12 weeks after injury.

Institute a program of active exercises to restore normal movement to ankle and tarsal joints.

ALTERNATE METHOD

This alternate method is employed when manipulative reduction fails to replace the fragment or redisplacement occurs after pressure is released from over the dorsal fragment.

Operative Reduction

1. Make a 3 inch incision parallel to the lateral margin of the anterior tibial tendon centered over the talonavicular joint.

2. Divide the deep fascia and the transverse crural ligament above and the cruciate ligament below.

3. Make a linear incision through the fatty layer and capsule.

4. By sharp dissection expose the dorsal fragment and the talus above and the first cuneiform below.

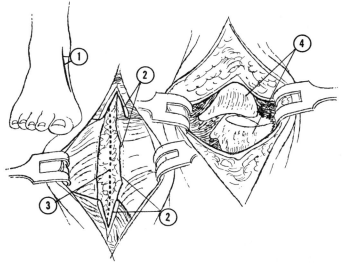

1. While the foot is plantar flexed and everted,

2. Make firm downward pressure on the dorsal fragment.

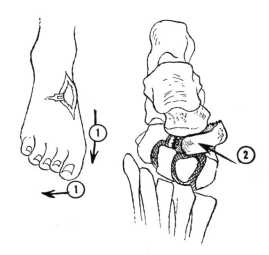

Operative Reduction (Continued)

This step is employed only when re-displacement of the dorsal fragment occurs upon releasing downward pressure.

1. While the fragment is held in place,

2. Pass a threaded wire obliquely through the first cuneiform, the dorsal fragment of the navicular, and the head of the talus.

3. Cut the wire just below the level of the skin.

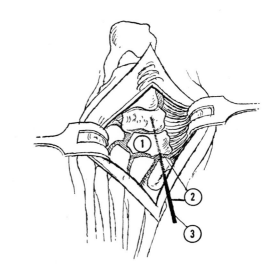

Postreduction X-Ray

1. The dorsal fragment is in its normal relation to the talus and the cuneiform bone.

2. A threaded wire secures the fragment in its normal position.

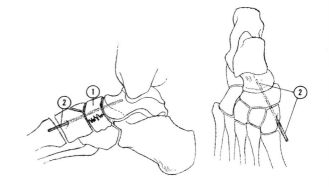

Immobilization

1. Apply a below-the-knee plaster cast.

2. The foot is slightly plantar flexed.

3. The foot is in neutral position as to inversion and eversion.

4. Mold the cast well under the longitudinal arch.

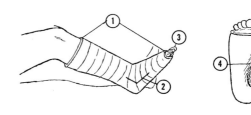

Page 1688

Postoperative Management

Allow the patient up on crutches with no weight bearing on the affected foot.

Change the cast every three to four weeks.

Remove the threaded wire six weeks after reduction.

After 10 to 12 weeks remove the cast and apply a cotton elastic bandage around the foot and lower leg.

Now begin weight bearing, first with crutches.

Institute an intensive program of active exercises to restore normal movements at the ankle and other tarsal joint.

CAUTION

Aseptic necrosis and osteoarthritis are common sequels of severe fractures of the navicular regardless of treatment.

Warn the patient of these possibilities.

When they occur, the treatment of choice is arthrodesis of the implicated joints.

FRACTURES OF THE CUBOID AND CUNEIFORM BONES

REMARKS

Generally fractures of these bones are associated with dislocation at the midtarsal or tarsometatarsal joint.

Isolated injuries may occur as the result of direct violence.

As a rule in isolated fractures there is little or no displacement of the fragments.

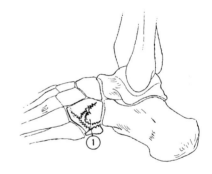

Appearance on X-Ray (Cuboid Fracture)

1. Comminuted fracture of the cuboid with minimal displacement.

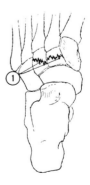

Appearance on X-Ray (Cuneiform Fracture)

1. Fracture of the second and third cuneiform bones with no displacement.

Immobilization

1. Apply a circular plaster cast from behind the metatarsal heads to the tibial tubercle.

2. The foot is at 90 degrees dorsiflexion.

3. The foot is in a neutral position as to inversion and eversion.

4. Mold the plaster well under the longitudinal arch.

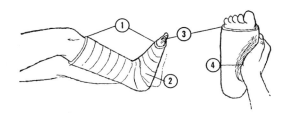

Management

Allow the patient up on crutches without weight bearing on the affected foot.

Remove the cast at the end of six weeks.

Fit the patient with a shoe with a Thomas heel and a longitudinal arch support.

DISLOCATIONS AND FRACTURE-DISLOCATIONS OF THE MIDTARSAL JOINT

REMARKS

The midtarsal joint comprises the talonavicular and the calcaneocuboid joints.

Severe torsional stresses either in abduction or adduction may produce partial or complete dislocations of this joint.

Fractures of some of the tarsal bones are frequent associated lesions, particularly fractures of the navicular or cuboid bones.

When fractures of the bones are concomitant lesions, displacement of the fragments is rarely great.

Generally the fractures can be ignored and attention is directed to reduction of the dislocation.

Occasionally severe disruption of the joints occurs, necessitating a primary surgical arthrodesis.

All dislocations must be reduced immediately.

Prereduction X-Ray

1. Inward displacement of the navicular and cuboid bones on the talus and calcaneus.

2. Anterior tarsal bones at the level of the midtarsal joint are displaced upward.

3. Fracture of the cuboid bone with minimal displacement.

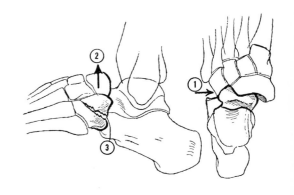

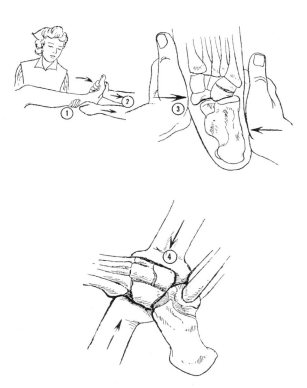

Manipulative Reduction

1. One assistant fixes the ankle.

2. Another assistant grasps the forefoot and makes strong forward traction.

3. The surgeon with the heels of his hands pushes the forefoot outward and the calcaneus inward; this reduces the inward displacement.

4. With the heels of both hands direct downward pressure is made on the anterior tarsal bone; this reduces the upward displacement.

Note: This same general pattern of manipulation is employed regardless of the direction of displacement.

Postreduction X-Rays

1. The navicular and cuboid bones are in normal relationship to the talus and calcaneus.

2. Fracture of the cuboid bone.

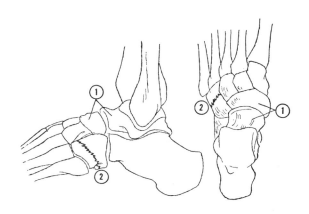

Immobilization

1. Apply a circular plaster cast from behind the metatarsal heads to the tibial tubercle.

2. The foot is at 90 degrees dorsiflexion.

3. The foot is in a neutral position as to inversion and eversion.

4. Mold the plaster well under the longitudinal arch.

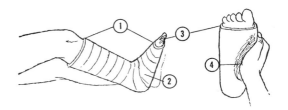

Postreduction Management

Allow the patient up on crutches without weight bearing on the affected foot.

Remove the cast at the end of eight weeks.

Fit the patient with a shoe with a Thomas heel and a longitudinal arch support.

Note: In the event that manipulative reduction fails, open reduction is justifiable; it may be necessary to transfix the bones with a threaded wire to maintain the correct position.

If pain due to traumatic arthritis persists after adequate treatment, surgical arthrodesis of the painful joints is indicated.

DISLOCATIONS AND FRACTURE-DISLOCATIONS OF THE TARSOMETATARSAL JOINT

REMARKS

These lesions may be produced by falls on the ball of the foot, direct violence or torsional stress.

All the metatarsals may be dislocated or one or more may be dislocated.

The displacement is affected by the direction of the force; the bones may be displaced upward, downward or laterally.

Fractures of the tarsal or metatarsal bones may be associated lesions.

Thrombosis or spasm of the large arteries of the foot may occur; check the circulatory status of the foot frequently both before and after reduction.

Reduction should be executed immediately.

Accurate replacement of the implicated bones is essential to attain a painless functioning foot.

If manipulative reduction fails, operative reduction and internal fixation with fine threaded wires is indicated.

Prereduction X-Ray

1. All metatarsals are displaced laterally.
2. The metatarsals are displaced upward.

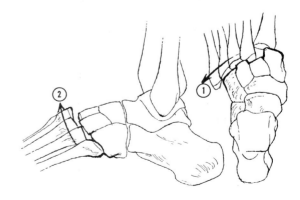

Page 1695

Manipulative Reduction

1. One assistant fixes the heel.
2. The second assistant makes strong steady traction on the forefoot.
3. While traction is maintained, the operator makes firm downward pressure on the bases of the metatarsal bones.

Note: The direction of the pressure is governed by the type of displacement; downward pressure is applied for upward displacement of the metatarsals and upward pressure for downward displacement.

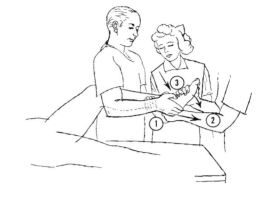

Postreduction X-Ray

1. The bases of the meatarsal bones are in normal relationship to the tarsal bones.

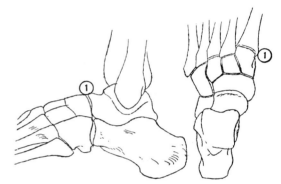

Immobilization

1. Apply a padded circular cast from the toes to below the knee joint.
2. The foot is at a right angle.
3. The foot is in the neutral position as to inversion and eversion.
4. Mold the plaster well under the longitudinal arch.

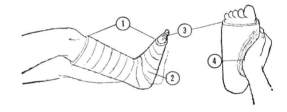

Postreduction Management

Elevate the limb on pillows.
Surround the foot with ice bags.
Check the circulation of the foot frequently.
After a few days allow the patient up on crutches without weight bearing on the affected foot.
Remove the cast after six to eight weeks; during this period allow no weight bearing on the limb.
Now fit the patient with a shoe with a longitudinal arch support and permit weight bearing.

Note: In some cases traumatic arthritis may develop later; if pain and disability is great, arthrodesis of the involved tarsometatarsal joints is indicated.

FRACTURE OF THE METATARSAL BONES

REMARKS

These lesions are usually the result of direct violent injuries; one or more bones may be involved.

Repeated stresses such as are produced by prolonged walking may cause a fracture in one or more metatarsal bones; usually the second or third metatarsal bones are involved. As a rule no displacement occurs. These are the so-called "march fractures."

Accurate reduction is essential in order to avoid serious disability of the foot; this is particularly true of fractures in the distal ends of the bones.

Most fractures can be treated by manipulative reduction; however, open reduction is justified if this method fails.

Fracture of the Metatarsal Bones without Displacement

Appearance on X-Ray (First Example)

1. Fracture of the shafts of the second and third metatarsal bones with minimal displacement.

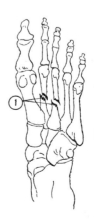

Appearance on X-Ray (Second Example)

1. March fracture of the third metatarsal; only a faint fine fracture line is visible.

2. Same fracture three weeks after onset of symptoms; note marked callus formation.

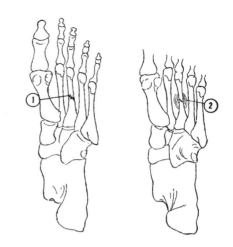

Immobilization

1. Apply a circular plaster cast from the toes to the tibial tubercle.

2. The foot is at a right angle.

3. The foot is neutral as to inversion and eversion.

4. Mold the plaster well under the longitudinal and transverse arch.

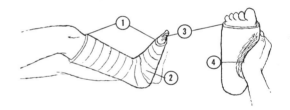

Management

Allow the patient up on crutches without weight bearing on the affected foot.

After 10 to 14 days, when swelling and pain have subsided, remove the plaster cast and apply another short leg plaster cast with a walking iron; the patient may now bear weight on the foot.

Remove the second cast six weeks after injury.

Avoid early mobilization and weight bearing in order to prevent formation of exuberant callus at the fracture sites.

After removal of the cast provide the patient with a stiff-soled shoe with a support for the longitudinal and transverse arches.

Fracture of the Metatarsal Bones with Displacement

REMARKS

Accurate reduction of these fractures is essential in order to prevent prolonged disability.

Most such fractures can be reduced by manipulative maneuvers.

Prereduction X-Ray

1. Fracture of the neck of the third, fourth and fifth metatarsals.

2. The distal fragments (heads of metatarsals) are displaced outward and downward.

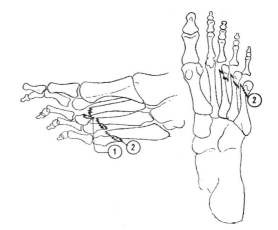

Manipulative Reduction

1. One assistant fixes the foot.

2. A second assistant makes steady traction on the toe by means of a loop of bandage around the toe.

3. The operator by direct pressure molds the fragments back into their anatomic position.

Note: This method is employed for each metatarsal fracture.

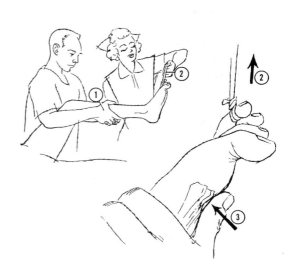

Postreduction X-Ray

1. The distal fragments of all three fractured metatarsals are in normal relation with the proximal fragments.

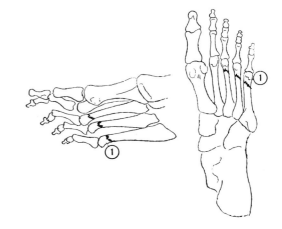

Immobilization

1. Apply a circular plaster cast from the toes to the tibial tubercle.
2. The foot is at a right angle.
3. The foot is in a neutral position as to inversion and eversion.
4. Mold the plaster well under the longitudinal and transverse arches.

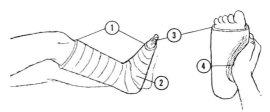

Management

Allow the patient up on crutches without weight bearing on the affected foot.

After 10 to 14 days, when swelling and pain have subsided, remove the plaster cast and apply another short leg plaster cast with a walking iron; the patient may now bear weight on the foot.

Remove the second cast six weeks after injury.

Avoid early mobilization and weight bearing in order to prevent formation of exuberant callus at the fracture site.

After removal of the cast provide the patient with a stiff-soled shoe with a support for the longitudinal and transverse arches.

ALTERNATE METHOD

REMARKS

Operative intervention is indicated when manipulative methods fail to achieve an accurate reduction.

Fractures just proximal to the heads are frequently difficult to maintain in normal alignment by conservative methods.

Prereduction X-Ray

1. Fractures of the shafts of the first, second and third metatarsal bones.

2. The distal fragments are displaced downward and backward into the sole.

Note: in this instance manipulative methods failed to achieve an accurate reduction.

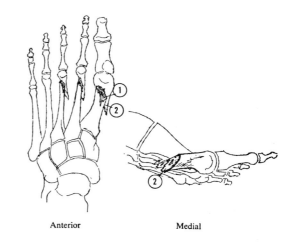

Anterior   Medial

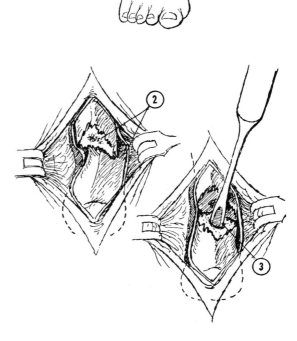

Operative Reduction

1. Make a 1 inch dorsal incision centered over the fracture site.

2. Expose the proximal and distal fragments by subperiosteal dissection.

3. With a small curette deliver the proximal end of the distal fragment into the wound.

Operative Reduction *(Continued)*

1. Dorsiflex the toe.

2. Pass a small Kirschner wire through the medullary canal of the distal fragment until it emerges from the skin.

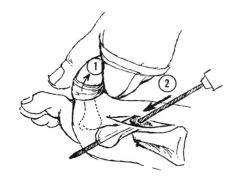

3. Reverse the drill and withdraw the wire until its proximal end is at the level of the fracture site.

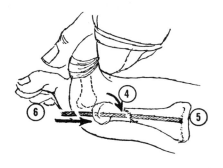

4. Appose the ends of the bone fragments.

5. Pass the wire proximally until its blunt end strikes the base of the metatarsal bone.

6. Cut the wire, leaving its end protruding ¼ inch above the level of the skin.

Note: This procedure is executed for each metatarsal fracture.

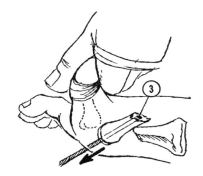

Postreduction X-Ray

1. All fragments are now in anatomic position.

2. A wire transfixes both fragments and maintains normal alignment.

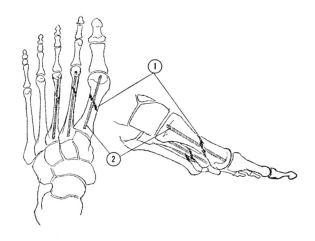

Immobilization

1. Apply a circular plaster cast from the toes to the tibial tubercle.

2. The foot is at a right angle.

3. The foot is in the neutral position as to inversion and eversion.

4. Mold the plaster well under the longitudinal and transverse arches.

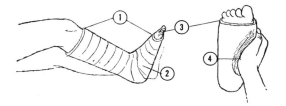

Postoperative Management

Elevate the foot on pillows.

Surround the foot with ice bags.

After three weeks remove the wire and apply a short leg plaster cast with a walking iron; again mold the plaster well under the longitudinal and transverse arches.

Six to eight weeks after operation remove the plaster cast and allow walking in a stiff-soled shoe with an arch support for the longitudinal and transverse arches.

Severely Comminuted Fractures of the Metatarsal Bones with Displacement

REMARKS

Often it is impossible to obtain and maintain reduction of severely comminuted fractures by simple conservative methods.

These lesions do not lend themselves to medullary wire fixation but can be reduced and length can be maintained by skeletal traction.

Prereduction X-Ray

1. Severe comminution with displacement of fragments and overriding.

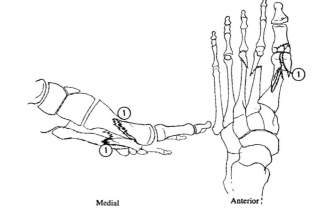

Medial   Anterior

Reduction by Skeletal Traction

1. With aseptic technique pass a small threaded wire transversely through the distal phalanx.

2. Apply a circular plaster cast from the tibial tubercle to just behind the metatarsal heads.

3. Incorporate a wire loop in the cast which extends 3 to 4 inches beyond the toes (use a wire coat hanger).

4. Use rubber bands to make continuous traction on the toes.

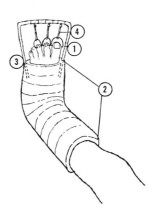

Note: Traction should not be too great lest the circulation of the toes is embarrassed.

Postreduction X-Ray

1. The length of the metatarsal has been restored.
2. Displacement of the distal fragments is corrected.

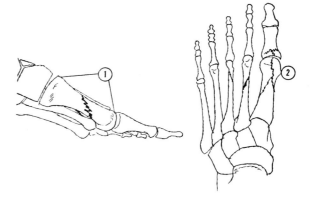

Management

Maintain traction for three weeks.
At the end of three weeks remove the wires.
Apply a circular plaster cast with a walking iron from the toes to the tibial tubercle.
After three more weeks remove the second cast.
Fit the patient with a stiff-soled shoe with arch supports for the longitudinal and transverse arches.

Fracture of the Base of the Fifth Metatarsal Bone

REMARKS

This is an avulsion injury caused by forcing the foot into inversion and plantar flexion.
The base of the fifth metatarsal is pulled off by the tendon of the peroneus brevis.
Displacement is never great, hence reduction is rarely necessary.

Page 1705

1. Avulsion of the base of the fifth metatarsal.

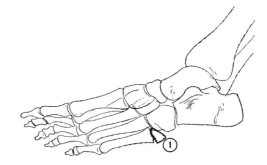

Immobilization

1. Apply a circular plaster cast from the toes to the tibial tubercle.
2. The foot is at a right angle.
3. The foot is in a neutral position as to inversion and eversion.
4. Mold the plaster well under the longitudinal and transverse arches.

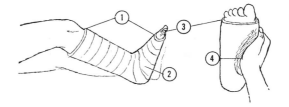

Management

Allow the patient up on crutches without weight bearing on the affected foot.

After 10 to 14 days, when swelling and pain have subsided, remove the plaster cast and apply another short leg plaster cast with a walking iron; the patient may now bear weight on the foot.

Remove the second cast six weeks after injury.

Avoid early mobilization and weight bearing in order to prevent formation of exuberant callus at the fracture sites.

After removal of the cast, provide the patient with a stiff-soled shoe with a support for the longitudinal and transverse arches.

DISLOCATIONS OF THE METATARSOPHALANGEAL JOINTS

REMARKS

These are rare lesions; the great toe is most commonly involved. Many are open lesions.

Immediate reduction is mandatory; a delay of several days may make it impossible to reduce the dislocation by closed methods.

Typical Deformity

1. The proximal phalanx is displaced upward and backward in the vertical position.

2. The head of the metatarsal is prominent.

3. The distal phalanx is flexed.

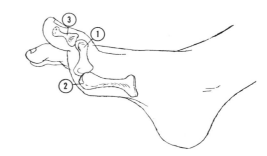

Prereduction X-Ray

1. The proximal phalanx rests on the dorsal aspect of the head of the metatarsal.

2. The distal phalanx is flexed.

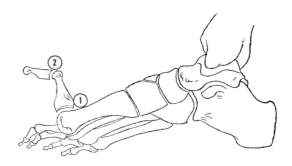

Page 1707

Manipulative Reduction

1. Pass a loop of bandage around the toe to make traction.

2. Make strong traction upward and backward (hyperextending the toe); this disengages the metatarsal head from the flexor tendons.

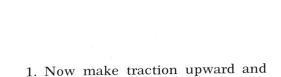

1. Now make traction upward and forward.

2. Place the thumb of the other hand behind the proximal end of the first phalanx and force the phalanx distally and downward over the metatarsal head.

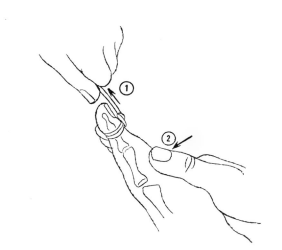

Immobilization

1. Apply directly to the skin a posterior plaster slab over the dorsum of the foot extending to the end of the great toe.

2. The toe is in the neutral position.

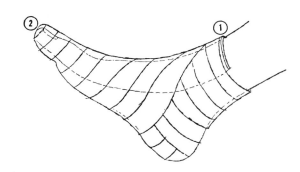

Management

Allow the patient up on crutches with no weight bearing on the affected foot.

Remove the plaster splint at the end of two weeks.

Provide the patient with a stiff-soled shoe.

FRACTURES OF THE SESAMOID BONES OF THE GREAT TOE

REMARKS

These lesions are rare and are the result of direct trauma applied to the foot, crushing the sesamoids between the head of the metatarsal and the ground.

The inner sesamoid is involved more often than the outer.

Fracture must be distinguished from a bipartite or tripartite sesamoid; in the former the line of division is sharp and irregular, in the latter it is smooth, regular and fragments are of equal size.

If pain and dysfunction persist after a period of immobilization and proper padding of the shoe, excision of the sesamoid is indicated.

Appearance on X-Ray

1. Fracture of the internal sesamoid.

2. The fragments are of unequal size.

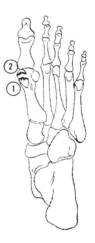

Immobilization

1. Apply a circular plaster cast from the toes to the tibial tubercle.

2. The great toe is moderately flexed.

3. A walking iron is incorporated in the cast.

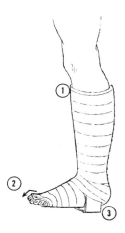

Management

Remove the cast at the end of four weeks.

Permit weight bearing in a shoe with an anterior bar placed on the sole of the shoe just behind the metatarsal heads.

For two or three more weeks immobilize the metatarsophalangeal joint with adhesive strapping.

If pain persists after several months of adequate treatment, excision of the sesamoid is indicated.

Excision is also indicated in cases of old untreated fractures causing pain and dysfunction.

FRACTURES OF THE TOES

REMARKS

These lesions are usually the result of crushing injuries; the great toe is most often affected.

Comminution of the phalanx occurs relatively frequently.

Many fractures are of the open type.

As a rule displacement of the fragments is minimal.

Fractures of the Toes with Minimal or No Displacement

Appearance on X-Ray (Proximal Phalanx of Fourth Toe)

1. Oblique fracture of the proximal phalanx of the fourth toe with minimal displacement. (No reduction required.)

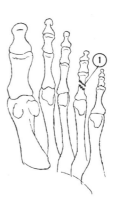

Appearance on X-Ray (Distal Phalanx of Great Toe)

1. Comminuted fracture of the distal phalanx of the great toe.

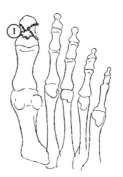

Immobilization (For Fractures of the Outer Four Toes)

1. Place a piece of felt between the toes.

2. Fix the fourth toe to the fifth toe with strips of adhesive.

3. Shoe with top cut out and a bar on the sole placed behind the metatarsal heads.

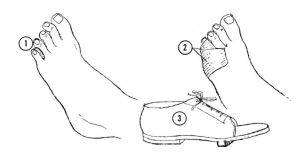

Management

For fractures of any of the toes allow the patient to bear weight in a shoe with the toe cap cut out and a metatarsal bar ½ inch high placed on the sole just behind the metatarsal heads.

In cases of severe swelling elevate the foot for two to three days before weight bearing is permitted.

Remove the adhesive strapping after two to three weeks and provide the patient with a stiff-soled shoe.

Immobilization (For Fractures of the Great Toe)

1. Place a piece of felt between the great toe and the second toe.

2. Bind the great toe to the second toe with strips of adhesive.

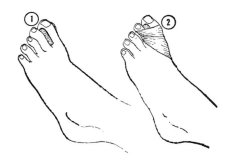

Fracture of the Toes with Displacement

REMARKS

Generally displacement can be corrected by simple traction on the toe.

Fractures of the proximal phalanges may exhibit forward angulation of the fragments.

If reduction is not stable and the deformity recurs after traction is released, continuous traction is indicated.

Prereduction X-Ray

1. Fracture of the proximal phalanx of the great toe with forward angulation of the fragments.

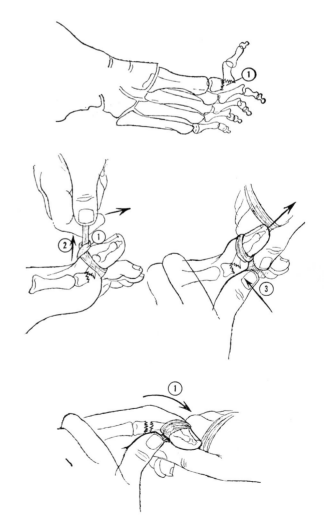

Manipulative Reduction

1. Pass a loop of gauze bandage around the toe.
2. Make direct traction upward and forward.
3. Place the thumb of the other hand over the apex of the angulation on the plantar aspect of the toe and make upward pressure.

1. While traction is maintained flex the toe.

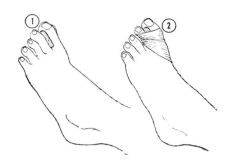

Immobilization

1. Place a piece of felt between the toes.

2. Bind the first toe to the second toe with strips of adhesive.

Alternate Method (Skeletal Traction)

(Employed if displacement recurs or reduction is not achieved by traction.)

1. Pass a small threaded wire transversely through the distal phalanx.

2. Apply a circular cast from behind the metatarsal heads to the tibial tubercle.

3. Incorporate a wire loop in the cast extending 3 to 4 inches beyond the toes.

4. Use rubber bands to make continuous traction on the toe.

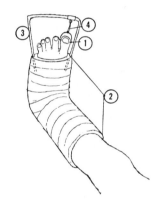

Management

Maintain traction for three weeks.

Remove the wire and immobilize the affected toe by fastening it to one of the adjacent toes with strips of adhesive.

Permit weight bearing in a stiff-soled shoe with the top cut out and a metatarsal bar on the sole of the shoe.

INDEX

INDEX